INTRO

A Guide to Communication Sciences and Disorders

INTRO

A Guide to Communication Sciences and Disorders

Michael P. Robb, PhD

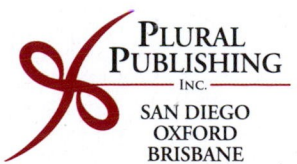

PLURAL PUBLISHING
INC.

SAN DIEGO
OXFORD
BRISBANE

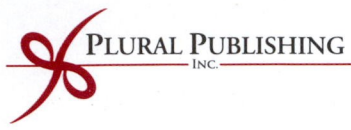

5521 Ruffin Road
San Diego, CA 92123

e-mail: info@pluralpublishing.com
Web site: http://www.pluralpublishing.com

49 Bath Street
Abingdon, Oxfordshire OX14 1EA
United Kingdom

Typeset in 11/13 Palatino book by Flanagan's Publishing Services, Inc.
Printed in Hong Kong by Paramount

Library of Congress Cataloging-in-Publication Data

Robb, Michael P.
 INTRO: a guide to communication sciences and disorders / Michael P. Robb.
      p. ; cm.
 Includes bibliographical references and index.
 ISBN-13: 978-1-59756-339-0 (alk. paper)
 ISBN-10: 1-59756-339-0 (alk. paper)
 1. Communicative disorders. 2. Speech therapy. 3. Audiology. I. Title. II. Title:
Guide to communication sciences and disorders.
 [DNLM: 1. Communication Disorders. 2. Hearing Disorders. WL 340.2 R631i 2010]
 RC423.R57 2010
 362.196'855—dc22

                                                    2009036445

CONTENTS

SECTION 4: AUDITION   321

12 Hearing Disorders   323

13 Auditory Rehabilitation   353

FOREWORD

Welcome to the fascinating and complex fields of speech and language pathology and audiology. These two professions are applied fields that draw on theory and knowledge from a variety of disciplines that support the practices devoted to prevention, assessment and evaluation, and treatment of disorders of speech, language, and hearing across the life span of human beings. This textbook provides the beginning student with an understanding of the basic conceptual and content knowledge and the vocabulary necessary to appreciate the complexity of human communication disorders. Within the crowded arena of introductory textbooks, there are a number of features of this text that make it particularly appealing, not the least of which is the sole authorship by Professor Robb. The distinct advantage of one author is that the perspective across the various topics is consistent and presented in a cohesive organization and level throughout. Capturing the right level is important for an introductory text and Professor Robb has done so based on his years of teaching the course for which this text is intended.

There are additional features of this text that add to its appeal. These features are in its contextualization. I applaud the approach the author takes to provide a context for both speech-language pathology and audiology within the broadly defined communication sciences. The scope of practice within each profession engages activities not directly targeted at communication, such as swallowing or intraoperative auditory assessment; however, the raison d'être of these professions is situated in human communication. The inclusion of historical referents within each chapter is another appealing feature, which gives the beginning student a perspective on how the contemporary fields have evolved from the contributions of earlier scholars working in different disciplines such as physics, engineering, phonetics, psychology, medicine, and philosophy. The historical references also allow the student to appreciate the tremendous advances in technology that assist the current speech and hearing scientists and practitioners to better understand and serve individuals with communication impairments. Finally, the text is written with full recognition that students around the world are preparing for careers in speech and language pathology and in audiology. Although the education and training will follow different models and the practice requirements might be different in various countries, the core substance of the fields is essentially the same. The text limits its discussion to the English-speaking communities, but clearly addresses the relevant multilingual/multicultural issues. Here the author brings his personal experience from teaching the introductory course in the United States and New Zealand.

A few observations about the communication context are in order. The overview of communication helps the reader appreciate the fundamental role of communication in all of nature. The most common definitions of communication involve some description of a mutual exchange of information or energy between two entities with varying degrees of elaboration of the process and its outcomes. A definition of this sort reminds us that communication is a universal among living entities ranging from the biochemical exchanges of unicellular organisms to complex symbolic systems such as language in humans.

The simple three-component model of communication (a sender, a communication channel, and a receiver) adapted from Shannon and Weaver has the advantage of identifying the major functional components involved in the act of communication. The model is an abstraction of the factors that influence and define the communication outcome. Applying this model to human communication and its disorders requires the specific knowledge of how the communication partners, who are both senders and receivers, acquire and use natural language abilities and what factors can impair the ability to acquire and use language for effective communication. That, of course, leads beyond the abstraction of a communication model to the primary content of this textbook. The content is an elaboration on the specifics of the human language user in a social milieu and the disorders that disrupt communication through problems that can originate anywhere within the communication dynamic. The human communicator is more than a "source code" generator and interpreter in an information system process and therein lies the nexus of communication sciences and disorders as a discipline of study.

Communicating with others is such a common experience that we give little thought to how it is accomplished. Because we are so familiar with being communicators, we generally are unaware of the learning and practice that went into developing the necessary communication skills that began as early as while still in the womb. We easily use different modes of communication available to us in our daily activities and only on occasion or in very limited circumstances do we experience the challenges of impeded communication. The situation is quite different, of course, for the person who has a communication disorder. The nature of the communication disorder and its consequences for the individual who experiences it depend on a host of interacting factors: organismic and environmental, developmental and acquired. The learning objectives stated for each chapter in this text appropriately focus on understanding the nature and consequences of the major disorders and their treatment in human beings.

Finally, it is appropriate to recognize the importance of the author's experience in the education of students at all levels of their apprenticeship in the field. Because he has taught beginning students in a career spanning several decades, he is familiar with the changing learning culture and mode of today's student. This experience is realized in the writing style and learning aids used throughout the text. In addition to his significant contributions as a teacher, Professor Robb has maintained an active research and scholarship agenda that gives him further credibility as an authoritative escort for beginning students in their introduction to the field. On a personal note, it is a unique pleasure for me as I approach the close of my academic career to acknowledge a treasured friend and former student for his achievement in producing a book that promises to stimulate the development of many future careers in communication science and disorders.

John H. Saxman, PhD
Professor and Chair
Department of
    Biobehavioral Sciences
Teachers College,
Columbia University

PREFACE

INTRO is designed for the beginning university-level student who has an interest in entering the field of communication sciences and disorders, or for a student who may be interested in entering one of the companion health professions. As is the case for any book claiming to be *introductory*, the aim is to paint a picture for the student using broad strokes. This book provides straightforward and essential information concerning a wide range of communication disorders found in children and adults.

The book is organized into four sections. Section 1 provides background information related to communication disorders. The chapters in this section cover the topics of communication science, the professions of audiology and speech-language pathology, and anatomy and physiology. Section 2 is concerned with developmental communication disorders, and includes chapters on child language disorders, child phonological disorders, fluency disorders, and cleft lip and palate. Section 3 covers acquired and genetic communication disorders. The chapters in this section describe voice disorders, neurogenic communication disorders, dysphagia, and genetic-based communication disorders. Section 4 addresses audition and contains chapters on hearing disorders and aural rehabilitation.

Unique aspects of the book include its use of an identical structure for each chapter to assist beginning students in grasping new vocabulary and concepts.

Each chapter provides a focus on "past and present." An introduction to each of the various disorders would not be complete without knowing some of the fascinating historical background surrounding each disorder, as well as up-to-date information concerning current theories and research. The book holds worldwide appeal and is written for an international audience. A portion of each chapter is dedicated to cultural aspects of communication disorders, as well as prevalence information about various communication disorders as found in English-speaking countries around the world, including Australia, Canada, the United Kingdom, the United States, and New Zealand. The chapters include a series of FYIs (for your information), which present interesting and novel information about the particular topic area. A number of Web sites are listed at the end of the chapters to provide students an opportunity to learn more about each topic. Many of these Web sites provide links to streaming video examples.

The sole authorship of the book ensures a balanced writing style that is missing from existing introductory texts. INTRO is a clear and concise primer for students wishing to obtain fundamental information about the myriad of communication disorders that occur across the life span. For some, this information will serve as a springboard for pursuit of a professional career in audiology and speech-language pathology. For others, my hope is that you will acquire an appreciation of the gift of communication that we so often take for granted.

I wish to thank the following reviewers for their comments on various chapters of the book: Kenn Apel, Maggie Lee Huckabee, Emily Lin, Greg O'Beirne, and Natalie Rickard. The book illustrations were made possible by the tireless work of Chia Pan. Finally, I am particularly indebted to Ray Kent who encouraged me to write a book of this kind and provided valuable oversight throughout its creation.

Michael P. Robb

To Jenne

Background to Communication Disorders

COMMUNICATION SCIENCE

OBJECTIVES

After reading this chapter, the student should be able to:

- Recognize the different forms and types of human communication.
- Recognize the importance of effective communication in various situations.
- Recognize that communication is a multifaceted process.
- Recognize that speech is an important tool for thinking, learning, and communicating.
- Recognize listening as an active, constructive process.
- Recognize that communication is an interactive process between sender and receiver.
- Recognize the role of culture in communication.
- Recognize the need for formal and informal oral communication.
- Recognize how theories of normal communication serve as a basis for the diagnosis and remediation of communication disorders.

INTRODUCTION

Communication involves the transfer of information between two living organisms. As humans, we are born with the physical attributes to communicate, although our earliest forms of communication are quite basic and revolve around fundamental needs and wants. The transfer of information is between infant and caregiver. As we grow, we learn to communicate more effectively by observing other people communicating. We model our communication on what we see, hear, and experience. Our communication skills grow in complexity and sophistication through formal education, and by practicing those skills and having them evaluated.

Communication science is an academic field of study that examines how people communicate as individuals, within a society, and in various cultures. Communication science is a field that has grown rapidly in large part due to advances in technology. Some of the greatest technologic advances that have occurred over the past decades are directly related to improvements in the way we communicate. Contemporary students of communication science draw on theories and practices common in the fields of linguistics, mass communication, political science, journalism, psychology, sociology, anthropology, and animal behavior. There are a variety of careers that can be pursued with a background in communication science. A listing of some of the many possible career choices is provided in Table 1.1.

The primary focus of this book concerns situations when the transfer of information between humans is somehow impaired. When communication fails, misunderstandings occur and sometimes people become frustrated, worried, or even angry. Some communication impairments are minor and can be easily corrected, whereas others are more severe and may require an extensive period of treatment. As a prerequisite to understanding various communication disorders, it is important to first have a grasp of normal communication. Knowledge concerning the normal process of communication serves as foundation for the identification and management of communication disorders. The aim of this chapter is to introduce concepts of normal communication that subsequently will serve as a platform for learning about various disorders presented in later chapters.

TERMINOLOGY AND DEFINITIONS

The word, communicate, is related to the word "common." The word has its origin in the Latin verb *communicare*, which means "to share" or "to make common." When we communicate we make things common. Communication is one of those activities that we take for granted. It seems to occur naturally and we spend the majority of our living hours engaged in some form of communication. Although we tend to think of communication as talking to someone, communication also occurs in other ways, like when we watch television or surf the Internet. We communicate to others by the way we dress, the style of our hair, and the tattoos we choose (or do not choose) to wear. At a fundamental level, communication can be defined as a two-way process in which a message is sent and received. The sender's

Table 1.1. Possible Career Options in the Various Fields of Communication Science	
Field of Study	*Career Choices*
Advertising	marketing specialist, sales manager
Communication Education	speech teacher, coach, professor
Journalism	reporter, editor, script writer
Radio/Television Broadcasting	disc jockey, announcer, news anchor
Public Relations	press agent, lobbyist, public opinion poller
Theatre/Performing Arts	actor, director, producer, model
Business	sales rep, negotiator, human resources manager
Education	college recruiter, teacher, researcher
Government/Politics	speech writer, press secretary, elected official
Health Careers	health care counselor, hospital administrator
International Relations and Negotiations	diplomat, foreign correspondent, foreign relations officer
Law	public defender, district attorney, legal secretary
Social and Human Services	social worker, recreational supervisor, human rights officer

role in the process of communication is to generate (or **encode**) a message. The receiver's role is to translate (or **decode**) this message. Communication is never a one-way process. Both the sender and the receiver need to participate. If the sender is unable to clearly encode a message, then a breakdown in communication occurs. Similarly, if the receiver is unable to successfully decode a message then communication is likely to fail. Excellent communicators are those who have mastered the process of both sending and receiving.

Communication is a phenomenon that is common to all living beings. All communication takes place by means of signs. A sign is something that stands for something else. These signs can take a variety of forms such as vocalizations, nonverbal gestures, physical movements, vibrations, smells, pictures, and letters. All of these signs serve the same purpose: to help with the exchange of information between sender and receiver. A branch of communication sciences that is concerned with the various types of signs used in communication is called **semiotics**.

It is estimated that 75% of a person's day is spent communicating in some way. Most of our daily communication involves speaking and listening to others. The remaining portion of the day is spent communicating via reading and writing. The face-to-face communication that occurs between people, usually in a private setting, is called **interpersonal** communication. For most of us, this is the type of communication where we feel most comfortable and at ease. **Group** communication relates to the exchange of information that takes place among a small collection of people. **Public** communication occurs on a larger scale than group communication and includes settings such as university lectures or formal presentations. **Organizational** communication takes place in environments such as workplace offices and corporations. Finally, **mass** communication is related to the exchange of information to a large public audience through some sort of medium, such as radio or television.

ANIMAL COMMUNICATION

Ethology is the study of animal behavior. The term is derived from the Greek word "ethos" meaning "character." Scientists, called ethologists, observe, record, and analyze how animals behave and interact with others. Ethologists are particularly interested in the way animals communicate. Two well-known ethologists are Charles Darwin and Jane Goodall (Figure 1.1). **Darwin** (1809–1882) is considered the first modern ethologist because of his extensive work examining the evolution of animal behavior and the expression of emotion. **Jane Goodall** (b. 1934) is a world-renowned ethologist and conservationist who has studied the vocalizations produced by

A

B

FIGURE 1.1. Famous ethologists Charles Darwin (**A**) and Jane Goodall (**B**). From Jeek at Wikimedia Commons. Permission granted through Creative Commons Attribution 2.5 License.

chimpanzees at Gombe National Park in Tanzania since the 1960s.

The ability to communicate is not unique to humans. Many species of nonhuman animals and even insects communicate with each other. Examples of the wide range of communication that occurs among nonhumans are provided in Table 1.2. Animals regularly send messages to each other and most of this communication is intraspecific (occurring between animals of the same species). The type of messages that are communicated within a species usually relate to basic matters such as signaling danger, marking territory, and sexual mating. The mode of animal communication is quite varied and may include: (1) auditory, (2) visual, (3) tactile,

Table 1.2. Some Forms of Communication Displayed by Nonhuman Species

Animal	Form of Communication
Bees	dance when they have found nectar
Chimpanzees	touch hands as a form of greeting
Dogs	stretch their front legs out in front of them and lower their bodies when they want to play
Dolphins	use vocalization and echolocation to communicate and navigate
Elephants	entwine their trunks as a show of affection
Fiddler crabs	wave their single giant claw to attract female fiddler crabs
Giraffes	press their necks together as a show of affection
Gorillas	express anger by sticking out their tongues
Horses	rub noses as a sign of affection
Kangaroos	thump their hind legs to warn others of danger
Swans	entwine their long necks when courting as well as fighting
Whales	breach (leap out of the water) repeatedly to send messages to other whales
White-tailed deer	show alarm by flicking their tail upward

or (4) chemical transmission. **Auditory communication** involves use of a variety of sounds for communication. A sound is uttered by one animal which is then heard and interpreted by other members of the same species. Animals make many different sounds to communicate. From the roar of a lion to the mew of a cat, sound is a way for animals to send messages to other animals. Another form of auditory communication used by animals is **echolocation**, which involves bouncing sound off objects to provide information about size, location, and movement of those objects. Echolocation is used at night or in environments that are perpetually dark, such as inside caves or deep in the ocean. **Visual communication** involves two types of communication: (1) badges, and (2) displays. **Badges** are the color and shape of the animal used to send a message to animals of the same species. For example, the size of male deer antlers sends a message to other males regarding its dominance (Figure 1.2). Badges can also help females pick a mate. The sex of many species of birds is often differentiated by color, with males being the more colorful. Male birds with the brightest color are perceived by female birds as being most healthy. **Displays** are related to animal body language and can be used to attract a mate or to warn off a predator. A dog will place its tail between its legs to display submission. A cat will arch its back to present a threatening profile. **Tactile communication** differs from other forms of communication because the sender of the message must be in physical contact with the receiver. Baboons are known to groom each other, which is a behavior pattern that serves to lessen tension between one another. **Chemical communication** is used by animals that have particularly keen senses of smell or taste. Dogs and cats rely primarily upon this sense for an awareness of events occurring around them. Many insects use chemical signals as well. Some animals release an odor containing **pheromones** (airborne chemicals) to send messages to others. The female gypsy moth produces a potent pheromone that can attract male moths from several miles away. The unique trail displayed by marching ants is a result of a pheromone laid down by ants that have gone ahead of others (see Figure 1.2).

HISTORY OF HUMAN COMMUNICATION

The ability to speak in a clear, eloquent, and effective manner has long been considered to be the hallmark of an educated person. Under the rubric (or label) of "**rhetoric**," the study of the theory and practice of communication dates back to the time of the ancient Greeks. **Plato** (428–347 BC) was a critic of rhetoric and suggested that it was simply a style of speaking and did not reflect substance or breadth of knowledge. He believed that one's speaking style is often used to deceive others because it does not distinguish between conviction and knowledge. **Aristotle** (384–322 BC) wrote extensively on the topic of rhetoric (Figure 1.3). He believed that good rhetoricians (i.e., good communicators) needed to develop five essential skills: (1) invention, which is the ability to generate ideas, (2) disposition, which is the ability to organize ideas, (3) style, which is use of appropriate language, (4) memory, which is the ability to recall facts and ideas, and (5) delivery, which is the use of voice and gestures.

A

B

FIGURE 1.2. Deer antlers provide a form of visual communication (**A**). From M. Karatay at Wikimedia Commons. A trail of ants reflect a form of chemical communication (**B**). From R. Whittle at Wikimedia Commons. Permission granted through Creative Commons Attribution 3.0 License.

Major advancements in the study of human communication occurred in England during the 18th century in what was termed the **Elocutionary Movement**. Elocutio was the Latin word for style but it literally means "speaking

FIGURE 1.3. Aristotle wrote extensively on the topic of rhetoric.

out." Its English derivative "elocution" was adapted as a term for reading aloud. This movement was concerned with the skill of communication in public settings, such as poetry readings, speeches, or plays. Correct elocution stressed the importance of vocal quality and inflection, force and projection, articulation and pronunciation, and gestures and facial expression. The movement also had a considerable influence on English education in the latter half of the century. The third U.S. president, **Thomas Jefferson** (1743–1826) was influenced by the elocutionary movement in his pursuit of the establishment of a democratic and free society in early America. The early 20th century saw a general melding of the concepts of rhetoric and elocution into what was called **speech communication**. This term was used to describe the discipline concerned with the act of speaking and making speeches. Use of the term communication or communication sciences has since become the preferred term because this encompasses the many forms of communication that are not exclusive to making public speeches.

A number of advancements have occurred in human communication over the centuries. They are too numerous to discuss here but a listing of some of the more significant advancements are provided in a time line format in Table 1.3. As new forms of communication have emerged, the old forms have become more specifically designed but not completely abandoned. For example, the radio did not vanish once the television was invented. Rather, these older forms of communication have become specialized. In regard to modern human communication, major advancements have occurred in media communications, or the methods used for communication. The history of these various methods of communication can be broadly categorized into two areas: (1) written communication and (2) telegraphy.

Written Communication

The earliest evidence of written communication dates back to our ancestors who lived in caves. As long ago as 25,000 BC, early humans painted pictures on cave walls that depicted events that happened in daily life such as hunting or planting. The earliest of these pictures were found in caves of southern France and Spain (Figure 1.4). It took primitive man thousands of years to create a written form of communication. Those civilizations that had written communication were the ones that

Table 1.3. Some Highlights in the Evolution of Communication

Date	Event
BC	
10,000:	An engraved antler with animals and plants portrayed is discovered in France.
2600:	Egyptian Book of the Dead
2200:	Oldest existing document written on papyrus paper
1400:	Oldest record of writing found on bones in China
400:	Chinese write on wood, bamboo, and silk
AD	
600:	Books printed in China
1200:	European monasteries create a letter system for communication
1450:	Johann Gutenberg creates a printing press
1565:	The pencil is invented in England
1609:	The first regularly published newspaper is produced in Germany
1639:	The first printing press is created in the American colonies
1755:	A regular mail ship sails between England and the American colonies
1785:	Stagecoaches carry mail between towns in the United States
1804:	The lithograph is invented in Germany
1815:	There are 3,000 post offices in the United States
1831:	Electric telegraph is invented in the United States
1835:	Creation of the Morse code for electronic communication
1868:	First modern style typewriter was invented
1876:	Alexander Graham Bell invents the telephone
1893:	The electric typewriter is invented called the Blickensderfer
1901:	Guglielmo Marconi transmits a radio signal across the Atlantic Ocean
1904:	A photograph is transmitted by wire in Germany
1905:	The postage meter is introduced in New Zealand
1919:	People are able to directly dial telephone numbers
1933:	Phonograph records are created with stereo sound
1938:	Allen DuMont markets a television for the home
1948:	Long-playing (LP) records are created on vinyl disks
1951:	Computers are sold commercially
1952	Bell Laboratories builds a primitive speech recognition system
1959:	Xerox manufactures a copying machine
1961:	FM stereo broadcasting begins
1965:	First communications satellite begins orbiting earth
1966:	Commercial distribution of FAX machines
1976:	Creation of Apple microcomputer
1979:	Japan creates first cellular phone network
1980:	Creation of CNN 24-hour news channel
1984:	Creation of portable compact disk player
1989:	Timothy Berners-Lee creates the framework for the World Wide Web
1991:	Video cassette recorders are found in 75% of U.S. homes
1996:	Over 9 million people use the Internet
2000:	AT&T develops the "How May I Help You" speech recognition system

A

B

FIGURE 1.4. Two forms of early written communication. A cave painting discovered in Lascaux, France, c. 15,000–10,000 BC (**A**) and an example of abbreviated hieroglyphic writing known as hieratic, c. 2000 BC (**B**).

developed most rapidly. Around 2000 BC the Egyptians developed a writing system that used **hieroglyphics**, which means, "the words of God," and is a form of writing in which the various symbols stood for certain sounds and words. It was used primarily by scribes, doctors, and priests to decorate the walls of temples and tombs. An abbreviated form of hieroglyphics, called **hieratic**, was used for more informal communication. This was a type of handwriting in which the symbols were abbreviated to the point of abstraction (see Figure 1.4).

Somewhere between 1700 and 1500 BC the **alphabet** was established as a form of written communication. The word is derived from the Latin origin, *alfabetum*, which combines the first two symbols of the Greek alphabet, "*alpha*"

and "*beta*." The use of alphabetic symbols was easier and faster to draw than pictures and was more universally recognized for their meaning. The use of an alphabet allowed for the creation of words and sentences. The Greek and Hebrew alphabets were established around 100 BC. The Greek alphabet became the source for the Latin alphabet created in 7 BC, which in turn became the source of the present day English alphabet. The Hebrew alphabet that is used today dates back to 600 BC. The Greek and Latin alphabets were designed to be written from left to right. These early alphabetic systems only used uppercase letters with lowercase letters introduced during the first century (Figure 1.5).

The invention of paper and writing instruments also played an important

FIGURE 1.5. The Hebrew, Greek, and Latin alphabets and the two forms of writing each alphabet.

role in the development of written communication. A form of writing paper known as **papyrus** was developed by the Egyptians around 3000 BC. The raw material of papyrus paper came from the plant *cyperus papyrus* that grew along the banks of the Nile, which was used to create rope, baskets, and boats. The method of paper production was kept secret by the Egyptians. The first widely used writing instrument that was predominant was the quill pen that was introduced around 700 AD. The quill is a pen made from a bird feather, and some of the strongest quills were those that were taken from living birds. Usually quill pens only lasted about a week before it was necessary to replace them.

Throughout the subsequent centuries, the written word became more accessible to large groups of people, but the process of writing was very laborious. The earliest books were primarily religious in nature, containing prayers and songs. To reproduce any written material, an individual needed to completely rewrite the document. A great deal of this work was completed by monks who spent long hours in monasteries making copies by hand of religious books and manuscripts. This approach to document reproduction came to an abrupt halt in 1450 with the invention of the movable-type printing press. **Johann Gutenberg's** (1398–1468) printing press was revolutionary, allowing for easier and faster reproduction of written material (Figure 1.6). The invention contributed to the creation of mass media communication and the free spread of ideas in an unprecedented fashion. The use of newspapers as a form of written communication became widespread with the introduction of the printing press. The essential features of the Gutenberg

FIGURE 1.6. Johann Gutenberg, inventor of the movable-type printing press.

printing press remained unchanged until the 19th century, when in the early 1800s a steam-powered printing press using continuous rolls of paper and iron (instead of wooden) machinery was created. This technologic advancement in printing made it possible for daily newspapers to be distributed at a fraction of the previous cost.

Telegraphy

Telegraphy refers to the long-distance transmission of written messages without the need to "physically transport" the message. Forms of telegraphy that have had a historical impact on human communication include the: (1) telegraph, (2) telephone, (3) television, and

The famous American novelist, **Mark Twain** (1835–1910) enjoyed and made use of new inventions during his lifetime. He was the first author to discard his pen and submit a typewritten manuscript to his publisher.

(4) internet. **Joseph Henry** (1797–1878) was an important American scientist of the 18th century. One of his discoveries occurred in 1830 when he demonstrated that an electrical signal could be transmitted over a wire that spanned the distance of one mile. This discovery led to the creation of the electric **telegraph**. Five years later, in 1835, **Samuel Morse** (1791–1872) formulated the **Morse code**, which is an alphabetic system that uses a combination of short and long clicks to create words (Figure 1.7). The combination of the electric telegraph, along

A

Morse Code Alphabet

A	.-	N	-.	0	-----
B	-...	O	---	1	.----
C	-.-.	P	.--.	2	..---
D	-..	Q	--.-	3	...--
E	.	R	.-.	4	....-
F	..-.	S	...	5	.....
G	--.	T	-	6	-....
H	....	U	..-	7	--...
I	..	W	.--	9	----.
K	-.-	X	-..-	Fullstop	.-.-.-
L	.-..	Y	-.--	Comma	--..--
M	--	Z	--..	Query	..--..

B

FIGURE 1.7. Samuel Morse (**A**) and his coded alphabet used for the telegraph (**B**).

with a simple to use alphabet system transformed the way we communicate. With the invention of the telegraph it became possible to transmit a message without the need for physical movement. This electric message traveled faster than people, horses, or trains. To this day, Morse code remains a viable means of providing reliable communications during difficult communication conditions.

The telegraph had been established for over 30 years before the development of another wire-based electrical communication system, the **telephone**. The telegraph was limited to sending a series of single electrical sounds along a wire. **Alexander Graham Bell** (1847–1922) determined a way to send a combination of electrical sounds (i.e., speech) along a wire (Figure 1.8). In 1876, Bell's famous first words to his assistant on the telephone, *"Mr. Watson come here I want to see you,"* ushered in a new form of communication, and signaled a demise in popularity of the telegraph. Since then, the telephone has become an integral part of our society, even leading to the establishment of an industry known as **telecommunications**. The invention of the telegraph and the telephone led to the eventual development of the **radio**. In 1901, an Italian inventor **Gugliemo Marconi** (1874–1937) sent and received the first radio signal, thus marking a new age of wireless communication (Figure 1.9). This technology has now been applied to telephones, which has contributed to a novel form of written communication known as **text messaging**.

The **television** has become a device that the majority of people cannot live without. Television is the transmission

FIGURE 1.8. Alexander Graham Bell, inventor of the telephone.

FIGURE 1.9. Guglielmo Marconi, inventor of the radio.

and reception of moving images by use of electrical signals. Around 1908, an English inventor by the name of **Alan Archibald (A. A.) Campbell-Swinton** (1863–1930) conceived the idea for an electrical method of scanning, or collecting an image, although it was not until the 1930s that the actual method using electron (or cathode) rays was developed by an American electrical engineer, **Allen B. DuMont** (1901-1965) (Figure 1.10). DuMont has been called the "Father of Television" and his invention of the picture tube still serves as the basic foundation for the type of televisions used today. Television is a mode of communication where TV viewers serve as decoders of information; its use has become the primary mode of communication to the mass media. For example, presidential elections today would be entirely different without the use of television.

Finally, the manner in which we communicate in this modern world has undoubtedly been transformed by computers. Two features of computer-based communication that have had wide sweeping influence are the **internet** and **speech recognition**. The internet is a worldwide network of thousands of computers and computer networks. The internet began in the early 1970s as a computer network that linked computers at several universities and research laboratories in the United States. As more and more universities began linking to the network, a software system was developed that allowed for anyone to roam, browse, or contribute to the internet. This software was developed in 1989 by English computer scientist **Sir Timothy Berners-Lee** (b. 1955) (Figure 1.11) for the European Organization for Nuclear Research (CERN) and became known as the **World Wide Web**. He is known as the "Father of the Internet." The internet has dramatically changed our world, allowing people to share information in spite of geographic barriers. By the early 1990s, e-mails had

FIGURE 1.10. Allen B. DuMont, known as the "Father of Television."

FIGURE 1.11. Sir Timothy Berners-Lee, known as the "Father of the Internet." From U. Bojars at Wikimedia Commons. Permission granted through Creative Commons Attribution 2.5 License.

FYI

Text messaging has led to the development of a unique shorthand form of written communication that makes sending messages quicker and easier. It is likely that many of these words will become so commonplace that they become candidates for inclusion in the *Oxford English Dictionary's* annual "new words" book. Examples of this shorthand include:

Word	Shorthand
Are	R
Why	Y
You	U
Please	PLS
Before	B4
Later	L8R
Excellent	XLNT
Tomorrow	2MORO
Please call me	PCM

---

replaced paper letters as the most common form of telegraphy. New forms of internet communication are developing rapidly with unique names to these various forms of communication such as **blogging, instant messaging, and microblogging** (e.g., Twitter). A description of forms of internet communication is provided in Table 1.4.

Speech recognition (also known as automatic speech recognition or computer speech recognition) is a process whereby the computer learns to understand discrete words and phrases. The earliest computer-based speech recognition systems were developed in the 1950s at Bell Telephone Laboratories in the United States. The challenge in developing such a system is that the computer must be able to decipher the wide degree of variability in the manner of speaking demonstrated from one person to the next. These differences encompass features such as age, sex, accent, and rate of speaking. Early systems were only able to recognize individual vowel or consonant sounds. This technology is rapidly evolving and is now entering the service industry. A current example is the automatic flight information system used by United Airlines. The system is referred to as "How May I Help You?" and is used for call routing of consumer help line calls. Although automatic speech recognition and speech understanding systems are far from perfect in terms of the word or task accuracy, they are becoming yet another form of communication used in society today.

Table 1.4. Some of the Currently Used Forms of Internet Communication

Electronic Mail (E-mail)	The process of typing a message and sending this message electronically across a computer network.
Internet Relay Chat (IRC)	A communications system that permits people from across the world to conduct online text based communication with one or more other users. IRC users normally see the text conversations of all users on the network.
Instant Messaging (IM)	A form of electronic communication that involves immediate correspondence between users who are all online simultaneously. IM tends to differ from IRC because the communication is typically only between two users.
Blogging	A blog is an online journal (a shortened form of Web log). Blogging is writing in one's blog for users on the Internet to openly view.
Skype	A software program that allows users to make telephone calls over the Internet.
Social Networks	A Web site, such as MySpace or Facebook that offers its viewer members the ability to share messages, media, and other information with each other.
Twitter	A social networking service that allows users to send one another a short message (or "tweets"; text-based posts, up to 140 characters long) to a person's personal Web site. Twitter is a form of microblogging.

FYI

The classic 1968 movie, *2001: A Space Odyssey* was possibly the first movie to introduce speech recognition technology into mainstream culture. One of the stars of the movie was an intelligent computer named *HAL* who spoke in a naturally sounding voice and was able to recognize and comprehend speech.

MODELS OF COMMUNICATION

The term **model** has a wide range of uses. It can refer to a type of product, a person who poses for photographers, or a miniature version of an object. From an academic standpoint, a model refers to an abstract idea. The **transmission model** of communication is an idea regarding the way in which humans communicate. This classic model was proposed in 1949 by Claude Shannon and Warren Weaver who were electrical engineers working for Bell Telephone

Laboratories in the United States. The essence of the model is that the successful transmission of a message requires both a sender and a receiver. A simplified version of the transmission model is shown in Figure 1.12; it views the process of communication as one in which a person affects the behavior or state of mind of another person. If the effect was smaller or different from what was originally intended, than a failure in communication takes place. A criticism of the model is that communication is viewed as a discrete event in which there is a simple beginning and end to the delivery and reception of a message. However, we know that communication is a much more complicated and sophisticated process that does not simply start and stop. Rather, communication is an ongoing and dynamically changing activity. Another criticism of the transmission model is that the model does not deal with the "meaning" associated with sending messages from the speaker to listener, simply the transmission of a message from one point to the other. Too often the message sent is not the message received, and the speaker's meaning does not come across to the listener.

A modification of the transmission model was proposed by Wilbur Schramm in 1954 through the inclusion of **feedback loops**. Feedback refers to the activity whereby information is sent back to the source from where the message came. As a reaction to this information, the speaker adjusts his or her message by strengthening, de-emphasizing, or changing the content or form of the original message. The feedback can come from either the speaker or the listener. As speakers, we are constantly monitoring our personal communication behavior and evaluating it. During the encoding of a message we may revise our message mentally before actually speaking, or we

may even choose to revise our message midstream to ensure the message is clearly presented. Feedback from the listener can take many shapes and forms. The listener may send nonverbal body language cues (e.g., eye contact) indicating that the message was understood, or the listener might simply state back to the original speaker that the message was not understood. The use of feedback is critical to the successful communication of messages. An example of the modified transmission model that includes feedback is shown in Figure 1.12.

The transmission model of communication is based on a single speaker and listener. This concept of communication is like a ball being tossed back and forth between two individuals. In reality, communication may involve more than two people. By simply introducing a third person into the communication setting it becomes apparent that communication involves many balls being tossed in both directions at the same time. The term **coregulation** is used to describe the exchange of information that occurs between individuals in a conversational setting. The manner in which each member of a conversational setting adjusts their speaking and listening behavior serves to affect the transfer of messages. These adjustments can help to improve overall communication among the group or lead to possible breakdowns in communication. An example of transfer of information that can occur among a group of three people is displayed in Figure 1.13. In this particular setting, there are at least five different communication interactions that can take place among the group (Brown & Van Riper, 1966). The arrows represent who can talk to whom and who can listen. If we were to assume that the three people were working together to solve a particular problem, such as

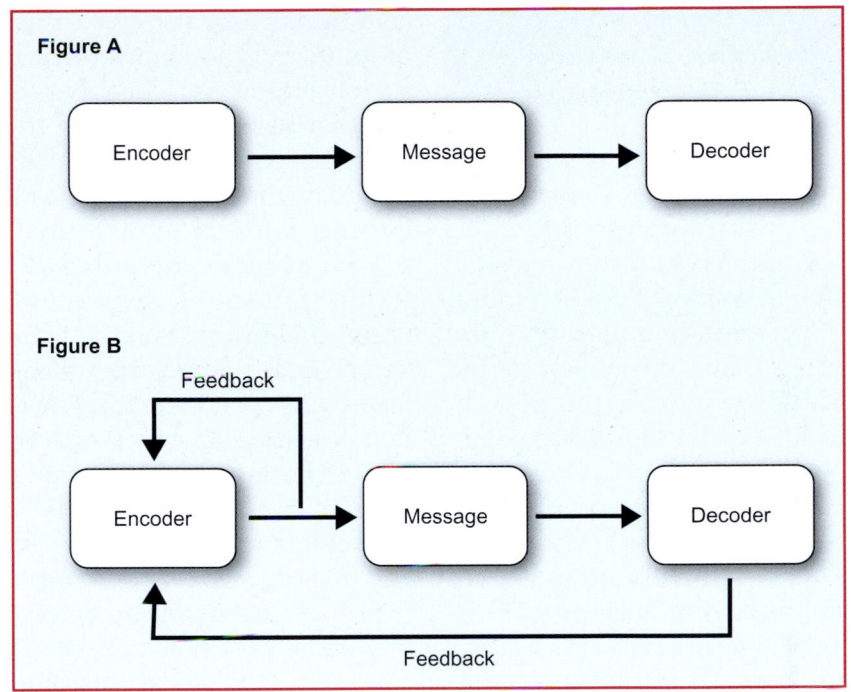

FIGURE 1.12. Classic transmission model of communication (**A**) and the revised transmission model that includes feedback loops (**B**).

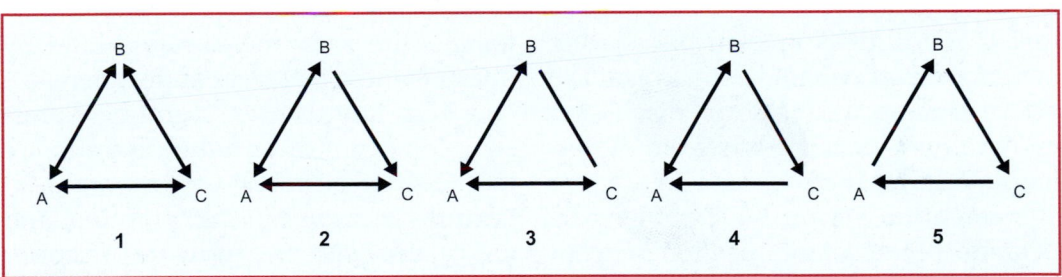

FIGURE 1.13. Communication nets composed of three people. The point of each arrow indicates the direction of communication.

determining the best driving route from Sydney to Melbourne, the following conclusions might be drawn:

- Condition 1 solves the problem with the greatest accuracy.
- Condition 5 solves the problem least accurately.
- Condition 5 gets the message through in the shortest time.

- Listeners are more confident in the two-way means of communication.
- Speakers are surer of themselves in the one-way means of communication.
- The group morale in condition 1 is likely to be the highest.
- Creativity is likely to be greatest in condition 1.
- Condition 1 is the noisiest and least orderly.

FORMS OF COMMUNICATION

The term **form** is defined as the shape and structure of anything, giving it individuality or distinctive character. This term can be applied to communication through two primary forms of communication: (1) verbal communication, and (2) nonverbal communication. **Verbal communication** is at the core of what most of us do; it is the expression of language using spoken words. Our verbal communication varies depending on the particular **communication act**, as well as the **formality** of communication. Acts of verbal communication include: (1) discussion, (2) dialogue, and (3) debate. **Discussion** is an act of verbal communication to make decisions. Discussions are likely to involve the exchange of facts and opinions between communicating partners. **Dialogue** refers to the free-flowing conversational exchange of ideas. These ideas involve the sharing of perspectives and understandings. The act of **debate** differs from discussion and dialogue because this form of verbal communication is used to achieve agreement on a topic which other participants of the communication may not share. We often think of debate as the verbal communication found in the political arena. One person states a point of view, which is subsequently challenged by an opposing view.

Verbal communication also varies in its formality. The level of formality can be found in the vocabulary and grammar characterizing spoken language. **Formal** verbal communication follows a specific code of communicating that might be found in settings such as classrooms, courtrooms, job interviews, or formal parties. Alternatively, **informal** communication also has a specific code of communication but allows for a much-varied manner of speaking. Situations such as "hanging out" with friends and informal parties are likely to reflect a markedly different form of verbal speaking compared to more formal settings.

Nonverbal communication refers to the features of communication that occur aside from what is actually spoken or heard. There are at least six different types of nonverbal communication that we use and experience on a daily basis. These include: (1) paralanguage, (2) sign language, (3) body language, (4) tactile communication, (5) proxemics, and (6) appearance. **Paralanguage** refers to factors such as tone of voice, loudness, inflection, and pitch. By altering these various parameters of voice, the message conveyed is likewise altered. A simple example would be to communicate an identically worded message, such as *Watch your step* in a soft comforting voice, versus a loud, alarming voice. A listener of this same message would likely interpret these messages quite differently.

Sign language is a form of expressive communication where words are replaced by gestures. Commonly used gestures include waving, pointing, and using fingers to indicate number amounts. There are also fully developed language systems that rely exclusively on signs, as often found in the Deaf community. This form of sign language is discussed further in Chapter 13.

Body language pertains to our use of facial expressions or postures to communicate information. Facial expressions are responsible for a huge proportion of nonverbal communication. One need simply smile or frown to communicate a clear nonverbal message. One way of concealing our communication via body language would be to put on a poker-face, which is a face that shows no emotion or change in expression. Expert card players are masters in the use of body language to prevent other card players from knowing the strength of their card hand.

Tactile communication refers to communication that occurs via touch. The use of touch can play a comforting role when paired with verbal communication such as consoling a grieving spouse. Use of touch between parent and child during the infancy period has also been shown to play an integral part in establishing social interaction. **Proxemics** concerns how space and time are used to communicate. A common example is our need for interpersonal space when communicating with others. The amount of personal space needed when having a casual conversation with another person usually varies between 18 inches to four feet. On the other hand, the personal distance needed when speaking to a crowd of people is around 10 to 12 feet. Finally, our **physical appearance** plays an important role in communication. Physical appearance such as clothes and hairstyle serves to convey a message regarding a person's attitude, mood, wealth, and cultural background, which subsequently affects the judgment and interpretations of others.

LEVELS OF COMMUNICATION

We communicate to people at a variety of personal levels, ranging from very superficial to deeply intimate. Powell (1969) identified five levels of communication that humans use to talk (or not to talk) to each other based on their familiarity with the other individual (Figure 1.14). His research was prompted

by the view that most people are initially hesitant about communicating openly with another person for fear of the other individual judging them negatively. The first or lowest level is the **cliché level**. This level of communication involves speaking to others with no real forethought or genuine intent. We use typical or routine questions (e.g., *"How's it going?"*) and give automatic answers (e.g., *"Fine"*) that may not be truthful. In reality, we would not expect an unfamiliar person to provide an elaborate and thoughtful response. The next level is the **fact level**, and involves communication concerning information or statistics about the weather, workplace, the news, and personal activities, such as, *"How do you think Manchester United will perform this year?"* This level of communication requires no in-depth thinking or feeling and does not reveal anything personal about ourselves.

The third level of communication is the **opinion level**. This is a level of communication that occurs between two people on a more personal level and includes comments, concerns, expectations, and personal goals. A question such as, *"Do you think the war will ever end?* would likely result in communication occurring at the opinion level of familiarity. The fourth level of communication is the **feelings level** and usually occurs between two people who know each other well and do not worry about communicating openly. Both individuals feel safe to share openly personal emotions. The highest level of communication is the **needs level**. This level communication occurs between two people who know one another intimately. We feel completely safe to reveal our unique needs with another person. We also may seem to know intuitively what the other person thinks.

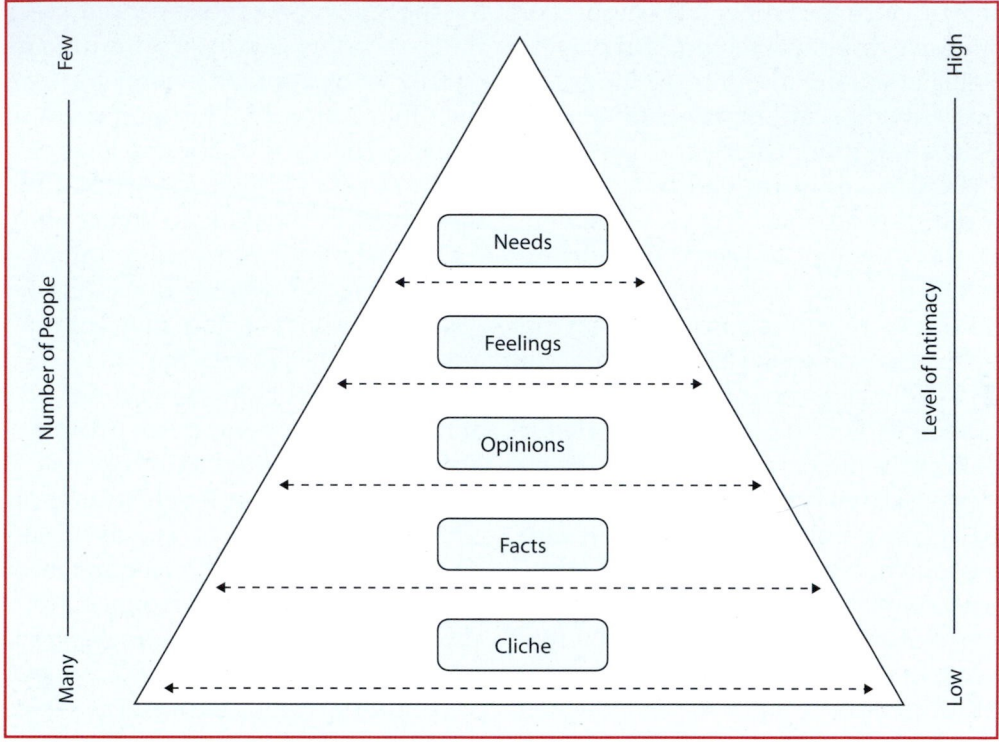

FIGURE 1.14. Five levels of communication according to the number of people and level of intimacy.

CURRENT RESEARCH IN COMMUNICATION SCIENCE

The field of communication sciences has grown enormously in recent decades and continues to evolve. The current areas of research in communication sciences can be summarized into four major themes: (1) technology, (2) culture, (3) discourse, and (4) practice. Communication **technology** is undeniably a rapidly evolving area of research. Advancements in computing technology are closely linked to the manner in which we communicate. Announcements concerning new innovative developments in communication and information technology are being made regularly. Less than 20 years ago, the telephone and television were two very distinct forms of technology used for communication. These two forms are rapidly merging, and 20 years from now we are likely to be exposed to a wide array of telecommunication devices that are an amalgamation of "listening" and "viewing" aspects of communication.

A second emerging area of research in communication sciences involves a focus on **culture**. As the notion of global communication and global interdependence becomes a reality, advances in communication are likely to impact one's culture. For example, access to the internet now allows for information transfer to some of the most remote and isolated parts of the world, although we know little about how this information influences various cultures. Currently, some

---

FYI

Communications satellites have a quiet, yet profound, effect on our daily lives. If you used your cell phone today, listened to the radio, or watched television, you accessed a communications satellite either directly or indirectly. These objects serve to link remote areas of the earth. A signal (such as a TV program) is sent from earth to the satellite, which then amplifies the signal and sends it to another point on earth. In this way, millions of people can watch an event, such as the Olympics, with only the smallest time difference in delay. There are over 800 satellites in space, and the United States owns more than half of these, followed by China and Russia.

---

countries strictly filter and ban various aspects of internet communication, while other countries are much less restrictive. The way in which communication technology converges with culture raises important questions about the effects of communication on the maintenance of cultural diversity.

A third area of research that is being explored in communication science is referred to as **discourse**. The term discourse refers to the act of conversational speaking and the meaning behind these conversations. On a larger scale, discourse refers to the common ideas and beliefs shared by a group of people. From a political standpoint, it is discourse that may separate supporters of the Republican Party from the Democratic Party. The musical fan base of Coldplay would also be a type of discourse community. Within this fan base, certain attitudes would be considered unacceptable and fall outside that of the community. For example, someone who did not hold the song, *Speed of Sound* in the same high esteem as other members of the discourse community might be summarily tossed out of the community. Examining the communication discourse of various communities allows researchers a unique opportunity to assess the shared beliefs held by groups of people.

Practice is a fourth area of research taking place in the area of communication science. Communication practice relates to the types of activities engaged in by people within various settings. A conversation that takes place among people sitting in Starbucks is a form of communication practice. The manner in which you use your cell phone by calling your grandparents every weekend is a form of communication practice. Some forms of communication practice may cross moral and ethical boundaries, such as pornography or political terrorism. These communication practices may not necessarily be good ways of communicating; however, they provide researchers with insight as to how people use communication in their everyday lives.

COMMUNICATION SCIENCES ON THE WORLD WIDE WEB

Listed below are Web sites that provide further information on the topic of communication sciences. At the time of publication each Web site was freely accessible.

Animal Communication Videos
http://www.pbs.org/saf/1201/video/watchonline.htm

Evolution of Communication Video
http://www.archive.org/details/ChiuShienZangRolandEvolvedCommunication

Exploring Nonverbal Communication
http://nonverbal.ucsc.edu/

History of Communication
http://www.historyworld.net/wrldhis/PlainTextHistories.asp?historyid=aa93

Human Communication Video Series
http://highered.mcgraw-hill.com/sites/0072560053/student_view0/new__video_series.html#

REFERENCES

Brown, C., & Van Riper, C. (1955). *Speech and man*. Inglewood Cliffs, NJ: Prentice-Hall.

Powell, J. (1969). *Why am I afraid to tell you who I am?* Niles, IL: Argus Communications.

Shannon, C., & Weaver, W. (1949). *Mathematical theory of communication*. Urbana: University of Illinois Press.

COMMUNICATION DISORDERS AND THE PROFESSIONS

OBJECTIVES

After reading this chapter, the student should be able to:

- Demonstrate an understanding of the audiology and speech-language pathology professions.

- Describe the various work settings for audiologists and speech-language pathologists.

- Demonstrate an understanding of developmental and acquired communication disorders.

- Demonstrate an understanding of organic and functional communication disorders.

- Demonstrate an understanding of epidemiology, including prevalence and incidence.

- Demonstrate an understanding of evidence-based practice.

- Demonstrate an understanding of the Code of Ethics.

- Describe sociocultural influences on normal and disordered communication.

INTRODUCTION

Communication is the process of speaking and listening. Most of us take communication for granted. We tacitly assume that when we speak, we will be understood or when someone speaks to us, we will understand them. Only when a breakdown in communication occurs do we realize how special and vital this act is. A communication disorder is one of the most common types of disabilities found throughout the world. Recall from Chapter 1 that the transmission model provides a useful way to conceptualize the act of communication, involving a speaker and a listener. A more detailed version of this model was proposed by Denes and Pinson (1973) with particular reference to the linguistic and physiological contributions to speaking and listening. They referred to this model as the speech chain (Figure 2.1).

According to speech chain model, the process of encoding a message occurs at three levels: (1) linguistic (2) physiological, and (3) acoustic. The linguistic level is the first step in the speech chain, whereby the message is organized in the brain. Once we determine the message to be spoken, various motor nerves required to produce the sounds and words of the message send impulses from the brain to the speech musculature. This physiological process represents the next link in the speech chain. Once these words leave our mouth, they become an airborne acoustic signal, thus representing the final link in the process of speech encoding. There is also a side, or "feedback," link in the process of speech encoding. We naturally listen to our own voices when talking. By doing so, the message spoken is compared to what was originally intended to be spoken. This occurs when we produce a **spoonerism** (or slip-of-the-tongue). The phrase, "mix up your words" spoken as, *wix up your mords*, is one such example. If we judge the message to be incorrectly spoken, the message can be modified. The remaining links of the speech chain are related to the process of decoding.

The steps involved in decoding the message occur in the reverse order of those just described for speech encoding. Our ears are exposed to the acoustic signal after it leaves the mouth of the speaker. At a physiologic level, the nerves vital to hearing transform this acoustic signal into electrical impulses along auditory (sensory) pathways leading to the brain. Once the sensory impulses reach the brain, they are deciphered into individual sounds, words, and sentences. This deciphering of the acoustic signal into a linguistic message represents the final link in the speech chain.

The speech chain model is useful to illustrate communication disorders. Any breakdown or disruption in the process of encoding that occurs along the pathway from the brain to the actual execution of speech can result in a communication disorder. Similarly, any breakdown in the decoding process in the chain between the outer ear and the brain can result in a communication disorder.

FYI

Many of the Looney Tunes cartoon characters were based on having a speech disorder. Porky Pig produced speech with a stutter. Daffy Duck, Tweety Bird, and Elmer Fudd all produced speech with some form of unique articulation disorder.

FIGURE 2.1. The process of communication depicted at linguistic, physiologic, and acoustic levels.

The focus of this chapter is to introduce the nature and type of communication disorders found in children and adults. As well, the professions dedicated to helping individuals with communication disorders are profiled.

TERMINOLOGY AND DEFINITIONS

A **communication disorder** is a diagnosed condition in which a person is unable to say correctly what she or he wants to say, and/or is unable to understand some or most of what is being said. Some individuals may have an isolated impairment in speech or hearing; others may have impairment in both domains. Simply stated, a communication disorder is any impairment in speaking or hearing that deviates from what might be considered normal.

Classification of Communication Disorders

Communication disorders can be grouped into two general categories (Figure 2.2). The first grouping is in regard to the timing of when the disorder first occurred. Specifically, did the disorder occur before or after birth? Any medical or health condition, including a communication disorder that occurs prior to birth, during birth, or shortly after birth, is referred to as a **developmental** or **congenital** disorder. An example of a developmental communication disorder is a child who is born with a cleft of the lip or palate (Figure 2.2A). This cleft, if left unrepaired, can greatly impair speech production. The second grouping of communication disorders pertains to whether the medical or health condition is found to occur later in life (i.e., after birth); if so, the disorder is referred to as an **acquired** disorder. Most often, an individual with

A

B

FIGURE 2.2. Examples of developmental and acquired communication disorders. (**A**) shows a child born with a cleft lip and palate. (**B**) depicts an individual with a head injury resulting from a motor vehicle accident.

an acquired communication disorder was demonstrating normal communication prior to experiencing the disorder. An example of an acquired communication disorder is an individual who suffers a traumatic brain injury following a motor vehicle accident (Figure 2.2B). As a result of this accident, the individual may experience a marked impairment in the ability to produce or understand speech. Prior to the accident, the person's communication most likely was normal.

Communication disorders can also be classified in regard to the cause (i.e., **etiology**) of the disorder. A medical or health condition with a known physical cause is called an **organic** disorder. In most cases, the physical condition is visible to the naked eye. Such is the case in a typical seven-year-old child who has lost her two front (central incisor) teeth. This condition is likely to pose a problem for the correct articulation of speech sounds that involve these physical structures (e.g., /s/ and /th/ sounds) (Figure 2.3). An organic disorder can also be invisible to the naked eye such as impairments resulting from brain abnormalities (e.g., stroke). If there is no known anatomic, physiologic, or neurologic basis for the observed disorder, the term **functional** disorder is used. A closely related term is **idiopathic** disorder, which denotes a condition that has an unknown cause. School-age children who mispronounce speech sounds, such as *"wabbit"* for *"rabbit,"* who show no apparent physical problems would be classified as showing a functional communication disorder. A number of communication disorders have no readily identifiable cause. Although we may not know the precise cause of these functional disorders, they still can be successfully treated. An illustration of the overlap of developmental and acquired disorders that have

FIGURE 2.3. Example of an organic communication disorder found in most normally developing children. The absence of upper central incisors is likely to affect speech sound production but only temporarily.

a functional or organic basis is shown in Figure 2.4.

A final comment about classifying communication disorders relates to the label we may place on a person who is demonstrating a disorder. In the past, it was common to place the disorder (or label) first and the person second. We might have referred to an individual as being a "cleft palate child." In other instances, an individual was simply labeled by the disorder, where we referred to the person as a "stutterer." These days, the more appropriate manner of referring to a communication disorder is to place the individual first and the disorder second. So, as professionals in the field of communication disorders we may encounter a child *with* a cleft palate or a person *who* stutters.

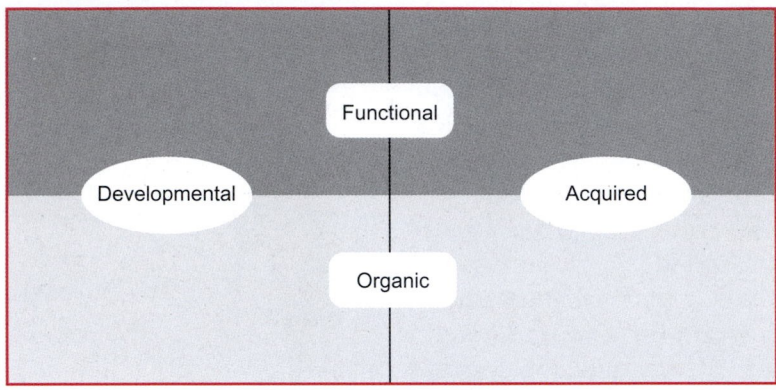

FIGURE 2.4. Categorization of communication disorders according to when the disorder occurred (developmental versus acquired) and how the disorder occurred (functional versus organic).

Occurrence of Communication Disorders

Epidemiology refers to the study of how often diseases and conditions occur in people and why. A common way of charting the occurrence of a disorder or disease is in reference to the overall population. **Prevalence** is a frequently used epidemiological measure of how commonly a disease or condition occurs in a population at a particular point in time. The prevalence is calculated by dividing the number of persons with the disease or condition at a particular time by the number of individuals examined. Prevalence often is expressed as a percentage. The **incidence** of a disease is another epidemiologic measure. Incidence measures the rate of occurrence of new cases of a disease or condition, and is calculated as the number of new cases of a disease or condition in a specified time period (usually 1 year) divided by the size of the population. So prevalence is a measure of all cases of disease at a point of time, and incidence is the measure of new cases of disease in a time period. In the context of communication

disorders, prevalence would refer to the estimated population of people who are managing communication disorders at any given time, whereas incidence would refer to the annual diagnosis rate of new cases of communication disorders.

The majority of epidemiology information on communication disorders relates to prevalence. Approximately one out of every seven individuals, or 12% of the population, has some form of communication disorder. This percentage encompasses disorders of either speech or hearing, ranging in severity from mild to profound. The prevalence of communication disorders in the United States is around 46 million people. Approximately 2.7 million Australians have a communication disorder. There are also prevalence data regarding certain types of communication disorders, as well as age groups. Specific prevalence information for various communication disorders is presented in the ensuing chapters. Some types of communication disorders occur more often than others. For example, there are estimates that 2.5 million people in the United Kingdom have speech and language disorders. Of this number, 800,000 have a disorder so severe that it is difficult for most people to understand them. The worldwide prevalence of communication disorders in children is approximately 25% of the population but lowers with increasing age. This lowering in prevalence presumably reflects a large number of children outgrowing or receiving treatment to alleviate the disorder.

Boys and Girls

A well-known fact is that boys tend to be more susceptible than girls for a large number of childhood diseases. This vulnerability is evident early in life with male infants showing significantly higher rates of premature birth and congenital abnormalities than female infants. In the first year of life, boys get sick and die more often than girls. In 2004, the infant mortality rate (deaths per 1,000 live births) in the United States was 7.4 for boys and 6.1 for girls. Developmental disorders such as autism are three to four times more common in infant boys than girls, and behavioral disorders are at least twice as common. The same is true for communication disorders. Take, for example, the condition of stuttering —boys are three times more likely to develop a stuttering disorder than girls. The precise reason as to why males are more prone to various health disorders remains unknown. Some genetics experts believe there probably is a biological difference that gives females a health advantage over males. One suggestion is that males are disadvantaged by not having the second "X" (sex) chromosome found in women. Having two "X" chromosomes may help to protect women against disease. This vulnerability is apparent in male mammals of all species, indicating a likely evolutionary explanation. It could well be that nature provides a health advantage to females because the survival of the species depends on them. Males simply may be more expendable than females!

THE PROFESSIONS

Speech-language pathology and audiology are health professions that collectively contribute to the field of human communication sciences and disorders. The profession of **speech-language pathology**, also referred to as speech-language therapy, encompasses the study of human communication, swallowing, speech and language development, and their disorders. The profession of **audiology** encompasses the study of human communication, normal processes of hearing, and hearing loss. A **speech-language pathologist** (SLP) is a professional educated in the study of human communication, swallowing, speech-language development, and its disorders. By evaluating the speech, language, and swallowing skills of children and adults, the SLP determines what communication or swallowing problems exist and the best way to treat them. An **audiologist** (AUD) is a professional educated in the study of human communication, normal hearing processes, and hearing loss. The AUD determines if a person has a hearing loss, the type of loss, and the best way to treat the loss. Speech-language pathology and audiology are distinct disciplines, but they have considerable overlap. To be fully skilled in either discipline, one should be familiar with both. Each discipline deals with impairments that disrupt the ability of the individual to communicate normally.

The audiology and speech-language pathology professions are found world wide but are not uniform across nations. A listing of some of the professional associations for AUDs and SLPs found around the world is shown in Table 2.1. There are approximately 110,000 SLPs and 12,000 AUDs currently working in the United States. Approximately 2,500 SLPs and 1,000 AUDs reside in Australia, and approximately 700 SLPs and 120 AUDs are found in New Zealand. There are around 2500 AUDs working throughout the United Kingdom and 11,000 SLPs currently practice in the United Kingdom. The combined number of SLPs and AUDs in India is approximately 2,000 and rapidly grow-

---

FYI

Most audiologists and speech-language pathologists engage in clinical practice. They often are referred to as *clinicians*. The people with communication disorders seen by these professionals are referred to as *clients*.

Table 2.1. Some of the Professional Associations in Audiology and Speech-Language Pathology

Australia	Audiological Society of Australia (ASA)
	Speech Pathology Australia (SPA)
Britain	British Academy of Audiology (BAA)
	British Society of Audiology (BSA)
	Royal College of Speech and Language Therapists (RCSLT)
Canada	Canadian Academy of Audiology (CAA)
	Canadian Association of Speech-Language Pathologists and Audiologists (CASLPA)
India	Indo-International Society of Communication and Hearing Sciences (IISCHS)
	Indian Speech and Hearing Association (ISHA)
Ireland	Irish Society of Audiology (ISA)
	Irish Association of Speech and Language Therapists (IASLT)
New Zealand	New Zealand Audiological Society (NZAS)
	New Zealand Speech-Language Therapists Association (NZSTA)
Singapore	Speech-Language and Hearing Association, Singapore (SHAS)
South Africa	South African Association of Audiologists (SAAA)
	South African Speech-Language-Hearing Association (SASLHA)
United States of America	American Academy of Audiologists (AAA)
	American Speech-Language-Hearing Association (ASHA)

ing. Both AUDs and SLPs are in high demand and there are an insufficient number to meet the demand, which is likely to increase since the number of people with communication disorders is predicted to grow. Members of the baby boom generation are now well into their middle age years and this large population is likely to contribute to an increase in the number of communication disorders that accompany old age. In addition, medical advances are resulting in improved survival rate for premature infants, as well as elderly stroke victims. The increase in survival rate will undoubtedly increase the number of individuals likely to require the services of an AUD or SLP.

FIGURE 2.5. John Thelwall, a pioneering speech scientist and orator.

HISTORY OF THE PROFESSIONS

The field of communication sciences and disorders has evolved over time. The first AUDs and SLPs were not given formal professional titles. They were researchers and teachers who took an interest in helping individuals with speaking and hearing difficulties. The foundation of the AUD and SLP professions was influenced by many disciplines including biology, psychology, medicine, physics, linguistics, rhetoric, and education. A number of individuals contributed to the field and some of the more noteworthy contributions are highlighted below.

John Thelwall (1764–1834) is recognized as a pioneering speech scientist and therapist in the United Kingdom (Figure 2.5). Thelwall was part of the Elocutionary Movement in the early 1800s that stressed high standards of education and high standards in the use of language. Thelwall was well known for giving radical political speeches. In addition to his oratory skills, he also published a number of works dealing with elocution, the acquisition of language, the anatomy of the speech organs, and the link between speech and mental illness. Thelwall noted that some children with speech defects respond better in therapy with a female compared to a male. He also was the first to classify speech disorders as being either natural (organic) or habitual (functional).

Alexander Melville Bell (1819–1905) and **Alexander Graham Bell** (1847–1922) were father and son who were both eminent English scientists and inventors. The family eventually settled in Canada and the United States. Although most know of the contribution made by Graham Bell to the development of the first practical telephone, few know of the contributions made by his father. Melville spent the majority of his life assisting others with their speech, whether it was formal elocution lessons or correction of speech disorders (Figure 2.6). His

FIGURE 2.6. A photo of Alexander Melville Bell (**A**) and a copy of his business (professional) card as published in his textbook *Visible Speech* in 1867 (**B**).

A

PROFESSIONAL CARD.

Mr A. MELVILLE BELL, Author of 'Visible Speech' may be consulted in all Cases of Impediment or Defect of Speech, Vocal Weakness, Monotony, Oratorical Ineffectiveness, &c.

STAMMERING AND STUTTERING.

The experience of upwards of Twenty-five years' Practice enables Mr A. MELVILLE BELL to undertake the permanent, and, in most cases, the speedy Removal of Stammering and other forms of Vocal Impediment.

References of the highest class are furnished to inquirers.

A limited number of Pupils can be accommodated as Boarders; but residence in the Establishment is not required in order to effect a Cure.

DEFECTS OF ARTICULATION.

In cases of Lisping, Burring, and other Single Elementary Defects, the entire Removal of the Faculty Habit rarely needs more than from Six to Twelve Lessons.

Children who are backward in acquiring the power of Speech are trained to the perfect use of their Vocal Organs. Parents or Governesses are invited to be present at the Lessons, and are directed in the means of carrying on the improvement, which is always rapidly commenced.

ELOCUTION.—PRONUNCIATION, READING, DELIVERY AND ACTION.

Clergymen, Barristers, Members of Parliament, and other Public Readers and Speakers, are Privately Instructed in the Principles and Practice of Effective Delivery, Oratorical Composition, &c.

Ladies and Non-professional Pupils, receive Special Lessons in the art of Reading, &c., according to individual requirements.

VISIBLE SPEECH—UNIVERSAL ALPHABETICS.

Pupils are practically initiated in the Physiology of Speech, and in the use of the Universal Alphabet, so as to be enabled to produce, and to record, all varieties of Native or Foreign Sounds.

Dialectic peculiarities are corrected; and Foreigners are taught to pronounce English with the characteristics of vernacular utterance;

TERMS.

Single Lessons in any Department, - - - - -	-	One Guinea.
Cure of Stammering, Stuttering, &c., -	(Twelve Lessons,) -	Ten Guineas.
Removal of Lisping, Burring, &c., - -	(Six Lessons,) -	Four Guineas.
Elocution, Reading, Delivery, &c., -	(Six Lessons,) -	Three Guineas.
Visible Speech,—Vocal Physiology, &c., -	(Six Lessons,) -	Three Guineas.

The following additional Establishments for the Cure of Stammering and for Elocutionary Instruction are conducted (in Edinburgh) by Mr MEVILLE J. BELL; and (in Dublin) by Mr D. C. BELL.

Edinburgh: No. 13 South Charlotte Street.
Dublin: No. 1 Kildare Place.

B

wife Eliza was severely hearing impaired, which influenced his own work, as well as that of his son. Melville Bell developed a transcriptional system known as "visible speech" that included drawings of the head and neck showing the physical movements behind the articulation of individual speech sounds. Following his father's death, Graham published the transcription system and taught it to teachers of the Deaf.

Henry Sweet (1845–1912) was a pioneer in modern transcriptional phonetics (Figure 2.7). He was an Oxford graduate and studied speech through an interest in the English language. He developed the Broad Romic symbol system that eventually led to the International Phonetic Alphabet. He established England as the birthplace of the science of phonetics. The 1913 play entitled, *Pygmalion* written by George Bernard Shaw (which later became the theatrical musical, *My Fair Lady*) is thought to be based loosely on the life of Henry Sweet (aka Henry Higgins).

One person who contributed to the development of the professions in Germany was **Hermann Gutzmann** (1865–1922). He helped to establish the field of logopedics, which is the science and study of dealing with speech defects in children. Gutzmann studied speech disorders from a medical point of view. He went on to create the Berlin School for Speech and Voice Therapy. The services provided by the Berlin school attained worldwide acclaim..

Wilhelm Wundt (1832–1920) was a German medical doctor, psychologist, physiologist, and professor who attended the Leipzig school in Germany (Figure 2.8). The Leipzig school was a research center in Germany that was responsible for training the first generation of psychologists. Sigmund Freud was influenced by the Leipzig school. The school also dabbled in techniques

FIGURE 2.7. Henry Sweet, an expert in phonetics (aka "Henry Higgins").

FIGURE 2.8. Wilhelm Wundt known as the "Father of Experimental Psychology."

for quantitatively measuring aspects of hearing and speech. Upon graduation, Wundt remained at the Leipzig school and developed a psychology laboratory. He is widely regarded as the "Father of Experimental Psychology." In particular, he is credited with developing the science of psychophysics, which forms the basis for the testing of hearing. Some of Wundt's students were influential in the field of communication disorders.

Edward Wheeler (EW) Scripture (1864–1945) graduated from Leipzig in 1888 under the supervison of Wundt. He was an American who developed skills in hearing measurement such as threshold testing and magnitude estimation. Scripture eventually developed a psychology laboratory at Yale University and wrote a book comparing stuttering to lisping or "super-energetic versus sub-energetic" speech production.

Carl Seashore (1866–1949), who was born in Sweden, traveled to America and studied under Scripture at Yale University (Figure 2.9). Seashore had interests in music, voice, and hearing. He built the first audiometer with the help of Scripture. He is also the individual who developed the concept of the decibel (dB) by separating loudness magnitude into units of 40 steps each. He later became the head of the psychology department at the University of Iowa.

In 1920, Seashore was approached by **Samuel Orton** (1879–1948) who was a physician interested in learning disabilities. Orton's daughter had difficulty in speaking and reading. He suggested to Seashore that someone should be specifically educated to work with individuals having these types of difficulties. Seashore selected the most promising student from the undergraduate psychology class at the University of Iowa and offered this specialized PhD to **Lee**

Edward Travis (1896–1987) (Figure 2.10). Travis received his PhD in 1924 and is recognized as the founding father of the

FIGURE 2.9. Carl Seashore, inventor of the audiometer.

FIGURE 2.10. Lee Edward Travis, known as the "Father of Speech-Language Pathology." (Reprinted with permission from Van Riper, C. [1981]. An early history of ASHA. *ASHA Magazine, 23*(11), 855–858.)

speech-language pathology profession in the United States. Travis established himself as a particular expert in the area of stuttering and had many well-known students who went on to establish educational programs across the United States, including Charles Van Riper, who established the program at Western Michigan University, and Max Steer, who established the program at Purdue University.

Around the same time that Travis was completing his studies, **Sara Stinchfield Hawk** (1885–1977) was awarded a masters degree in 1920 from the department of psychology at the University of Iowa (Figure 2.11). Her thesis topic pertained to the area of stuttering. In 1922, Hawk became the first person in America to receive a PhD degree specifically designated in the area of speech pathology, awarded from the University of Wisconsin. Both Hawk and Travis were founding members of the American Speech and Hearing Association established in 1925.

Raymond Carhart (1912–1975) is referred by many to be the "Father of Audiology" in the United States (Figure 2.12). He is credited with coining the word "audiology" to designate the science of hearing. Carhart was a professor of speech at Northwestern University. When World War II broke out, he was commissioned as an officer in the U.S. Army where he developed an aural rehabilitation program for individuals who were deafened as a result of war exposure. His wartime efforts working with thousands of hearing-impaired soldiers served as the basis for the development of a new discipline that is now audiology. Upon conclusion of the

FIGURE 2.11. Sara Stinchfield Hawk. The first person to obtain a PhD in speech-language pathology.

FIGURE 2.12. Raymond Carhart, known as the "Father of Audiology."

war, he returned to Northwestern and proceeded to develop a specific program in audiology.

Finally, the efforts of **Hallie Quinn Brown** (1849–1949) have been overlooked by many historians in regard to her contributions to speech-language pathology in the United States (Figure 2.13). She was a renowned American elocutionist and educator in the late 19th century and a significant figure in the history of speech-language pathology in the United States. She was born the daughter of two former slaves, and taught elocution and literacy training to children, most notably for African Americans and women, during a period in history when it was not fashionable to do so.

FIGURE 2.13. Hallie Q. Brown, American elocutionist and educator in the late 19th century.

EDUCATIONAL PREPARATION

People who choose to become either AUDs or SLPs are entering a clearly defined field of professional practice. So what does it mean to be a *professional*? A professional can be defined as a person who is trained to do a special job in exchange for payment. This often is the case when considering people in the sports world, where it is easy to distinguish a professional athlete from an amateur athlete, through their being paid. Another form of professionalism is in regard to occupations that require education or training pertinent to a specialized field, as distinguished from general education. Training for professionals who work in communication disorders has developed from different starting points and within different philosophical contexts in various countries. The educational requirements to become an AUD compared to an SLP are not identical. There also are differences between countries in regard to the educational requirements for each profession. The differences between countries can be broadly categorized as reflecting an **American model** or **British model** of education. These models are presented separately.

The American Model

A primary feature of the model of education used in the United States is the emphasis on a liberal arts education at the undergraduate level followed by a period of intensive and concentrated education at the graduate level. To become eligible to practice as either an AUD or SLP in the United States, a graduate-level education is required. An example of the typical educational

FYI

There are hundreds of university programs worldwide that educate audiologists and speech-language pathologists. Many countries offer no formal educational programs, requiring residents of these countries to travel abroad to obtain their professional qualification. One of the newest communication disorders programs is the University of Kuwait. Students receive academic coursework in English and apply this to the clinic setting speaking Arabic.

model for both degrees is provided in Table 2.2. As undergraduates, students pursue a bachelor's degree in a major usually called Communication Disorders. This major encompasses fundamental aspects of both audiology and speech-language pathology. The first 2 years of undergraduate education involve coursework covering a wide range of general education courses. These courses serve to satisfy the liberal arts foundation for the bachelor's degree. The final 2 years of undergraduate education focus more specifically on coursework in audiology and speech-language pathology. The majority of this coursework centers on normal aspects of hearing and speech and an introduction to some of the more common communication disorders such as child language disorders and phonological disorders. Upon graduation, the student holds a **preprofessional** bachelor's degree in communication disorders. To satisfy the educational requirements to become an AUD or SLP professional, the student must obtain a graduate degree. Students are allowed to choose freely whether to pursue graduate education in audiology or speech-language pathology.

For those wishing to pursue a clinical career in audiology, the requisite degree is a Doctor of Audiology (AuD) degree, which ranges from 3 to 4 years of study, depending on the particular curriculum established by the university. The first 2 years of graduate study involve detailed coursework and on-site clinical education in audiology and hearing science. The final year involves an extensive off-campus full-time clinical experience (an externship), and in many cases a research project is required.

For those wishing to become a SLP, the requisite degree is a master's degree, which takes 2 years of full-time study to

FYI

Universities that offer educational degrees in audiology and speech-language pathology usually have their own clinic, which provides diagnostic and therapy services to the local community and an opportunity for students to work alongside experienced clinicians as part of their clinical training.

Table 2.2. American Model for the Education of Audiologists and Speech-Language Pathologists

Audiology	Speech-Language Pathology
Undergraduate Education	**Undergraduate Education**
4-year Bachelor's (BSc or BA) Degree	4-year Bachelor's (BSc or BA) Degree
Years 1 and 2 "related" areas of study	Years 1 and 2 "related" areas of study
Years 3 and 4 "major" areas of study	Years 3 and 4 "major" areas of study
Minimal fieldwork	Minimal fieldwork
Graduate Education	**Graduate Education**
3–4 year Doctor of Audiology (AuD) Degree	2-year Master's (MSc or MA) Degree
Years 1–3 Audiology coursework	Years 1–2 Speech-Language Pathology coursework
600 hours of fieldwork	400 hours of fieldwork
Year 4 Externship	3 one-semester Externships
Clinical Fellowship Year (CFY)	Clinical Fellowship Year (CFY)
National Examination	National Examination
Obtain CCC-A	Obtain CCC-SLP

complete. Across the 2 years of study, students complete coursework in communication disorders and engage in a mix of on-campus and off-campus clinical experiences. Students who complete either the AuD or master's in SLP are eligible to work after graduation. The first year of professional employment is referred to as the **clinical fellowship year** (CFY). During the CFY, the individual works in his or her respective profession; however, periodic oversight is provided by a work colleague who holds professional membership status in the American Speech-Language-Hearing Association (ASHA). Membership status is designated by the acronym CCC, which refers to the Certificate of Clinical Competency. Individuals who complete the 1-year CFY make a formal application to ASHA to be awarded the CCC. All AUDs and SLPs working in the United States generally are expected to hold the CCC in order to practice in their respective professions. Working without this credential is a violation of professional ethics.

The British Model

The British model of AUD and SLP education is in widespread use in the United Kingdom, Australia, India, Ireland, New Zealand, and South Africa. The British model places less emphasis on a liberal arts education compared to the American model. Instead, education is more concentrated on the essential coursework and clinical competencies for becoming either an SLP or AUD. The education required to become a SLP is based on a 4-year undergraduate degree, with students entering the major during the first year of university study. By the conclusion of the 4-year degree, students are likely to have taken the same number of courses in speech-language pathology as an American student, and gained the same amount of clinical experience. The British model for the education of audiologists allows for two educational paths. One path is similar to that established for SLP, whereby the degree can be completed as part of 4-year undergraduate education. The second path involves completion of a 2-year Master's degree in audiology. To obtain a Master's degree in audiology it is not mandatory to hold a Bachelor's degree in communication disorders but rather a degree that is compatible with audiology such as psychology, biology, engineering, or business. Similar to the United States requirement, most countries require AUD graduates to complete a CFY as part of the first year of professional experience prior to becoming full-fledged members of their respective professional associations. Examples of the typical British educational models for the SLP and AUD degrees are provided in Table 2.3.

Qualities of an AUD and SLP

Professionals who work as either AUDs or SLPs interact with individuals of all ages and backgrounds. One of the prime attributes of becoming a successful professional is having good people skills, such as knowing how to interact effectively with others who have various disorders and a range of backgrounds. People are individuals, with as many similarities from one person to the next

Table 2.3. British Model for the Education of Audiologists and Speech-Language Pathologists

Audiology	Speech-Language Pathology
Path 1: Undergraduate Degree	**Undergraduate Degree**
4-year Bachelor's Degree	4-year Bachelor's Degree
Year 1 "related" areas studied	Year 1 "related" areas studied
Years 2–4 Audiology coursework	Years 2–4 Speech-Language Pathology coursework
300 hours of fieldwork	300 hours of fieldwork
3 one-semester externships	3 one-semester externships
Path 2: 2-year Masters Degree	
Bachelor's degree in related areas (psychology, biology, linguistics)	
Years 1–2 Audiology coursework	
300 hours of fieldwork	
3 one-semester externships	
Clinical Fellowship Year	
National Examination	
Obtain CCC	

as there are differences. An effective AUD or SLP is able to relate to a wide range of clients and bring out their best performance, whether it is related to testing the hearing of an elderly individual or promoting language development in a young nonverbal child. The two professions are not physically demanding but they can be emotionally and intellectually demanding. These professionals must be able to approach problems objectively and provide support to their clients and families. Many disorders are complex and not fully understood, so professionals must be able to tolerate challenge and uncertainty. Because a client's progress may be slow, AUDs and SLPs must have patience and compassion. Another quality of being a good AUD or SLP is to have sharp listening skills and exceptional observational skills. They also should be able to effectively communicate test results and possible treatment choices to their clients in a manner that is easily understood.

PROFESSIONAL WORK SETTINGS

SLPs and AUDs can be found in a range of work settings. In some instances, the professionals work side by side. Alternatively, some forms of professional practice have quite unique work settings. A description of some of the more common work settings is provided below.

Education

By far, the largest employer of SLPs are public and private schools, and specialized schools such as those designated for hard of hearing and deaf children.

The type of work performed by a SLP in educational settings may involve employment at a single school or serving as an **itinerant** SLP that entails traveling between many schools and having a caseload of clients in each school. Some AUDs are employed in deaf education centers or in public school systems, where they may be involved in performing routine audiologic assessments on students. Higher education settings such as colleges and universities also employ AUD and SLP lecturers and professors to teach students pursuing a career in communication disorders. Approximately 50% of the SLP workforce and 10% of the AUD workforce can be found in educational settings.

Hospitals

Approximately 40% of SLPs and 60% of AUDs are employed in health care settings, including hospitals and residential or nonresidential health care facilities. The two primary hospital settings are: (1) acute care and (2) rehabilitation care. An **acute care hospital** is one where the patient has recently been admitted because of a planned surgery or an accident/trauma. The type of patient seen by the SLP in an acute setting may involve someone who has had their larynx removed as a result of throat cancer, or possibly an individual who recently experienced a stroke, or motor vehicle accident. In these situations, the SLP often will first visit the patient in the hospital bed shortly after the medical condition has been treated. The SLP will diagnose whether a communication disorder exists, as well as the severity of the disorder. A patient may eventually transfer from an acute care hospital to a **rehabilitation hospital** where she or he is now being managed on a longer term basis. The SLP typically is employed to provide treatment to the patient to assist with their eventual discharge from the hospital and transitioning to communicating in the outside environment. Once discharged, the individual may still have a communication disorder and likely would receive services via a residential (e.g., nursing home) or non-residential facility. The type of client seen by an AUD in a hospital setting may be an individual who receives a hearing assessment as part of a routine physical examination. Sometimes AUDs can be found in the operating room of hospitals, where they may monitor a patient's hearing during delicate operations that can affect the hearing mechanism.

Private Practice

Individuals engaged exclusively in private practice account for approximately 5% of the SLP workforce and 20% of the AUD work force. The type of client seen by a SLP private practitioner is generally one who is not in a medically acute condition. Rather, the SLP may see children with mild communication disorders that typically do no qualify for therapy services in a school setting. Or the SLP may offer a unique or specialty type of service, such as working exclusively with individuals who have voice problems, or individuals who may speak English as a second language and are receiving assistance with reducing the strength of their foreign accent. AUDs may work independently or with other private practitioners such as ear, nose, and throat (ENT) physicians. A major facet of this type of job setting is the prescription and fitting of hearing aids. Some AUDs hold full-time employment in another setting but also engage in a minimum level of private practice.

Research

A small percentage (approximately 5%) of SLP and AUD professionals work exclusively in research settings. These individuals are not engaged in clinical practice or education, but rather in scientific investigations of basic and applied aspects of communication sciences and disorders. One well-known institution in the United States is the Boys Town National Research Hospital in Omaha, Nebraska that focuses on childhood deafness, visual impairment, and related communication disorders. A well-known hearing research laboratory in Melbourne, Australia is the Bionic Ear Institute.

Industry

One particular work setting that is unique to AUDs is their employment in the hearing aid industry. Around 5% of

---

FYI

There is a severe shortage of audiologists and speech-language pathologists world wide. In addition to this overall shortage, less than 25% of the work force is made up of males. This sex imbalance is also found in other allied heath professions such as nursing, physiotherapy, and occupational therapy.

AUDs work in industry and may serve as sales representatives for large hearing aid companies. These individuals are experts on current hearing aid devices on the market and provide consultation to practicing AUDs about the latest product advancements.

PROFESSIONAL CODE OF ETHICS

To be a professional involves behaving with dignity and in an ethical manner, and in such a way that people trust your judgment. **Ethical** behavior refers to doing the right thing and encompasses attributes such as (1) honesty, (2) respect, and (3) responsibility. Being honest involves truthfulness and refraining from lying and cheating. Respect involves tolerance and openness toward others regardless of personal or cultural differences. Responsibility means taking your professional duties seriously and accepting culpability for your decisions. Many professional organizations have established a series of behavioral guidelines that govern the day-to-day activities of a professional. These guidelines are referred to as a **code of ethics**, and are a list of common sense rules and regulations that refer to doing the right thing when practicing as a professional.

Most professional associations will establish an ethics board that is designed to handle any complaints raised against individual members. Individuals who are found to be in violation of any of the established codes may run the risk of being sanctioned by their professional association. The level of sanctioning can range from a reprimand that could involve payment of a fine, to the temporary suspension of professional licensure, or in extreme cases, to being handled by state or national law enforcement agencies.

The AUD and SLP professions adhere to a code of ethics, an example of which is established by the American Speech-Language-Hearing Association as provided in Appendix 2-A. There are slight differences in the code of ethics developed by AUD and SLP associations world wide but some of the common tenets are that AUDs and SLPs:

1. Should safeguard the welfare of the clients they serve.
2. Should maintain high standards of professional competence.
3. Should maintain accurate and up-to-date information about the nature, management, and treatment of communication disorders.
4. Should uphold the dignity of the profession and accept the profession's self-imposed standards.

CULTURAL CONSIDERATIONS AND COMMUNICATION DISORDERS

Population centers throughout the world are becoming increasingly diverse both culturally and linguistically. In order to effectively meet the needs of a diverse population, AUDs and SLPs need to be sensitive to issues that can influence both the identification and management of communication disorders. Multilingual and culturally diverse clients are those who use languages and dialects other than that of the AUD or SLP or do not share the same cultural background as the AUD or SLP. Clients may belong to a different culture and communicate in a language different from the AUD or SLP, or may share the same language to some degree while belonging to a different culture. If misunderstood or misinterpreted, the AUD or SLP may inadvertently mistake certain communication behaviors as signs of a disorder. There also are cultural differences in beliefs about health, disability, and delivery of clinical services. The differences can influence how an individual would either perceive a communication disorder or accept certain treatment for the disorder. Professionals providing services to individuals from different cultural backgrounds need to be aware of unique perspectives or communication styles common to those cultures. The complexities of communication in a multicultural environment are demonstrated in Figure 2.14. Some observations about different cultural styles that should be considered by AUDs and SLPs when communicating with individuals of differing cultural and linguistic backgrounds include the following (Roberts, 2001).

Sharing Space

People from different cultures share physical space differently. In some cultures, it is quite acceptable for people to

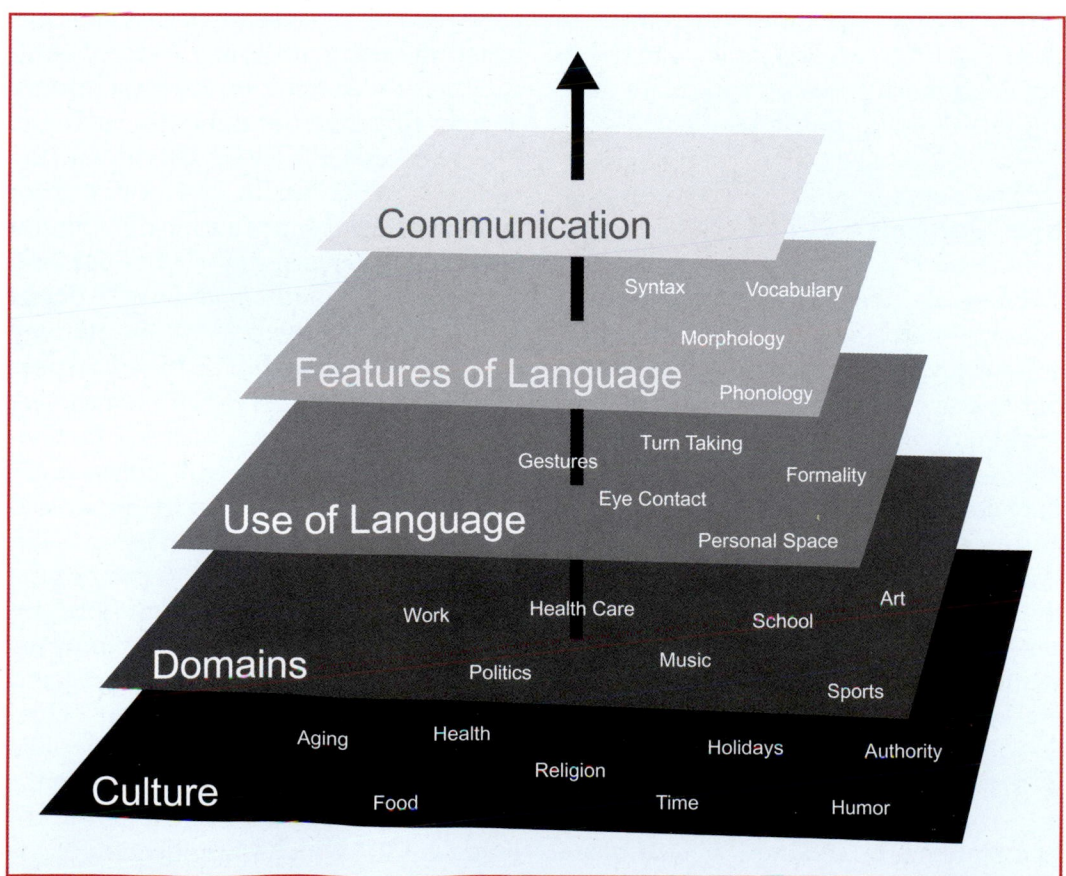

FIGURE 2.14. Depiction of the various layers of communication within a cultural context.

stand in close proximity to one another while talking, whereas in other cultures people like to keep farther apart. For example, Hispanics might view Americans as being distant because they prefer more space between speakers. On the other hand, Americans often view individuals who come too close as invading their private space.

Touching

The rules for touching others vary from culture to culture. In Hispanic and other Latin cultures, two people engaged in conversation often are observed touching and individuals usually embrace when greeting each other. In other cultures, people are more restrained in their greetings. Most Arabic cultures do not customarily shake hands with individuals of the opposite sex.

Eye Contact

The simple act of looking at another person when speaking can have different cultural connotations. Avoidance of direct eye contact is sometimes seen as a sign of attentiveness and respect, whereas sustained direct eye contact may be interpreted as a challenge to authority. Among African Americans, it is not unusual for the listener to avert their eyes, whereas European Americans prefer to make direct eye contact while listening.

Time Ordering

The statement, "business before pleasure" refers to the belief that we must take care of our responsibilities before enjoying ourselves. The notion of completing one activity at a time is called *monochronic* and many mainstream cultures perceive time in this manner. However, some cultures are *polychronic* where several activities occur at the same time. Many Polynesian cultures are polychromic with social interactions interwoven throughout a work activity.

CURRENT ISSUES IN THE PROFESSIONS

Evidence-Based Practice (EBP)

The notion of **evidence-based practice** (EBP) has its origins in the field of medicine where it is known as evidence-based medicine. EBP is a form of clinical decision-making by the practitioner to help improve the patient's outcome. The need for EBP was driven by the desire to shift health care away from basing decisions primarily on opinion and past practices, many of which had not been sufficiently examined to determine their effectiveness. A simple way of conceptualizing EBP is based on asking the questions, *"Why am I practicing this way?"* and *"Is there evidence that can guide me to a better outcome in my practice?"* The processes of EBP can be illustrated in the shape of a triangle (Figure 2.15). Two points on the triangle represent the professional's search for best practice based on their personal experience as well as that found in the academic and research arena. The third point of the triangle represents the professional's acknowledgement of his or her client's needs and values. The center of the triangle is EBP, which is a collection of the three points that should guide the professional's practice.

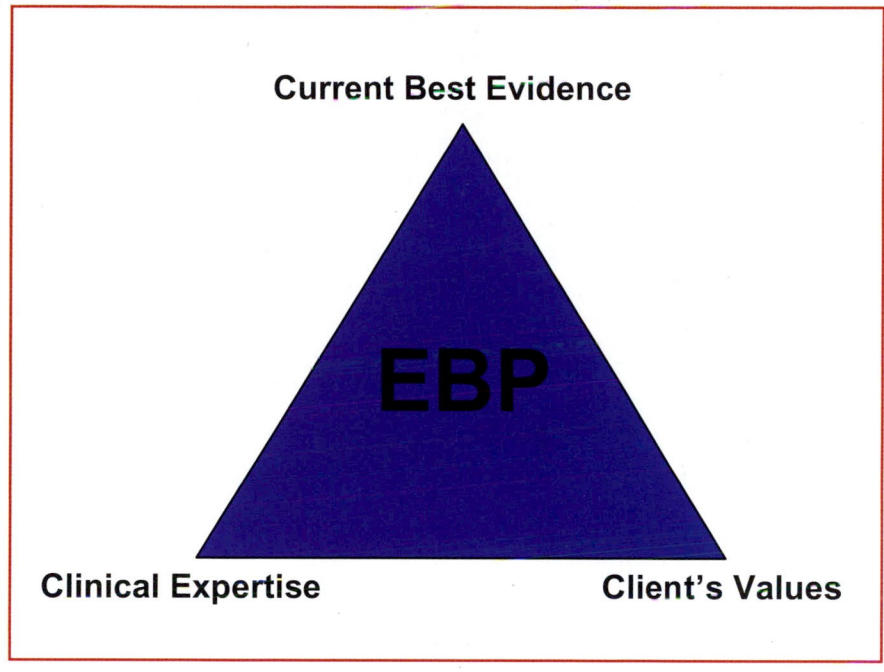

FIGURE 2.15. Evidence-based practice (EBP) triangle illustrating the processes and responsibilities of professionals who adopt EBP.

Two types of evidence guide professional practice. The first is evidence that demonstrates effective treatment approaches (i.e., what to do). The second type of evidence demonstrates ineffective treatment approaches (i.e., what not to do). Both are equally important in helping to improve the patient's outcome. The implementation of EBP in the field of communication disorders is only just beginning, as it is in most professions. Similar to what has been found in medicine, AUDs and SLPs cannot rely on what they learned several years ago (e.g., as students) to carry them through a lifetime of professional practice. On average, research in any particular area of health can be expected to double every 10 years. Keeping this in mind, in order for practice to be effective, the information we base our practice on needs to be constantly updated.

As expert clinicians, AUDs and SLPs should consistently seek new information to improve therapeutic effectiveness (Ratner, 2006).

Professional Licensure

Whenever we try to help others we inevitably risk harming them. Most health professions, namely in medicine, are practiced with tight regulations imposed by local and national governments. These regulations are designed to safeguard the public from potential harm, whether it is emotional, physical, or financial. They attempt to ensure that professionals work within a well-defined scope of practice in which the education and training of the professional is suited to the health problem at hand. The concepts of **beneficence** and **nonmaleficence**

FYI

Audiologists and speech-language pathologists who choose to work in a private practice usually are required to purchase professional liability (or malpractice) insurance. These insurance policies are designed to protect the client from an audiologist or speech-language pathologist who fails to exercise a competent degree of skill and care in the performance of their duties.

---

are used to determine whether a particular profession should require licensure. Beneficence refers to "doing good," and implies that positive steps are taken by the professional to prevent harm to the patient or to remove the patient from harm. Nonmaleficence refers to an obligation by the professional "not to harm" the patient. Beneficence and nonmaleficence can be seen as two ends of the same continuum of patient care.

Health care workers are committed to helping others, and should therefore consider the principles of beneficence and nonmaleficence. This has prompted many countries to license (or regulate) various health care professions in a manner similar to what is found in medical practice. At present, there is surprisingly little worldwide consistency toward the regulation of the AUD and SLP professions by government bodies. Yet, it would appear that both professions have the potential for causing patient harm. Table 2.4 provides examples of some of the harm that can occur to patients who have a communication disorder and are seen by an incompetent AUD or SLP. The United Kingdom and South Africa require professional licensure of all AUDs and SLPs, whereas Australia, Canada, and the United States vary in regard to the total number of states or provinces that require licensure. At present, neither profession is regulated in New Zealand, although steps are being taken

to mandate licensure. Currently, a conviction for practicing as an AUD or SLP without a license is a minor misdemeanor in countries where no professional licensure is required.

Professional Reciprocity

The professions of AUD and SLP are practiced throughout the world. A question that often arises is whether it is possible to work outside one's home country. The answer is yes, but each country may have its own unique requirements. Generally, the first step in seeking employment in another country is to contact the professional association of the specific country. A list of the various professional associations in AUD and SLP found in various English-speaking countries is provided in Table 2.1. The association will determine whether the applicant's education and professional experiences are equivalent to that found within the country. The process of **reciprocity** is a situation whereby two countries accept the validity of professional credentials granted by the other country. This can be a lengthy process that involves providing evidence of language proficiency, educational background, and clinical experience. There are few, if any, countries that allow for immediate reciprocity. Although there is a common universal thread to these professions, namely, to

Table 2.4. Examples of Harm That Might be Caused by Unqualified or Incompetent Audiologist or Speech-Language Pathologist

Audiologist Error	Potential Harm
Misdiagnosis of brainstem tumor.	Failure to treat the problem resulting in the worsening of tumor.
Misdiagnosis of newborn hearing loss.	Delayed/disordered speech, cognitive, learning outcomes.
Failure to identify conditions of chronic otitis media in preschool children with speech and language difficulties.	Permanent sensorineural hearing loss, poor educational achievement.
Taking of deep ear impressions.	Serious physical and mental harm can be caused if the deep ear impression is performed incorrectly.
Failure to provide necessary environmental support for communicatively impaired patients who have demonstrated physical weakness (stroke, paralysis).	Injury due to fall.
Purchase of unnecessary hearing aids.	Financial harm.
Speech-Language Pathologist Error	**Potential Harm**
Initiation of feeding too soon or inserting objects into the mouth during dysphagia treatment.	Patient choking and/or aspirating leading to aspiration pneumonia and possible death.
Providing therapeutic services to an individual with a perceived voice problem without first referring to an otolaryngologist.	Overlooking possible cancer of the larynx, resulting in surgical removal of larynx and possible death.
Failure to identify seizure activity in speech disordered clients, such as those with traumatic brain injury, or cerebral palsy.	Permanent brain damage, coma, death.
Incorrect choice of augmentative devices for nonverbal patients.	Limitation of communication competence if choice is below the patient's abilities. Frustration, withdrawal, decreased motivation to attempt communication. Inappropriate educational and vocational placement.

improve communication abilities, there are some subtle and not so subtle differences across countries.

A worldwide effort is now under-way to streamline the process for SLPs to work abroad. A case in point is the recent pact between a handful of countries referred to as the **Mutual Recognition**

Agreement (MRA). The MRA was originally established in 2004 and currently includes the American Speech-Language-Hearing Association (ASHA), the Canadian Association of Speech-Language Pathologists and Audiologists (CASLPA), the New Zealand Speech-Language Therapists Association (NZSTA), the Irish Association of Speech and Language Therapists (IASLT), the Royal College of Speech and Language Therapists (RCSLT), and Speech Pathology Australia (SPA). The premise of the MRA is that under certain terms and conditions an individual's credentials are deemed substantially equivalent. Each country may still require applicants from another country to achieve certain competencies prior to the start of employment; however, the steps toward working in the country of interest are *fast tracked*. No such agreement is currently available for the AUD profession. That is not to say that an AUD educated in one country cannot work in another, but rather the steps toward having one's credentials recognized in another country are likely to take a bit longer than for an SLP.

An additional resource for those interested in working in another country is the International Directory of Communication Disorders (IDCD). The IDCD is a compilation of Internet resources focusing on communication disorders, including national associations, international associations and groups, educational programs, and employment opportunities (Bleile et al., 2006). The IDCD also contains personal accounts of international experiences of persons in the profession, sample Code of Ethics, and examples of volunteering and employment opportunities. The purpose of the IDCD is to facilitate international connections between professionals in AUD and SLP. The IDCD is a free resource for persons in the professions (http://www.comdisinternational.com/purpose.html).

THE PROFESSIONS OF AUDIOLOGY AND SPEECH-LANGUAGE PATHOLOGY ON THE WORLD WIDE WEB

Listed below are Web sites that provide further information on the professions of audiology and speech-language pathology. At the time of publication each Web site was freely accessible.

A Guide to Internet Resources in Audiology
http://www.aud.org.uk/

A Guide to Internet Resources in Speech Pathology
http://www.abacon.com/internet guides/spath/weblinks.html

American Speech-Language-Hearing Association
http://www.asha.org/students/

Audiology and Speech-Language Pathology Professions video
http://education-portal.com/directory/category/Medical_and_Health_Professions/Communication_Disorders_Sciences/Audiology_and_Speech-Language_Pathology.html

Multilateral Mutual Recognition Agreement
http://www.asha.org/about/membership-certification/MultilateralMRA.htm

Speech Therapist Shortage video
http://www.webmd.com/video/speech-therapist-shortage

REFERENCES

American Speech-Language-Hearing Association. (2003). *Code of ethics* [Ethics]. Available from http://www.asha.org/policy

Bleile, K. M., Ireland, L., & Kiel, T. (2006, Dec. 26). The professions around the world: New Web-based directory goes global. *ASHA Leader, 11*(17), 8–9, 26–27.

Denes, P., & Pinson, E. (1973). *The speech chain: The physics and biology of spoken language.* New York: Anchor Books.

Ratner, N. B. (2006) Evidence-based practice: An examination of its ramifications for the practice of speech-language pathology. *Language, Speech, and Hearing Services in Schools, 37,* 257–267.

Roberts, P. (2001). Aphasia assessment and treatment for bilingual and culturally diverse patients. In R. Chapey (Ed.), *Language intervention strategies in adult aphasia* (3rd ed.). St. Louis, MO: Lippincott, Williams & Wilkins.

Robertson, S., Kersner, M., & Davis, S. (Eds.). (1995). *A history of the college 1945–1995.* London: Royal College of Speech and Language Therapists.

Van Riper, C. (1981). An early history of ASHA. *ASHA Magazine, 23*(11), 855-858.

APPENDIX 2-A

ASHA Code of Ethics (2003)

PREAMBLE

The preservation of the highest standards of integrity and ethical principles is vital to the responsible discharge of obligations by speech-language pathologists, audiologists, and speech, language, and hearing scientists. This Code of Ethics sets forth the fundamental principles and rules considered essential to this purpose.

Every individual who is (a) a member of the American Speech-Language-Hearing Association, whether certified or not, (b) a nonmember holding the Certificate of Clinical Competence from the Association, (c) an applicant for membership or certification, or (d) a Clinical Fellow seeking to fulfill standards for certification shall abide by this Code of Ethics.

Any violation of the spirit and purpose of this Code shall be considered unethical. Failure to specify any particular responsibility or practice in this Code of Ethics shall not be construed as denial of the existence of such responsibilities or practices.

The fundamentals of ethical conduct are described by Principles of Ethics and by Rules of Ethics as they relate to the conduct of research and scholarly activities and responsibility to persons served, the public, and speech-language pathologists, audiologists, and speech, language, and hearing scientists.

Principles of Ethics, aspirational and inspirational in nature, form the underlying moral basis for the Code of Ethics. Individuals shall observe these principles as affirmative obligations under all conditions of professional activity.

Rules of Ethics are specific statements of minimally acceptable professional conduct or of prohibitions and are applicable to all individuals.

PRINCIPLE OF ETHICS I

Individuals shall honor their responsibility to hold paramount the welfare of persons they serve professionally or participants in research and scholarly activities and shall treat animals involved in research in a humane manner.

Rules of Ethics

1. Individuals shall provide all services competently.
2. Individuals shall use every resource, including referral when appropriate,

Reprinted with permission from American Speech-Language-Hearing Association. (2003). Code of Ethics [Ethics]. Available from www.asha.org/policy

to ensure that high-quality service is provided.

3. Individuals shall not discriminate in the delivery of professional services or the conduct of research and scholarly activities on the basis of race or ethnicity, gender, age, religion, national origin, sexual orientation, or disability.

4. Individuals shall not misrepresent the credentials of assistants, technicians, or support personnel and shall inform those they serve professionally of the name and professional credentials of persons providing services.

5. Individuals who hold the Certificates of Clinical Competence shall not delegate tasks that require the unique skills, knowledge, and judgment that are within the scope of their profession to assistants, technicians, support personnel, students, or any nonprofessionals over whom they have supervisory responsibility. An individual may delegate support services to assistants, technicians, support personnel, students, or any other persons only if those services are adequately supervised by an individual who holds the appropriate Certificate of Clinical Competence.

6. Individuals shall fully inform the persons they serve of the nature and possible effects of services rendered and products dispensed, and they shall inform participants in research about the possible effects of their participation in research conducted.

7. Individuals shall evaluate the effectiveness of services rendered and of products dispensed and shall provide services or dispense products only when benefit can reasonably be expected.

8. Individuals shall not guarantee the results of any treatment or procedure, directly or by implication; however, they may make a reasonable statement of prognosis.

9. Individuals shall not provide clinical services solely by correspondence.

10. Individuals may practice by telecommunication (for example, telehealth/e-health), where not prohibited by law.

11. Individuals shall adequately maintain and appropriately secure records of professional services rendered, research and scholarly activities conducted, and products dispensed and shall allow access to these records only when authorized or when required by law.

12. Individuals shall not reveal, without authorization, any professional or personal information about identified persons served professionally or identified participants involved in research and scholarly activities unless required by law to do so, or unless doing so is necessary to protect the welfare of the person or of the community or otherwise required by law.

13. Individuals shall not charge for services not rendered, nor shall they misrepresent services rendered, products dispensed, or research and scholarly activities conducted.

14. Individuals shall use persons in research or as subjects of teaching demonstrations only with their informed consent.

15. Individuals whose professional services are adversely affected by substance abuse or other health-related conditions shall seek professional assistance and, where appropriate, withdraw from the affected areas of practice.

PRINCIPLE OF ETHICS II

Individuals shall honor their responsibility to achieve and maintain the highest level of professional competence.

Rules of Ethics

1. Individuals shall engage in the provision of clinical services only when they hold the appropriate Certificate of Clinical Competence or when they are in the certification process and are supervised by an individual who holds the appropriate Certificate of Clinical Competence.
2. Individuals shall engage in only those aspects of the professions that are within the scope of their competence, considering their level of education, training, and experience.
3. Individuals shall continue their professional development throughout their careers.
4. Individuals shall delegate the provision of clinical services only to: (1) persons who hold the appropriate Certificate of Clinical Competence; (2) persons in the education or certification process who are appropriately supervised by an individual who holds the appropriate Certificate of Clinical Competence; or (3) assistants, technicians, or support personnel who are adequately supervised by an individual who holds the appropriate Certificate of Clinical Competence.
5. Individuals shall not require or permit their professional staff to provide services or conduct research activities that exceed the staff member's competence, level of education, training, and experience.
6. Individuals shall ensure that all equipment used in the provision of services or to conduct research and scholarly activities is in proper working order and is properly calibrated.

PRINCIPLE OF ETHICS III

Individuals shall honor their responsibility to the public by promoting public understanding of the professions, by supporting the development of services designed to fulfill the unmet needs of the public, and by providing accurate information in all communications involving any aspect of the professions, including dissemination of research findings and scholarly activities.

Rules of Ethics

1. Individuals shall not misrepresent their credentials, competence, education, training, experience, or scholarly or research contributions.
2. Individuals shall not participate in professional activities that constitute a conflict of interest.
3. Individuals shall refer those served professionally solely on the basis of the interest of those being referred and not on any personal financial interest.
4. Individuals shall not misrepresent diagnostic information, research, services rendered, or products dispensed; neither shall they engage in any scheme to defraud in connection with obtaining payment or

reimbursement for such services or products.

5. Individuals' statements to the public shall provide accurate information about the nature and management of communication disorders, about the professions, about professional services, and about research and scholarly activities.

6. Individuals' statements to the public —advertising, announcing, and marketing their professional services, reporting research results, and promoting products—shall adhere to prevailing professional standards and shall not contain misrepresentations.

PRINCIPLE OF ETHICS IV

Individuals shall honor their responsibilities to the professions and their relationships with colleagues, students, and members of allied professions. Individuals shall uphold the dignity and autonomy of the professions, maintain harmonious interprofessional and intraprofessional relationships, and accept the professions' self-imposed standards.

Rules of Ethics

1. Individuals shall prohibit anyone under their supervision from engaging in any practice that violates the Code of Ethics.

2. Individuals shall not engage in dishonesty, fraud, deceit, misrepresentation, sexual harassment, or any other form of conduct that adversely reflects on the professions or on the individual's fitness to serve persons professionally.

3. Individuals shall not engage in sexual activities with clients or students over whom they exercise professional authority.

4. Individuals shall assign credit only to those who have contributed to a publication, presentation, or product. Credit shall be assigned in proportion to the contribution and only with the contributor's consent.

5. Individuals shall reference the source when using other persons' ideas, research, presentations, or products in written, oral, or any other media presentation or summary.

6. Individuals' statements to colleagues about professional services, research results, and products shall adhere to prevailing professional standards and shall contain no misrepresentations.

7. Individuals shall not provide professional services without exercising independent professional judgment, regardless of referral source or prescription.

8. Individuals shall not discriminate in their relationships with colleagues, students, and members of allied professions on the basis of race or ethnicity, gender, age, religion, national origin, sexual orientation, or disability.

9. Individuals who have reason to believe that the Code of Ethics has been violated shall inform the Board of Ethics.

10. Individuals shall comply fully with the policies of the Board of Ethics in its consideration and adjudication of complaints of violations of the Code of Ethics.

ANATOMIC PROCESSES OF SPEECH AND HEARING

OBJECTIVES

After reading this chapter, the student should be able to:

- Label major anatomic structures and systems for speech, language, and hearing.

- State the physiologic functions of these structures and systems.

- Identify individuals who have made historic contributions to understanding the anatomy of speech and hearing.

- Describe the essential physiologic processes involved in the production of speech.

- Describe the essential physiologic processes involved in hearing.

- Understand how impairments in one or more systems can cause communicative disabilities.

- Relate the anatomy and physiology of these structures and systems to the professional responsibilities of the audiologist and speech-language pathologist.

INTRODUCTION

Anatomy is the study of the structure of organisms and the relations of their parts. The word **anatomy** comes from the Greek *ana-* meaning "up" or "through," and *tomie* meaning "a cutting." Anatomy was once a "cutting up" because the structure of the body was originally learned through **dissection** of human cadavers. However, less invasive methods are now available to examine the living body, using such devices as endoscopic cameras and body scans (e.g., CAT-scan, MRI-scan). **Physiology** is the study of the functions of living organisms and their parts. This word is also Greek in origin with *physis* meaning "nature," and *logia* meaning "to speak." So physiology involves describing the nature of things. **Gross** anatomy and physiology involves examination of the structure and function of body parts that can be seen with the naked eye. **Cellular** anatomy and physiology (or **histology**) entails examining those body parts best seen under the microscope. Traditionally, both gross and cellular anatomy and physiology are foundation courses that beginning medical students are required to take. This is no different for students of the audiology and speech-language pathology professions. To fully appreciate the nature of normal communication and disorders of communication, knowledge about the structure and function of the speech and hearing mechanism is essential. This chapter provides some introductory exposure to speech and hearing anatomy and physiology. The material presented is referred to in later chapters concerning communication disorders resulting from anatomic and physiologic abnormalities of the speech and hearing mechanism.

SPEECH ANATOMY

The human anatomy involved in the production of speech is grounded in biological structures and processes used for doing nonspeech things such as breathing, swallowing, and coughing. These structures can be divided into three subsystems: (1) respiratory, (2) laryngeal, and (3) articulatory. As human beings, we have learned to exploit these structures that were originally designed for basic survival, and to use these structures to communicate with other human beings. A survey and description of the structure and function of the respiratory, laryngeal, and articulatory systems is provided.

Respiratory System

The respiratory system consists of the lungs, trachea, pharynx, oral and nasal passages, diaphragm, and rib cage. The general location of each of these anatomical structures is shown in Figure 3.1. The respiratory system is divided into the **upper respiratory tract** (including the oral and nasal cavities, pharynx and trachea), and the **lower respiratory tract** (the lungs and bronchi). Air is inhaled primarily through the nostrils into the **nasal cavities**. The nasal cavities are lined with mucous membranes which are covered with tiny hairs known as cilia. These features within the nasal cavity serve to warm, moisten, and filter the air of possible contaminants. For most

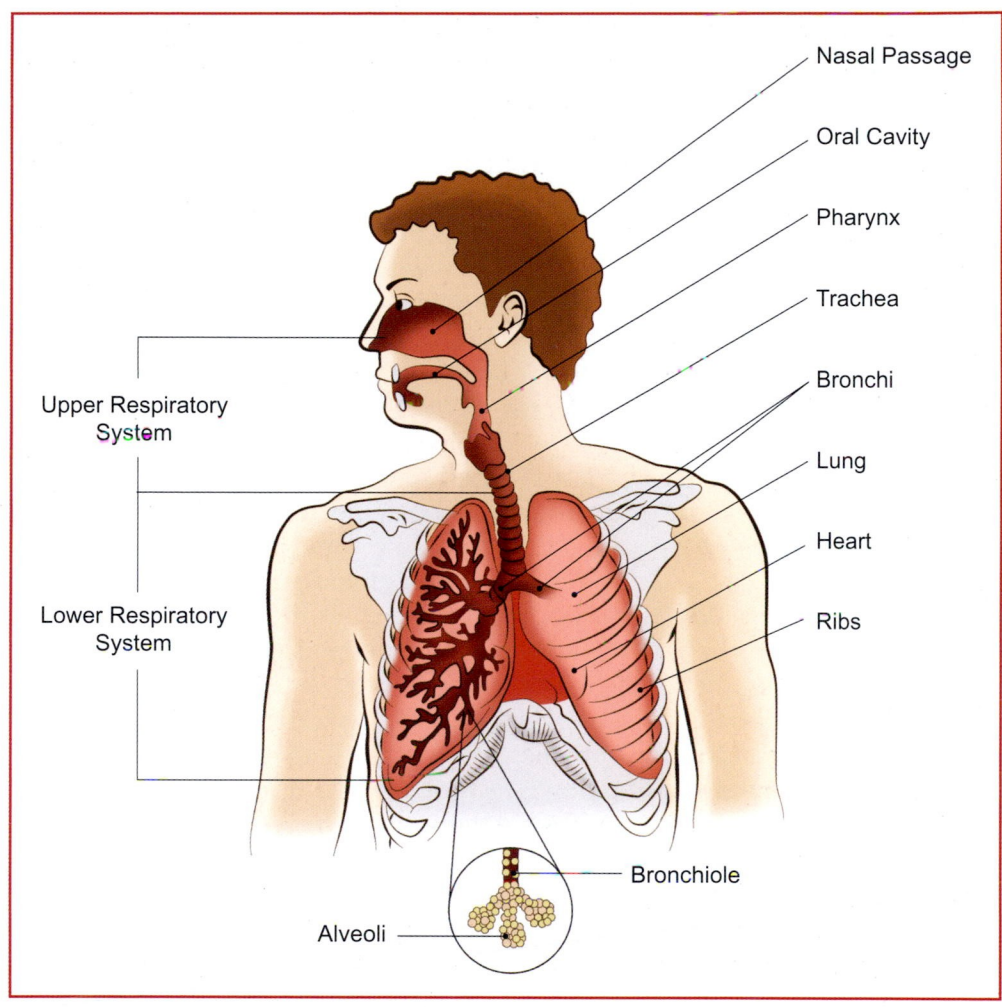

FIGURE 3.1. Anatomic features of the human respiratory system.

of us breathing is breathing and it does not matter whether it is from the mouth or nose. **Mouth breathing** may appear to be a harmless form of breathing; however, there are many negatives associated with breathing through the mouth. Excessive mouth breathing is problematic because air is not filtered and warmed as much as when inhaled through the nose, as it bypasses the nasal cavity. The dust and dirt deposited in the membranes cannot be disposed of as they are by the nasal cavity, and therefore remain to produce irritation and inflammation. Mouth breathing is thought to contribute to a higher than average occurrence of upper respiratory infections, and may also exacerbate the occurrence of asthma. Excessive mouth breathing may also be indicative of situations in which the nasal cavity is obstructed, thereby preventing nasal breathing to occur naturally. In cases such as this, mouth breathing is done out of necessity. Situations like enlarged adenoids can lead to excessive mouth breathing. **Adenoids**

> **FYI**
>
> At rest, a healthy adult breathes about 14 to 16 times per minute. After exercise it could increase to over 60 times per minute. New babies at rest breathe between 40 and 50 times per minute. By age five, it decreases to around 25 times per minute.

(e.g., tonsils) consist of a paired mass of tissue in the back of the nasal cavity that serve to filter out debris that is inhaled through the nose.

The **pharynx** is a hollow tube about 5 inches long that starts behind the nose and ends at the top of the trachea. The tube is made of muscles that encircle the throat. At the bottom of the pharynx the tube splits with one tube running down the front of the neck, called the **trachea** (i.e., windpipe). The second tube running down the back of the neck is called the **esophagus** (i.e., food tube). The pharynx serves a twofold purpose. When food enters the oral cavity and readied for swallowing, it is directed down the pharynx. The muscles surrounding the pharynx contract and push the food toward the esophagus and onward to the stomach. During the process of breathing, air inhaled through the nose is directed toward the pharynx and down through the trachea.

The trachea is the principal tube that carries air to and from the lungs and is made up of elastic tissues and about 20 rings of cartilage. It is designed to be flexible so that we can twist and turn our head and neck while at the same time being able to breathe normally. The trachea branches into two main tubes

supplying air to the right and left lung, respectively. These are called **bronchial tubes**. An inflammation of these airway tubes is called bronchitis. The tubes continue to divide again and again becoming narrower and narrower, referred to as **bronchioles**. The very end of these airway tubes look like spongy sacs known as **alveoli**. Tiny blood vessels surround each of the alveoli. It is at this point in the process of breathing when oxygen that is inhaled into the lungs is delivered to the bloodstream and carried to the rest of the body. Each cell in the body needs oxygen at all times. At the same time, these tiny sacs remove carbon dioxide from the blood, which is exhaled from the body.

Collectively, the bronchial tubes, bronchioles, and alveoli serve to make up the lungs. The **lungs** are so large that they occupy most of the space in the chest. The lungs are cone shaped. Although the lungs come as a pair, they are not exactly the same size as is often found for other paired anatomic structures such as our eyes or nostrils. Instead, the lung on the left side of the body is a bit smaller than the lung on the right. This extra space on the left leaves room for the heart to occupy space within the chest. The lungs are protected by 12 sets of rib bones creating the **rib cage**. Beneath the lungs is the **diaphragm** muscle, which extends across the bottom of the rib cage. The diaphragm is the principal muscle of respiration. When we inhale to take a breath, the diaphragm is drawn downward and the rib cage is expanded and elevated. The combined actions of the rib cage and diaphragm serve to enlarge the overall chest area, and air then passes into the lungs to fill the larger space. We rely heavily on the diaphragm for our respiratory function so that when the

---
FYI

Lung cancer is the leading cause of cancer death in both men and women. It occurs most commonly between the ages of 45 and 70, and has become more prevalent in women in the last few decades because more women are smoking cigarettes. In 2007, over 160,000 people in the United States died of lung cancer—about 90,000 men and 70,000 women.

---

diaphragm is impaired, it can seriously compromise our breathing.

The primary functions of the respiratory system are to help sustain life through the exchange of gases. When a person takes a breath, the air taken in is composed of several gases. The mixture is mostly comprised of oxygen, nitrogen, and carbon dioxide. Oxygen is an odorless gas that makes up about 20% of air and is essential to life because it is used for chemical reactions that occur in the cells of the body. Oxygen is brought in and utilized by the body, while carbon dioxide and nitrogen are expelled from the body.

A **respiratory cycle** consists of two phases, an **inhalation phase** and an **exhalation phase**. During the inhalation phase, the muscles are used to expand the size of the lungs so that outside air naturally flows inward toward the lungs. The process of inhalation is viewed as an **active** muscular process. During the exhalation phase, the lungs recoil back to their original size and naturally expel air out toward the oral/nasal cavities. The process of exhalation is viewed as a **passive** muscular process. During quiet, restful breathing, the amount of time dedicated to each phase of the respiratory cycle is approximately equal. During the process of speaking, the respiratory cycle is dramatically altered. The inhalation phase comprises only 10% of the cycle, while exhalation comprises 90% of the cycle (Figure 3.2). The reason for this is obvious; we need to prolong exhalation in order to produce strings of words and sentences on one breath. Two ways in which we are able to prolong the exhalation phase are to: (1) inhale a larger amount of air during quiet breathing, and (2) prolong expiratory airflow using vocal tract resistance. The balloon analogy is useful to consider in regard to vocal tract resistance (Figure 3.3). Blowing up a large balloon is analogous to inhaling a large amount of air into the lungs. Upon releasing air from the balloon, one could either let the balloon naturally deflate or pinch the end of the balloon (i.e., create resistance) to prolong the expiratory airflow. Ways in which we prolong expiratory airflow for speech include vocal fold resistance (vibration) and oral cavity resistance (consonant articulation). In addition, the respiratory muscles relax gradually so that the air is not pushed out of the lungs in a short rush.

Laryngeal System

The anatomic structures comprising the laryngeal system include cartilages, muscles, and bone. The **larynx** (pronounced "lare-rinks") is not a single structure but rather a framework of

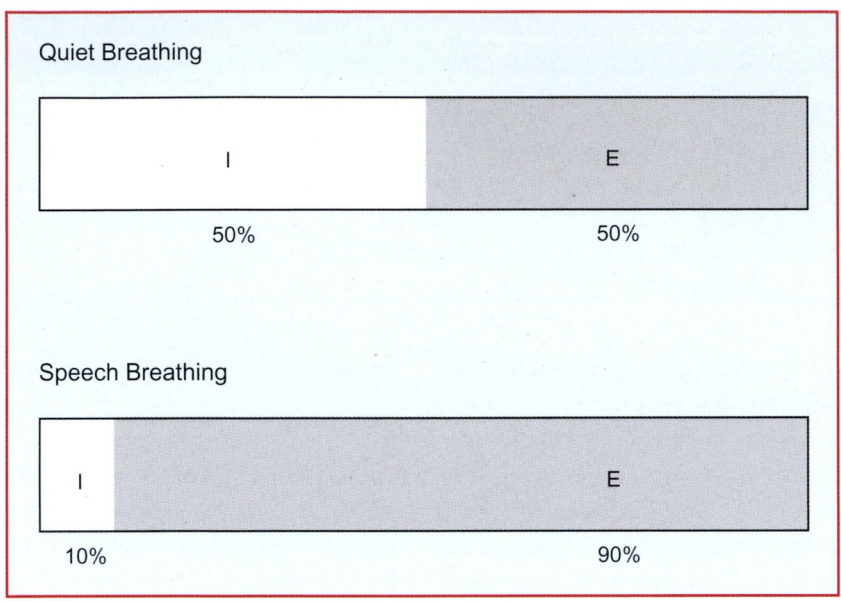

FIGURE 3.2. Comparison of the inspiratory and expiratory proportions of the respiratory cycle required for quiet breathing and speech breathing.

A   B

FIGURE 3.3. Balloon analogy for breathing during quiet and speech production. (**A**) shows no resistance during expiratory airflow, and (**B**) shows resistance to airflow resulting in longer expiratory airflow.

many structures; these major structures are shown in Figure 3.4. The largest of these is the **thyroid cartilage**, which is approximately in the middle of the larynx. The thyroid cartilage is formed by two large plates that are joined ante-

A

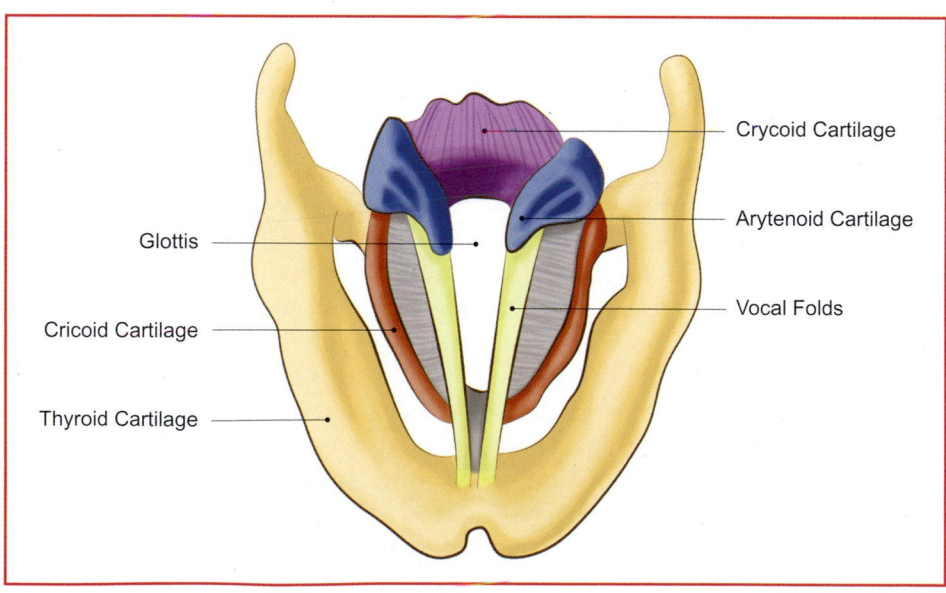

B

FIGURE 3.4. Anatomic features of the human laryngeal system presented as a side (*lateral*) view (**A**) and view from above (*superior*) (**B**).

riorly (in the front) to create a slight bump in the neck. This bump is called the laryngeal prominence (or Adam's apple) and is most visible in adult males. The thyroid cartilage has nothing to do with the thyroid gland, which is also located in the neck. A leaf-shaped cartilage that arises from above the laryngeal prominence is the **epiglottis**. This structure does not play an important role in producing speech, although during swallowing, the tip of the epiglottis helps to direct food away from the lungs and toward the stomach. Located above the thyroid cartilage is the **hyoid bone**, which is shaped like a horseshoe and situated very high in the neck. This bone serves as a point of attachment for muscles of the tongue (from above) and for muscles of the larynx (from below). It is sometimes called a "floating bone" because it has no direct attachments to other bones. At the base of the larynx lies the **cricoid cartilage**. The cricoid cartilage is ring-shaped and rests directly on top of the trachea. Collectively, the hyoid bone, thyroid cartilage, and cricoid cartilage comprise the structural framework of the larynx from top to bottom.

Inside the laryngeal framework lie the **vocal folds** (i.e., vocal cords). The technical name for the vocal folds is the thryoarytenoid muscle. The name of the muscle specifies the precise location of the vocal folds within the larynx. This is a paired muscle that makes up the right and left vocal folds. The vocal folds are attached at the front of the larynx at a point inside the thyroid cartilage (just below the Adam's apple). The vocal folds are attached at the back of the larynx to the **arytenoid cartilages**, which sit on top of the cricoid cartilage. The arytenoid cartilages swivel to allow the vocal folds to open and close, as well as shorten and lengthen. During quiet breathing, the vocal folds remain open to allow air to flow in and out of the lungs. The space between the open vocal folds is called the **glottis**. In most cases, the vocal folds remain in an open position; otherwise, we would be unable to breathe. The primary reason for closing the vocal folds is to either swallow or speak. During swallowing, the vocal folds close to prevent food and liquid from entering the trachea. These materials need to be directed into the esophagus. During the production of speech, we inhale air and close the vocal folds. The vocal folds lie stretched across the top of the trachea. As we begin to exhale, air pressure is built up under the closed vocal folds. When a sufficient amount of pressure is achieved, the vocal folds are forced open and vibrate rapidly during expiratory airflow. Think of how you can make a squealing noise by blowing through two blades of grass held between your thumbs—it is a similar action. The process of converting the air pressure from the lungs into audible vibrations is called **phonation**. The basic rate at which the vocal folds vibrate is referred to as the **fundamental frequency** (F_0) of voice. It is the F_0 of our voice that is perceived by others as being our voice pitch. For young children, F_0 is approximately 350 cycles per second (or hertz, Hz). For women and men, the average F_0 is around 240 Hz and 120 Hz, respectively. The reason for the lowest F_0 being found among men is due to the fact that the vocal folds are large and bulky and naturally vibrate at a slower rate compare to those that would be short and thin, as found in women and children (Figure 3.5). A visual depiction of vocal fold vibration is found in Figure 3.6.

Articulatory System

The term **articulation** refers to movement of one structure against another. Speech articulators are those structures that are in contact with another struc-

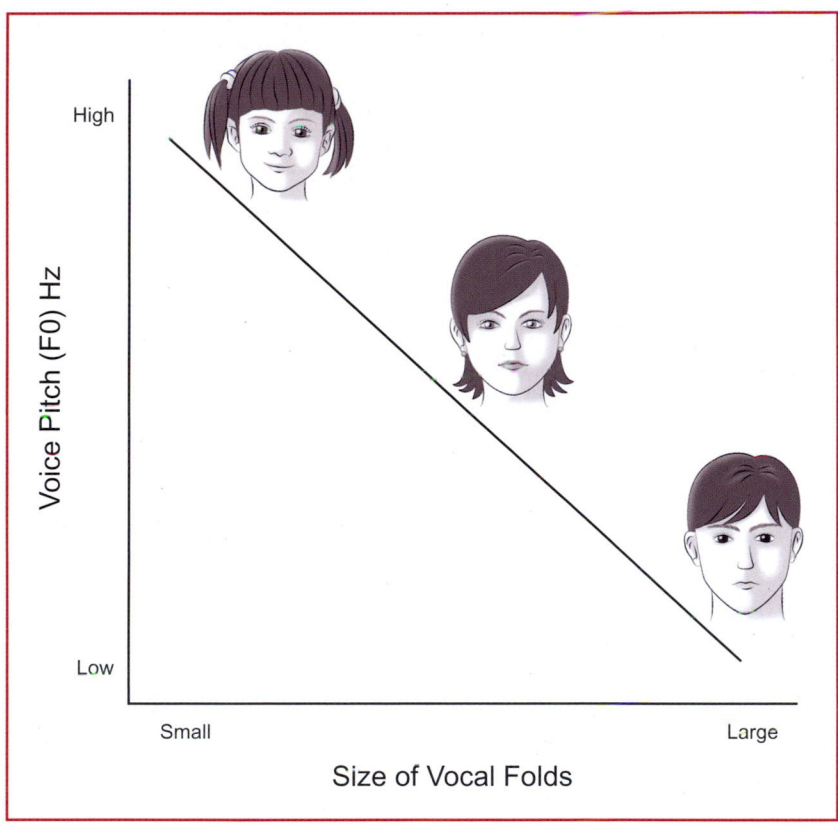

FIGURE 3.5. Relationship between vocal fold size and voice pitch (F_0).

ture for the purpose of creating the sounds of speech. The major structures comprising the articulatory system are shown in Figure 3.7. The system runs from the larynx to the lips and includes a combination of cavities, muscles, and boney structures. The entire articulatory system is contained within the **vocal tract**. The term **tract** refers to an extended area of land or space. In this case, vocal tract refers to an extended area of space within the body that is used for vocalization. The vocal tract consists of three cavities: (1) the mouth or **oral cavity**, (2) the nose or **nasal cavity**, and (3) the throat or **pharyngeal cavity**. Each of these cavities plays a role in the production of speech and also in the process of

respiration, as noted earlier. The articulators within the vocal tract can be categorized as either movable or fixed.

Movable articulators are those that make contact with either another movable structure or a permanently fixed structure. The movable articulators include the lips, tongue, soft palate, pharynx, and mandible. The **lips** are two folds of tissue that surround the mouth and play a role in eating, speaking, and of course kissing. The lips are required to produce consonant sounds such as /p/, /b/, and /m/. An exception to this might be found in **ventriloquism**, which is the art of speaking without moving the lips, so that an illusion of the voice coming from another source is created.

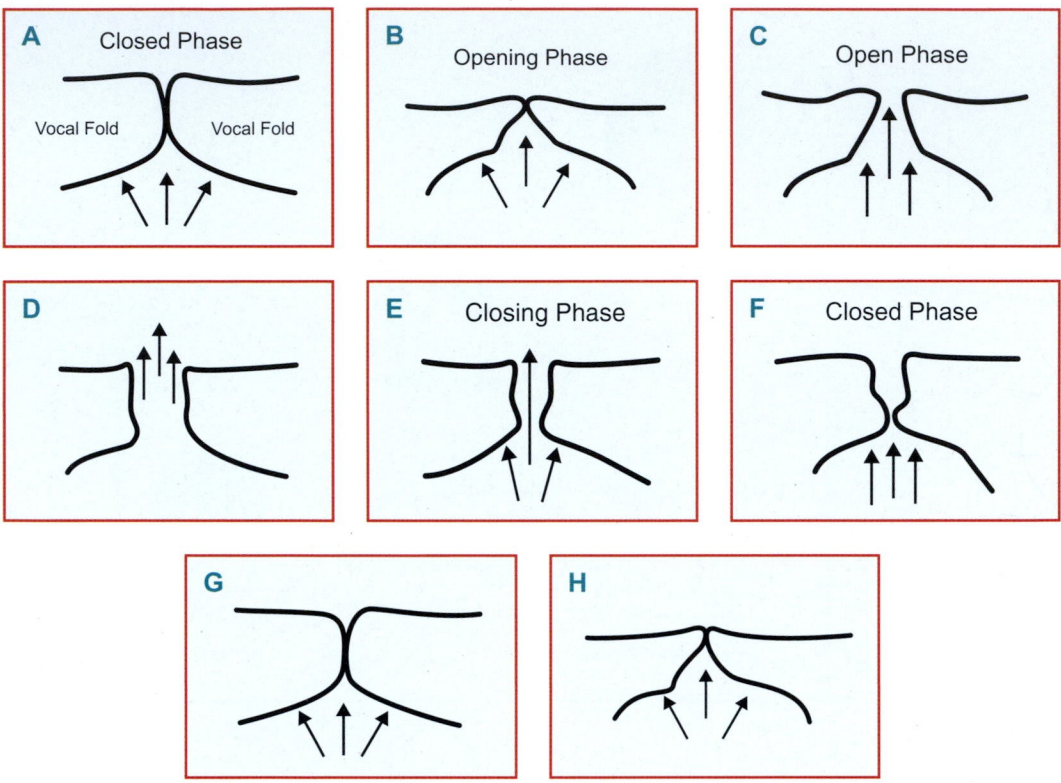

FIGURE 3.6. Frontal view of the vocal folds showing the sequential steps involved in the process of vocal fold vibration. The arrows indicate the buildup and direction of airflow from the trachea through the vocal folds.

The **tongue** probably is the most important speech articulator. This muscle is extremely strong, as it must move food around in our mouths as we chew. The tongue is required for the production of all vowel sounds and a majority of consonants such as /s/, /l/, and /th/ (e.g., the consonants in the word "sloth"). The **soft palate** (or **velum**) is the soft tissue located at the back of the roof of the mouth. The soft palate is distinguished from the hard palate at the front of the mouth in that it does not contain bone. The very tip of the soft palate is called the **uvula**, which is a tiny "punching bag" of flesh. The soft palate serves to close off the oral and nasal cavities by articulating with the back of the pharynx. This

process is known as **velopharyngeal closure**. All vowels and consonants, with the exception of /m/, /n/, and /ng/ (e.g., the consonants in the word "meaning") involve velopharyngeal closure. That is, the sounds are only articulated within the oral and pharyngeal cavities. If the soft palate was to remain lowered during the production of consonant and vowels, our speech would become highly nasalized because the flow of speech would be simultaneously directed through the oral and nasal cavities. The **pharynx** is not only a cavity within the vocal tract but a movable articulator. The muscular walls of the pharynx move to assist with velopharyngeal closure. The **mandible** forms

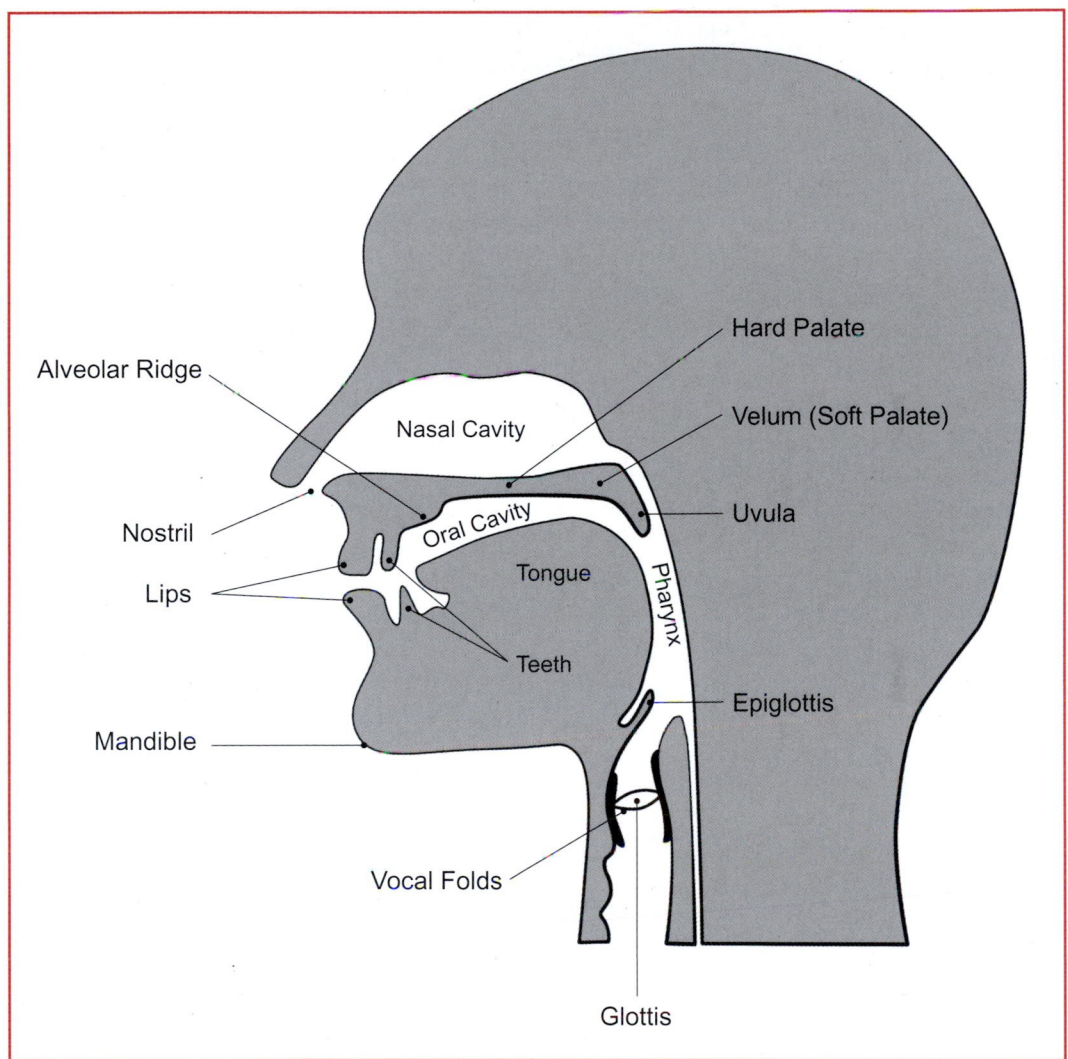

FIGURE 3.7. Anatomic features of the human speech articulatory system.

the lower jaw and holds the lower teeth in place, and works as a bilateral hinge with a connection to the temporal bone on each side of the skull. It serves as a "fine tuner" of speech articulation and moves continuously during typical speech production. Although it is not imperative for the mandible to move to produce speech, when it does, the quality of speech markedly improves. An example of this fine tuning is demonstrated in what is known as **pipe speech**. Pipe speech (speaking with a tobacco pipe clenched between the teeth) imposes constraints on jaw movement although speech can still be articulated. Once the pipe is removed from the mouth, speech becomes noticeably clearer.

Fixed articulators are those that cannot be moved by muscles. They include the hard palate, alveolar ridge, and teeth. The **hard palate** is the front portion of the roof of the mouth that is

---

FYI

The term **glossectomy** refers to surgical removal of all or part of the tongue. A glossectomy is performed to treat cancer of the tongue. Removing the tongue is indicated if the patient has a cancer that does not respond to other forms of treatment. In most cases, however, only part of the tongue is removed (partial glossectomy). Many people are still able to produce speech even when a considerable portion of the tongue is removed.

---

made of bone, and also serves as the base of the skull. It is used for the articulation of sounds such as /sh/ (as in the word "shoe"). The **alveolar ridge** is located on the roof of the mouth between the upper teeth and hard palate. It contains the sockets of the teeth, and can be felt with the tongue in the area right behind the upper teeth, where there is a change in the angle of the roof of the mouth. Speech sounds such as /t/, /d/, and /z/ (e.g., the consonants in the phrase "tie dyes") are articulated with the tongue at the alveolar ridge. The **teeth** are also involved in the articulation of speech sounds. The upper and lower central incisors (i.e., front teeth) are necessary for articulation of consonants such as /v/, /f/, and /th/ (e.g., as in the words "vie" and "faith").

THE PROCESS OF SPEECH PRODUCTION

As noted in Chapters 1 and 2, the process of speech production involves the encoding of a message. The starting point for speech encoding is the brain. The centers of the brain responsible for generating language organize the message to be spoken and send neural commands to the anatomic structures involved in speech production. The details of brain anatomy and the nervous system are provided in Chapter 9; however, it is important to recognize that without the brain's control of the respiratory, laryngeal, and articulatory systems, speech production would be impaired, if not impossible.

The normal process of speech production entails a transformation of aerodynamic into acoustic energy. The anatomic and physiologic processes involved in the generation of speech can be depicted in the formula **S * T = P**. The S symbol refers to the **source**. In order to produce speech, there needs to be a source of energy that provides the driving force behind the act of uttering a sound. The anatomic system that provides the source for speech production is the **respiratory system**. The T symbol refers to a **transfer function**. The concept of a transfer function is similar to that of a filter, in which the original source is altered or transformed. In the case of speech production, the original source (i.e., the air flowing upward from the respiratory system) is transformed by movements from the **laryngeal system** and the **articulatory system**. The final symbol in the formula, P, refers to the **product** in the generation of speech. The end-product reflects the contributions of the respiratory system, laryngeal system, and articulatory system to the acoustic generation of sound.

This acoustic energy is ultimately perceived by a listener as words and sentences. An anatomical representation of S * T = P is provided in Figure 3.8.

HEARING ANATOMY

The act of hearing is referred to as **audition**. The anatomic aspects of audition can be divided into two main components, the **peripheral auditory system** (PAS) and the **central auditory system** (CAS). The PAS consists of structures spanning from the outer ear to the auditory nerve. The CAS begins at a point beyond the auditory nerve and terminates at the auditory centers in the

FIGURE 3.8. The process of speech production according to the S * T = P formula. S refers to the source of speech, namely, the respiratory system. T refers to the transfer function of the vocal tract involving the laryngeal and articulatory systems. P is the end product of the contributions from the various systems.

> **━━━ FYI ━━━**
>
> The auditory nerve is also known as the acoustic nerve, the eighth cranial nerve, and the vestibulocochlear nerve. The nerve is essential for both hearing and balance.

brain. A basic survey and description of the structure and function of the PAS and CAS is provided.

PAS

Outer Ear

A depiction of the outer ear, as well as the entire PAS is shown in Figure 3.9. The outer ear consists of two parts: (1) auricle, and (2) the ear canal, or the external auditory meatus. The **auricle**, sometimes called the **pinna**, is the most visible part of the entire auditory system and is comprised of elastic cartilage (Figure 3.10). Some of the prominent landmarks of the auricle include the **helix**, which is the outer rim. The **tragus** is the small cartilaginous notch that is in front of the external opening of the ear. The **lobule** is the dangling fleshy part of the auricle and is the location where ears are normally pierced. The auricle serves two purposes. The first is to protect the middle ear from damage, particularly the eardrum. The auricle also serves to help eliminate **front-back confusion** by assisting in distinguishing sounds that arise from in front of the listener from those that arise from behind the listener. Movement of the auricle is particularly advanced in several types of animals, which developed as a means of detecting predators. One need simply

FIGURE 3.9. Cross-sectional view of the peripheral auditory system showing some anatomic detail of the outer, middle, and inner ear structures.

FIGURE 3.10. Landmarks of the auricle.

watch the ears of a dog or cat when presented with sounds coming from various directions. As humans, our auricles have evolved into fixed, immobile structures. However, it is not uncommon to find an individual who is hard of hearing to cup a hand behind the ear as an aid to improved localization of sound. The **external auditory meatus** is a 2.5-cm canal that runs from the auricle to the eardrum. The term meatus refers to a natural opening or canal. The outer one-third of the canal, that is nearest to the auricle, is made of elastic cartilage. The inner two-thirds of the canal are carved into the **temporal bone** of the skull. The entire canal is lined with skin and very fine hair. The ear canal also contains glands known as ceruminous glands. These glands secrete a substance called **cerumen**, commonly referred to as earwax. Cerumen plays an important role in preventing the ear canal from drying out. Cerumen also has been found to be useful in preventing intruders, such as insects, from entering the ear because they find this waxy substance to be noxious. The function of the external auditory meatus is to funnel sound toward the eardrum. In addition, the general shape of the external auditory meatus serves to provide a slight "boost" in loudness for high frequency sounds, which are found to resonate in the canal.

Middle Ear

The middle ear is an air-filled space located entirely within the temporal bone. The major structures of the middle ear include the tympanic membrane, three miniature bones, two muscles, and the eustachian tube. The **tympanic membrane** (or eardrum) is a thin, tough, fibrous membrane that spreads out across the ear canal. The tympanic membrane is a very durable and tightly stretched membrane that vibrates as incoming sound pressure waves reach it. Suspended within the middle ear space is a

---

FYI

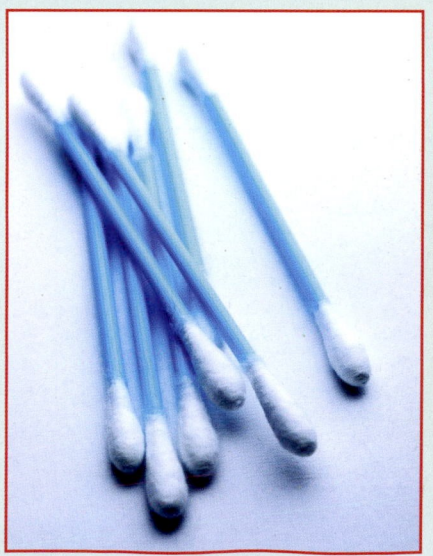

Cotton swabs are not designed for cleaning ears. Rather, they are meant to be used for household use, as well as for applying first aid. Using cotton swabs in ears can do more damage than good. Attempts to use cotton swabs to remove cerumen can result in impacting cerumen deeper into the ear canal. This can lead to ear infections, tympanic membrane damage, as well as hearing loss.

series of three small bones that form a bridge between the tympanic membrane and the inner ear. These three bones are the **malleus** (or hammer), **incus** (or anvil), and **stapes** (or stirrup). They are the smallest bones in the human body and make up what is known as the **ossicular chain** and each bone is an ossicle (from the Latin word *ossiculum* for diminutive bone).The malleus is in contact with the tympanic membrane. At the other end of the chain, the stapes is inserted into the oval window of the cochlea (inner ear). Collectively, these bones provide a mechanical link between the outer ear and the inner ear.

Two tiny muscles are located within the middle ear and make contact with the ossicular chain. The **tensor tympani** muscle runs from the front wall of the middle ear cavity and attaches to the malleus bone. The **stapedius** muscle runs from the back wall of the middle ear cavity and attaches to the stapes bone. These muscles provide a form of protection to the inner ear by stiffening the ossicular chain in the presence of very loud sounds, typically in excess of 90 dB. In essence, the ossicular chain is immobilized from functioning normally and causes a decrease in the loudness of sounds entering the inner ear. The contraction of these middle ear muscles is involuntary and known as the **acoustic reflex** (see also Chapter 13). The **eustachian tube** runs from the middle ear space down towards the upper region of the pharynx (Figure 3.11). The func-

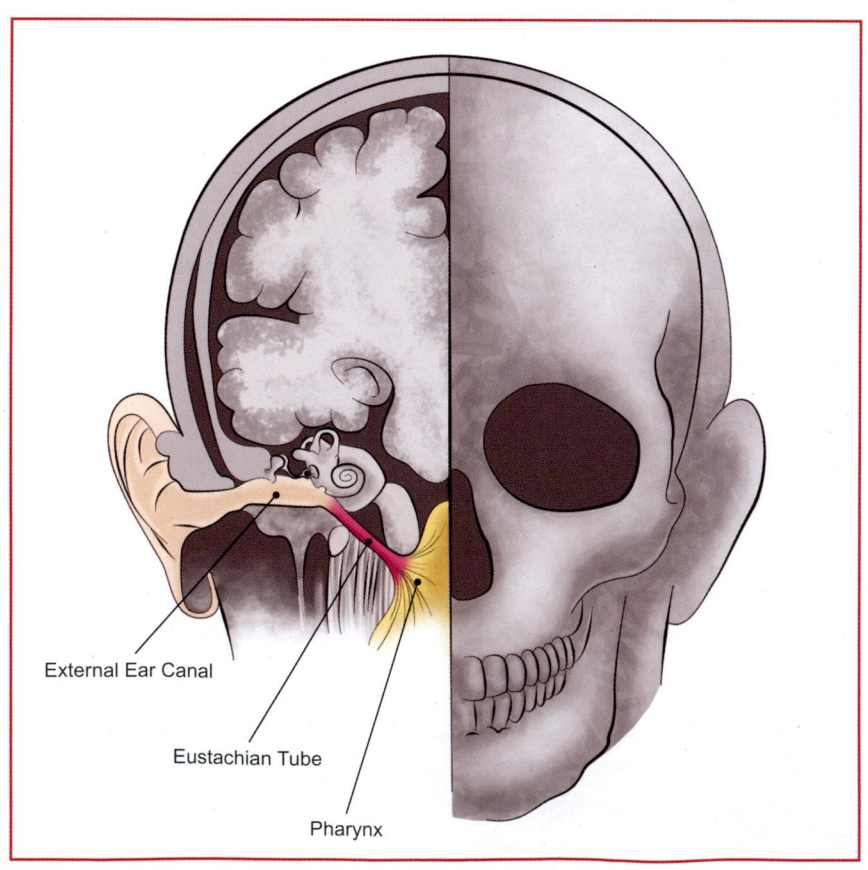

External Ear Canal

Eustachian Tube

Pharynx

FIGURE 3.11. Depiction of the anatomic location of the eustachian tube.

tion of the eustachian tube is to protect, aerate, and drain the middle ear. It also serves to equalize middle ear air pressure with environmental air pressure. The eustachian tube is normally closed and opens only under changes in pressure. When your ears "pop" on an airplane, the reason is that the eustachian tube has opened and equalized air pressure. In adults, the eustachian tube is approximately 35 mm long and runs from the middle ear to the pharynx along a 45° angle. In young children, the tube measures only 17 mm and is nearly horizontal in angle. This nearly flat angle in young children makes for poor drainage of fluid from the middle ear, and predisposes young children to middle ear infections.

Inner Ear

Similar to the middle ear, the inner ear is housed entirely within the temporal bone of the skull. Whereas the middle ear is an air-filled space, the inner ear is a fluid-filled space. The inner ear consists of two main organs. The **vestibular apparatus** serves as the body's balance organ and the **cochlea** serves as the body's hearing organ. A key structure in the vestibular apparatus is the **semicircular canals**, which work with the brain to sense, maintain, and regain balance and a sense of where the body and its parts are positioned in space. Most causes of dizziness are inner-ear problems associated with the vestibular apparatus. Specialty occupations such as astronauts or fighter pilots require an unusually intact vestibular apparatus that allows them to function during potentially dizzying environmental situations.

The cochlea has an appearance that is somewhat like that of a small snail. Indeed the term cochlea is Greek for the word snail shell. The cochlea has approx-

FYI

Empedocles, the Greek philosopher known for numbering the four basic elements (fire, air, earth, and water), was the first to describe the cochlea. He called the structure, "κσΧλΟς" the name of a seashell found in the Mediterranean region. However, his discovery fascinated him more for the perfect shape of the anatomic structure than its function or relation to hearing.

imately 2¾ turns in humans. The largest turn (that nearest the stapes) is the **basal end** of the cochlea and the smallest turn is called the **apical end**. A helpful way to visualize the cochlea is to examine the structure from the inside. A cross-sectional view (Figure 3.12) reveals that the cochlea consists of three compartments. The upper compartment is called

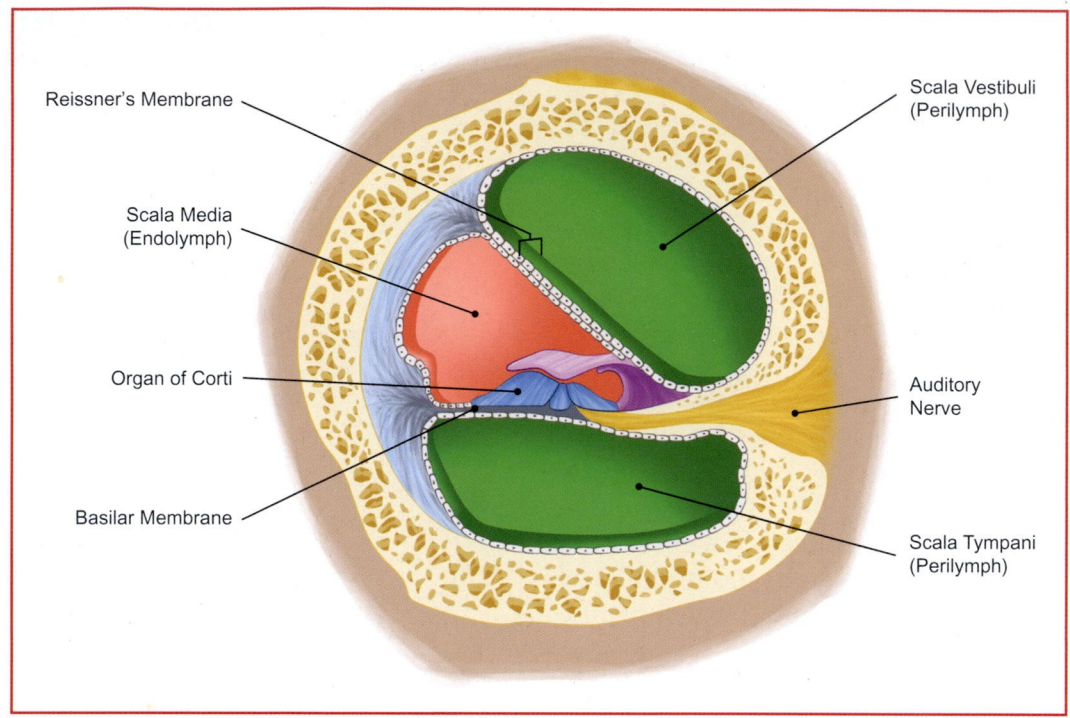

FIGURE 3.12. Cross-sectional view of cochlea and associated landmarks.

the **scala vestibuli**, the lower compartment is the **scala tympani**, and the middle compartment is the **scala media** (or cochlear duct). At the apex of the cochlea is a small hole called the **helicotrema**, which connects the scala vestibuli and scala tympani compartments. Both compartments are filled with a fluid called **perilymph**. Perilymph is a fluid that is comparable in density to plasma or cerebrospinal fluid. The scala media is filled with a thick fluid substance called **endolymph**, which is a unique fluid unlike that found anywhere else in the body.

The **organ of Corti** lies within the scala media of the cochlea. This organ is responsible for converting the mechanical sound energy of the middle ear into electrical impulses. The organ of Corti sits on one side of the **basilar membrane**, which is the wall that separates the scala tympani from the scala media. The organ of Corti consists of four rows of **hair cells** that run the entire length of the cochlea from basal to apical ends. In total, there are approximately 20,000 hair cells. At the top of each cell, a minute fiber from the auditory nerve is attached. These hair cells sense the sounds received from the middle ear and transmit the signals to the auditory nerve that, in turn, forwards the signal to the brain. A fascinating feature of the organ of Corti is its **tonotopic organization** (Figure 3.13). When sounds of varying pitch (Hz) enter the cochlea, the hair cells in the cochlea do not all respond in the same way as different regions of the cochlea are selectively responsive to different frequencies of sound. The basal end of the cochlea

FIGURE 3.13. Schematic representation of tonotopic organization found within the cochlea (basilar membrane).

vibrates most at high-frequency tones and the apical end vibrates most at low-frequency tones. Assuming that each hair cell reflects a specific frequency, the normal range of hearing extends from 20 Hz up to 20,000 Hz. Research has shown that humans are unable to perceive sounds lower than 20 Hz. The **auditory nerve** is a bundle of over 30,000 nerve fibers that carries hearing and balance information from the inner ear to the brain. The nerve consists of the cochlear branch, carrying information about hearing, and the vestibular branch, carrying information about balance. The fibers from the auditory nerve extend into the brainstem, where its fibers make contact with the cochlear nucleus, the next stage of the auditory system.

FYI

Echolocation, also called biosonar, is the process of determining the distance and direction of objects by using sound. Animals such as bats, shrews, dolphins, and whales emit pulses of high-frequency sound that bounce off things in their surroundings like insects, branches, or fish. The reflected sounds, or echoes, are picked up by their sensitive ears to locate food or obstacles in darkness, such as in caves and in the ocean.

CAS

Once the electrical impulses generated in the cochlea are transmitted through the auditory nerve, the nerve fibers carry information about the sound to the brainstem. Figure 3.14 shows a simplified diagram of the CAS. All of the nerve fibers from the auditory nerve terminate at the **cochlear nucleus** which is located in the medulla region of the brainstem. The cochlear nucleus is one of the most studied structures of the CAS in humans and animals and reflects a high concentration of neurons. Beyond the cochlear nucleus, the auditory system is characterized by a neural pathway in which a majority of the nerve fibers cross the midline of the brainstem. Prior to this crossing over, sound that entered one ear involved anatomic structures on the same side of the head. The auditory pathway courses upward through higher regions of the brainstem, including the pons and midbrain. At various locations along the way, the pathway terminates at clusters of **brainstem nuclei**. Eventually, the auditory path-

FIGURE 3.14. Simplified depiction of the anatomic structures comprising the central auditory system.

way exits the brainstem and enters the temporal lobe of the brain. The precise location in the temporal lobe where the final process of hearing takes place is the **auditory cortex** (or Heschl's gyrus). Sound entering the left ear is ultimately processed in the auditory cortex of the right hemisphere and vice versa.

THE PROCESS OF HEARING

Each part of the ear serves a specific purpose in the act of detecting and interpreting sound. The usual manner by which humans hear is via an airborne signal. Once sound is generated, it travels through the air in a disturbance called a sound wave. The outer ear serves to collect and channel the sound wave towards the middle ear. Thus, its function is to act as a **transmission** line in carrying the signal from one point to another. The sound is then **transformed** into mechanical energy by the tympanic membrane of the middle ear and the ossicular chain. The mechanical vibrations in the middle ear are an exact copy of the original airborne sound wave vibrations. As the vibrations reach the last bone in the ossicular chain (stapes), they enter the fluid-filled inner ear via the oval window of the cochlea. The vibrations of the stapes at the oval window are then **transduced** into a hydraulic wave, called a traveling wave. This wave enters the cochlea and displaces (stimulates) hair cells within the cochlea. The stimulation of specific hair cells is converted to nerve impulses that are an exact match to the frequencies comprising the original airborne sound wave. The transduction of mechanical energy to nerve impulses continues all the way

to the brain. The physical characteristics of the original sound are preserved at every energy change along the way until the sound becomes one the brain can recognize and process. Figure 3.15 provides a simplified breakdown of the process of hearing. Although this process is viewed as a linear (left to right) one, it is worth noting that there are various points in the hearing process where the original sound is channeled backward. However, this is beyond the scope of this introductory chapter.

HISTORIC ASPECTS OF ANATOMY AND PHYSIOLOGY

Henry Gray (1827–1861) was an English anatomist and surgeon (Figure 3.16). His most famous accomplishment occurred in 1858, when he published *Gray's Anatomy: Descriptive and Surgical*. Intended for medical students, physicians, and surgeons, the first edition of the book contained 750 pages and 363 figures. **Henry Vandyke Carter** (1831–1897) assisted Gray by providing the illustrations for the book. In 1861, at the age of 34, Gray contracted smallpox from his nephew and died. *Gray's Anatomy* has lived on as the authoritative anatomy text and an indispensable teaching tool. The book has more than double the number of pages from its first appearance in 1858. Gray accomplished much as a young man; imagine what he could have accomplished had he lived a full life.

Gray's contribution to the fields of anatomy and physiology were immense and covered the entire range of the human body. A number of individuals made contributions that more directly impacted the fields of audiology and

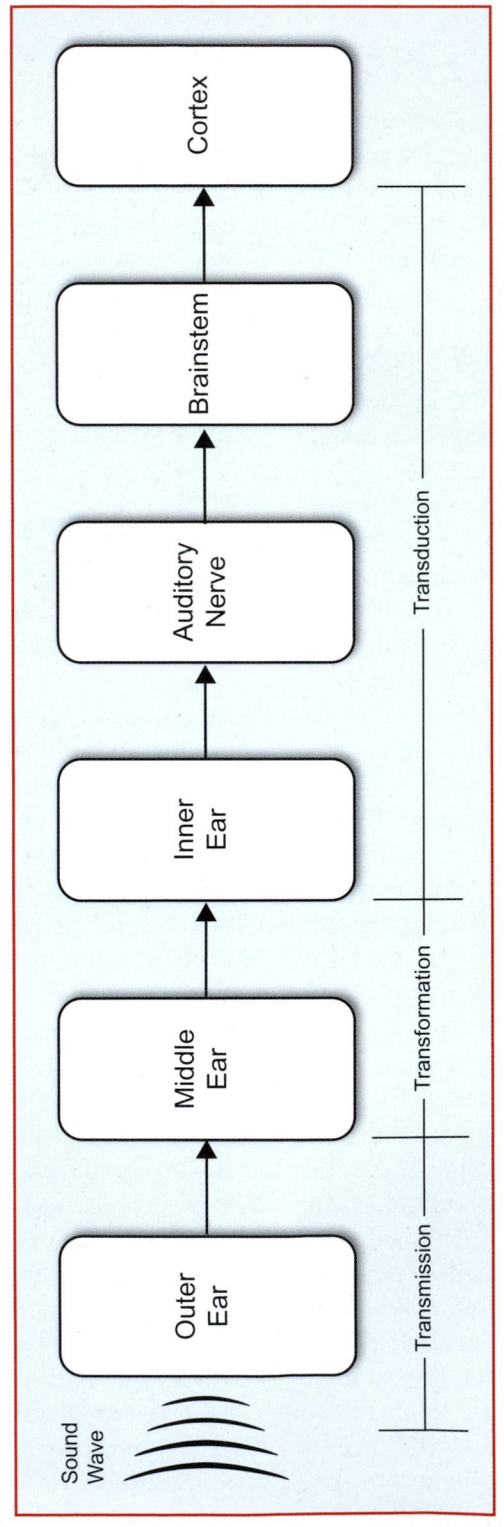

FIGURE 3.15. Process of hearing showing the flow of sound through the entire auditory system.

FIGURE 3.16. Henry Gray, an accomplished anatomist and surgeon in the early 1800s.

FIGURE 3.17. Bartolomeo Eustachi, the 16th-century Italian physician who studied anatomic features of the ear.

speech-language pathology. For example, **Bartolomeo Eustachi** (1510–1574) was a 16th-century Italian physician (Figure 3.17). In 1562 and 1563 he produced a remarkable series of reports (treatises) on various parts of the body including the kidneys, teeth, and the ear. In his report concerning the ear, he provided an accurate description of the tensor tympani and stapedius muscles, as well as the *tuba auditiva*, that has since been referred to as the eustachian tube. The discovery by Eustachi of the connection between the middle ear and the pharynx is thought to have later inspired Shakespeare to write his play *Hamlet*, a story in which Hamlet's father is killed by poison poured into his ear.

Antoine Ferrein (1693–1769) was a French anatomist who was the first person to coin the term **vocal cords**. In 1741, while dissecting corpses, he discovered in the center of the larynx two

muscular shelves that ran horizontally (front to back). He concluded that speech and song were produced entirely by the vibration of these bands of muscles caused by air being blown outward from the lungs. He compared the structures to that of a violin, in which the strings or "cords" work to produce sound. Vocal fold is the modern term for vocal cord; the change in terminology came about because of a better understanding of the anatomy and function of the larynx. Rather than looking and functioning like a stringed instrument, the vocal folds more closely resemble a lip of tissue.

Alfonso Corti (1822–1876) was born in Italy (Figure 3.18). As a medical student he enrolled first at the University of Pavia, and later at the University of Vienna where he became interested in the field of anatomy. Corti began his scientific career studying the cardiovascular

FIGURE 3.18. Alfonso Corti provided detailed anatomic descriptions of the inner ear.

FIGURE 3.19. Sir Victor Negus, a pioneer in detailing the anatomy of the human and animal larynx.

systems of reptiles. Later he turned his attention to the mammalian auditory system. In the years 1850-1851 he worked in the laboratory of Albert von Kölliker at the University of Würzburg (Germany) and examined more than 200 cochleas from cats, dogs, pigs, sheep, rabbits, and rats. It was there that he developed new coloring techniques in microscopic anatomy, which enabled him to describe individual components inside the cochlea. Prior to this time, it was notoriously difficult to preserve inner ear structures because they quickly deteriorated once removed from their fluid-filled compartments. In 1851, he published a paper describing a structure located on the basilar membrane of the cochlea containing hair cells that convert sound vibrations into nerve impulses. This structure came to be known as the organ of Corti. His work was the starting point of our knowledge of the cochlea.

Sir Victor Negus (1887–1974) was born in London and received his medical education in laryngology at King's College Hospital in 1912 (Figure 3.19). He had a long and meritorious career in laryngology. He was a pioneer in detailing the anatomy of the human and animal larynx. In 1929 he published a monumental work entitled *The Mechanism of the Larynx* that had a profound influence on laryngologists, anatomists, and many other scientists throughout the world. In this publication, he was able to demonstrate which structures of the human larynx serve to differentiate man from other species.

The work of Negus on the structure of the larynx eventually contributed to the development of theories regarding the evolution of man and speech. In particular, Phillip Lieberman and Edmund Crelin (1971) argued that man's need to produce a wide range of sounds for communication led to the development of a unique **two-tube** (oral and pharyngeal) vocal tract. The two tubes are reflected in a clear separation between the oral cavity and the larynx, which rests low in the neck. All other animal species have a **single-tube** vocal tract, reflected by close approximation between the oral cavity and larynx (Figure 3.20). This single-tube anatomy allows for easy ingestion of food and drink with no danger of food entering the lungs. This anatomical configuration also permits breathing to occur simultaneously. Anthropologists believe a single-tube vocal tract is a form of "survival" anatomy that allows animals to smell danger while eating. The two-tube vocal tract of adult humans is less efficient for eating, and actually makes humans more susceptible to choking because of the large gap between the oral cavity and the esophagus. Additionally, adult humans cannot breathe and drink simultaneously. Interestingly, human infants do not show a two-tube vocal tract at birth but rather a single-tube vocal tract. With the larynx located high in the neck it is not possible for liquids to enter the airway, which is what makes it possible for an infant child to suckle the nipple while still being able to breathe. As the child grows, the larynx slowly descends to form a two-tube vocal tract. Among animals, the single-tube vocal tract does not permit the production of a wide range of sounds, although the two-tube vocal tract allows for a wide range of speech sounds, prompting theorists that the lowering of the larynx in man is an "anatomic specialization" for human speech.

Willard R. Zemlin (1929–1998) (Figure 3.21), born in Minnesota, made an enormous contribution to the field of speech and hearing science through his work in basic anatomy and physiology. Zemlin was a faculty member in the Department of Speech and Hearing Science at the University of Illinois. He was the first speech-language pathologist in the world to develop a textbook on the anatomy and physiology of the speech and hearing mechanism that was designed for students in communication disorders. Based on his own dissection work, Zemlin set about detailing essential anatomy, using line drawings and photographs. The result was the publication

A   B   C

FIGURE 3.20. Comparison of the vocal tract anatomy of an adult human, nonhuman primate, and human infant. Only adult humans have a distinct two-tube vocal tract, whereas nonprimates and human infants have a sloping one-tube vocal tract.

FIGURE 3.21. Willard Zemlin, who was interested in the anatomy and physiology of the hearing and speech mechanisms. (From the Willard R. Zemlin Memorial Web site. Permission granted by Eileen Zemlin.)

of the classic textbook, *Speech and Hearing Science, Anatomy and Physiology*, first published in 1964. The book continues to be in widespread use.

CULTURAL CONSIDERATIONS AND ANATOMY AND PHYSIOLOGY

It is no surprise that people come in all shapes and sizes. This observation led to the development of **anthropometry**, which is the scientific study of the measurements of the human body. The field was established to assist in understanding human physical variations and aid in anthropological classification. The term is derived from the Greek terms *anthropos*, meaning man, and *metron*, meaning measure. Anthropometry was first introduced in the late 19th century to the field of criminology, as a supposedly useful means of identifying criminals based on their physical characteristics. A Paris police clerk, Alphonse Bertillon, (1853–1914) devised a system that was used to identify people held in police custody, based on classification of facial and bodily characteristics, and the description of scars and tattoos. Eventually, it was discovered that use of physical characteristics as a form of criminal profiling was not effective and served to perpetuate social racism. Probably the most infamous abuse of anthropometrical research occurred in the years leading up to, and surrounding, World War II. Anthropometric studies performed by German Nazis were used in the classification of Aryan and non-Aryan races, and lead to the decimation of countless individuals who did not fit into established categories.

Putting these extreme examples of anthropometric misuse aside, contemporary anthropometry studies continue to be conducted for various purposes (Figure 3.22). One particular body measurement that is currently used in criminology is fingerprinting. Academic anthropologists often investigate the evolutionary changes in human body shape and size, stemming from ancestors from different environmental settings. For example, there is undisputable evidence that human populations exhibit similar climatic variation to other large-bodied mammals, such as the finding that indigenous individuals who reside in colder climates tend to be larger than individuals residing in warmer climates and that individuals in cold climates will tend to have shorter, thicker limbs than those in warm climates. Health practi-

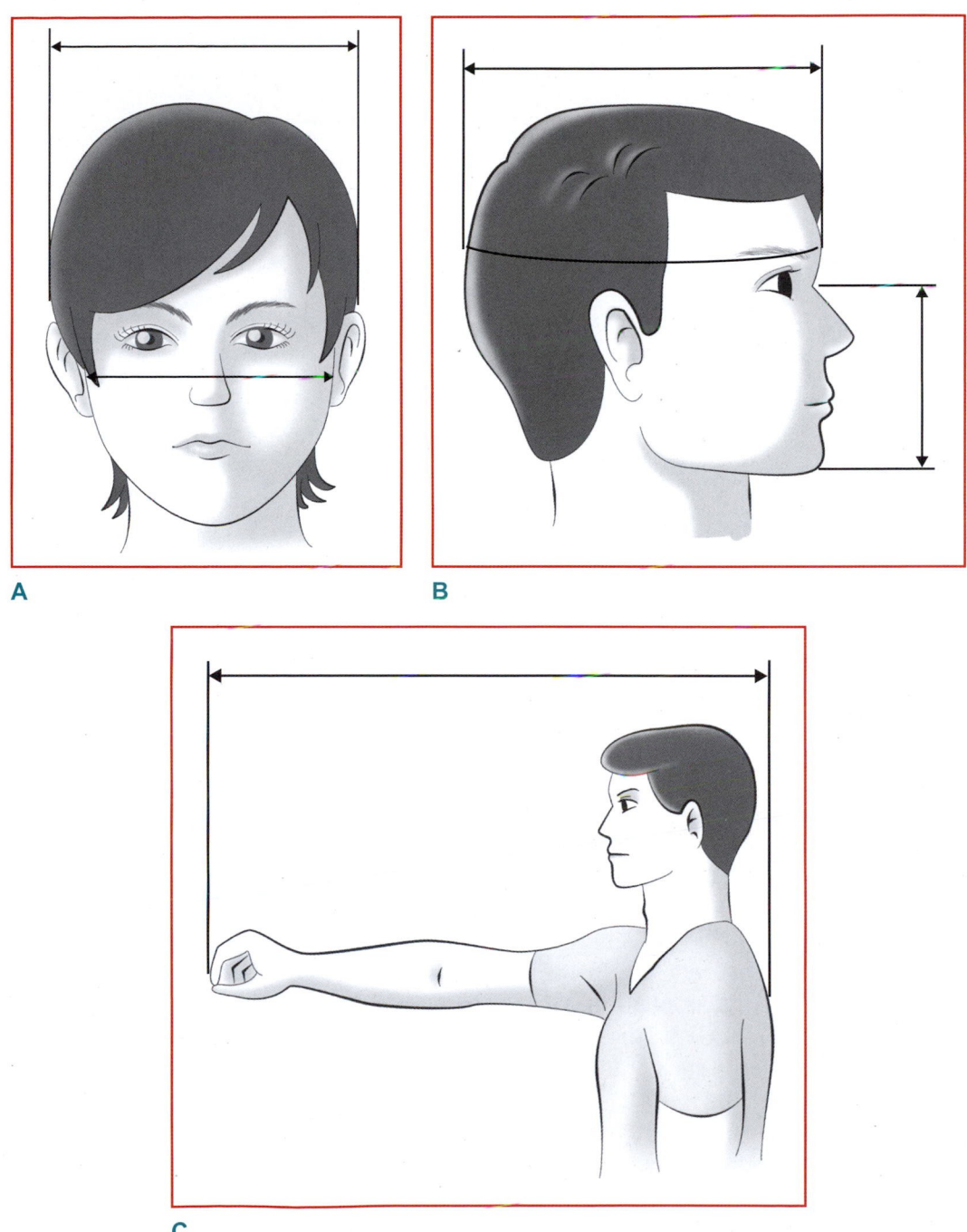

A

B

C

FIGURE 3.22. Examples of anthropometry for various parts of the body. *continues*

tioners use body measurements as an index of physiologic development and nutritional status. For example, determining a child's weight at a given age provides information about the child's overall nutritional status. Measuring a

D   E

FIGURE 3.22. *continued*

child's weight and height can be used to detect acute malnutrition. Measuring mid-upper arm circumference provides an index of muscle wastage. Measurement of skin fold thickness is related to the amount of subcutaneous fat as an index of over- or undernutrition.

Differences in body shape and size are also a consideration in the field of disabilities, including communication disorders. Anthropometry of people with disabilities, such as those confined to a wheelchair, is important in the design of home facilities, as well as work spaces. Anthropometry has been used with increasing frequency to characterize syndromes and to establish ranges of variation within syndromes. For example, there is research revealing that approximately one-third of children with autism have macrocephaly (i.e., large skull) and indicates that autism is sometimes associated with abnormal physical development (Woodhouse et al., 1996). Noting anatomic differences in the structure and function of a person's oral-peripheral speech mechanism is a routine consideration in the SLP's assessment of communication disorders. Finally, audiologists are routinely confronted with anatomic differences in ear anatomy that are a major consideration in the appropriate fitting of hearing aids. Clearly, anatomic and physical differences between people across all walks of life are the norm rather than exception. Anthropometry has evolved to serve a useful role in the clinical evaluation and management of individuals with known and suspected disabilities.

CURRENT RESEARCH IN SPEECH AND HEARING ANATOMY AND PHYSIOLOGY

Vocal Tract Development

Since the initial anatomic observations made by Negus, and later by Lieberman and Crelin (1971), we have known that the vocal tract of very young children is not a smaller replica of the adult vocal tract but is quite different in overall configuration. The human infant vocal tract more closely resembles that of a non-human primate rather than that of an adult human. There is surprisingly little research that has charted the developmental changes that occur as a young child matures. Research is now underway examining vocal tract growth from infancy through early childhood and adolescence (Vorperian & Kent, 2007). Based on magnetic resonance imaging (MRI), we know now that vocal tract growth is not uniform. As the child's vocal tract changes from a one-tube to two-tube vocal tract, the various anatomic structures do not grow at a similar rate. In particular, the tongue, which is the primary speech articulator, seems to grow in "spurts." A major goal of this research is to determine how these changes in vocal tract reconfiguration affect speech acquisition in normally developing children, as well as those who show atypical speech development.

Ossicular Chain Replacement

One of the continuing goals of scientists and engineers is to develop technolo-gies that reduce the severity of physical disabilities. An example of this technology can be found in regard to hearing loss resulting from middle ear defects. In severe cases, the treatment of middle ear defects can now be treated with either a partial or total ossicular replacement prostheses (PORPs and TORPs, respectively). The ability to replace existing middle ear bones with artificial bones was made possible through the development of the surgical microscope and the development of ear-microsurgery. The various design aspects of ossicular prostheses have presented their own unique challenges to the engineers involved in the development of these products. Currently, the primary consideration that goes into the PORP or TORP is that they be of approximately the same weight as the original ear bones, as this is of vital importance for a prosthesis to function properly. Such implants typically result in substantial improvement in the hearing of those who receive them, although current technology does not allow for the complete restoration of a person's hearing. Through continued development, it is possible that use of ossicular implants might some day completely correct one's hearing.

Hair Cell Regeneration in the Cochlea

As noted earlier, a key anatomic feature of the cochlea is the thousands of hair cells that run along the entire length of the basilar membrane. These hair cells serve to transmit electrical impulses to the brain that represent frequencies as high as 20,000 Hz. At present, once cochlear hair cells are damaged, their function cannot be restored, so the death of a hair cell ultimately results in an irreversible hearing loss. The greater the number of hair cells destroyed, the greater the hearing loss. The loss of hair cells can result from prolonged exposure to loud noise, drugs, or disease. However, it has been known for 20 years that hair cells can be regenerated in cold-blooded vertebrates. Researchers discovered that, after being exposed to loud sounds, birds have the remarkable ability to regenerate and replace dead hair cells and return their hearing to near normal, leading to the question, "Why can't humans also regenerate damaged hair cells?" Unfortunately, hair cell regeneration is not as simple as it might seem. Human ears are very complex organs, so it is no surprise that hair cell regeneration is also a complex process. The most promising area of research is the controversial method of using stem cells to replace the destroyed hair cells (Izumikawa et al., 2005). Human stem cells would be most effective for this process by coaxing new hair cells to grow. Currently, stem cell research pertaining to hair cell regeneration is being carried out on mice that will ultimately be tested to see if the results are replicable to humans.

ANATOMY AND PHYSIOLOGY ON THE WORLD WIDE WEB

Listed below are Web sites that provide further information on the topic of anatomy and physiology of speech and hearing. At the time of publication each Web site was freely accessible.

Bartleby.com edition of Gray's Anatomy of the Human Body
http://www.bartleby.com/107/

W. R. Zemlin Memorial Web Site
http://zemlin.shs.uiuc.edu/

How the Ear Functions Video
http://www.archive.org/details/HowtheEa1940

The Larynx and Voice Video
http://www.archive.org/details/larynx_and_the_voice

REFERENCES

Izumikawa M., Minoda, R., Kawamoto, K., Abrashkin, K. A., Swiderski, D. L., Dolan, D. F., et al.. (2005). Auditory hair cell replacement and hearing improvement by Atoh1 gene therapy in deaf mammals. *Nature Medicine, 11*, 271–276.

Lieberman, P., & Crelin, E. S. (1971). On the speech of Neanderthal man. *Linguistic Inquiry, 2*, 203–222.

Vorperian, H. K., & Kent, R. D. (2007). Vowel acoustic space development in children: A synthesis of acoustic and anatomic data. *Journal of Speech, Language, and Hearing Research, 50*, 1510–1545.

Woodhouse, W., Bailey, A., Rutter, M., Bolton, P., Baird, G., & LeCouteur, A. (1996). Head circumference in autism and other pervasive developmental disorders. *Journal of Child Psychology and Psychiatry, 37*, 665–671.

Developmental Communication Disorders

CHILD LANGUAGE DISORDERS

OBJECTIVES

After reading this chapter, the student should be able to:

- Distinguish between speech, language, and communication.

- Differentiate elements of language (phonology, morphology, syntax, semantics, pragmatics).

- Understand basic concepts of each element of language, such as "morpheme" or "phoneme."

- Explain the course of normal spoken language development.

- Understand the distinctions between different disabilities that are characterized by a language disorder, including specific language impairment, intellectual disabilities, and autism spectrum disorders.

- Know the difference between language disabilities and cultural language differences.

- Understand the definition and implications of a language disorder.

- Understand basic principles of formal, standardized language assessment.

- Understand basic principles of informal language assessment.

INTRODUCTION

Language is the expression of human communication through which information can be experienced, explained, and shared. This sharing is based on a system of signs, sounds, and gestures that convey meaning. Language provides the foundation upon which communication, problem solving and synthesizing knowledge take place. A disorder of language, therefore, can have a profound impact on a person's ability to learn and function competently in the world. A language disorder is impairment in the ability to understand and/or use words in a communicative context. Some characteristics of language disorders include improper use of words and their meanings, inability to express ideas, inappropriate grammatical patterns, reduced vocabulary, and an inability to follow directions. Children may hear or see a word but not be able to understand its meaning. They may have trouble getting others to understand what they are trying to communicate. Concern regarding a child's language development is one of the most common reasons for parents of preschool children to seek the advice of their family doctor. Although some children initially may take longer than normal to acquire language they may show rapid improvements. For other children, their language difficulties may be more persistent, requiring intervention by an SLP. A long-term deficit in language can adversely affect an individual's academic progress, as well as social relationships. The focus of this chapter is to provide background on normal aspects of language development and then to use this information as a basis for describing child language disorders.

TERMINOLOGY AND DEFINITIONS

Language is complex and involves multiple domains, such as nonverbal language, oral language (i.e., listening and speaking), and written language (i.e., reading and writing). A classic framework for describing the various strands of language was proposed by **Lois Bloom** and **Margaret Lahey** in 1978 (Figure 4.1). They divided language processes into three areas of skill that contribute to overall communicative competence. These skills consist of: (1) language **form**, (2) language **content**, and (3) language **use**. The form of language is created through the features of phonology, morphology, and syntax. **Phonology** refers to the knowledge a person has of the consonant and vowels sounds in the

FIGURE 4.1. Lois Bloom developed a framework for describing the various strands of language. (Permission granted by L. Bloom.)

language. Although the number of sounds that exist in a language is limited, a nearly endless number of words can be constructed from these sounds. **Morphology** refers to the smallest meaningful unit of language. Morphology involves the stringing together of sounds (phonemes) and includes such structures as prefixes and suffixes. Morphemes are of two types, free morphemes and bound morphemes. A **free morpheme** is a stand-alone word. Examples of free morphemes are *play*, *safe*, and *elephant*. Each of these words contains only one morpheme because they cannot be divided into smaller units and still retain their meaning. Examples of **bound morphemes** include prefixes and suffixes, such as those attached to the words: *playing*, *unsafe*, and *elephants*. Each of these words contains two morphemes and each morpheme within the word contributes uniquely to the word's overall meaning. However, the morphemes "ing," "un," and "s" have no meaning in and of themselves unless they are attached, or bound, to a free morpheme. **Syntax** refers to the rules used in combining words to make a sentence. As with the sounds of language, the rules for combining words to structure a sentence in a particular language are finite. For example, the rules of English require that a noun occurs before a verb in a sentence, such as *"He is running,"* as opposed to *"Running is he."*

The content of language includes the meanings of individual words and words in combination. Another name for language content is **semantics**. The words we use symbolize concepts. If there was no meaning to what was being said, there would be no point in using language. The meaning of words constrains how words may or may not be used together. For example, the sentence *"I saw the tree swimming in the lake"* would make little sense, although it is syntactically correct. Content involves knowledge of vocabulary and the relationships between words. Words can have denotative or connotative meaning. **Denotative**, is the literal (dictionary) mean of a word. **Connotative**, involves use of words for a meaning other than their literal meaning. For example, the denotative meaning of the word, *mother* is female parent. The connotative meaning of mother could evoke alternative meanings such as *love* and *security*. Other nonliteral aspects of language content can be found in **idioms**, such as, *"If the shoe fits, wear it"* or *"It's raining cats and dogs."*

The final component in the Bloom and Lahey model is language use. Another term for language use is **pragmatics**. The pragmatic functions of language involve the use of language in context for a particular purpose or reason. Pragmatics entails three major communication skills:

1. **Using** language for different purposes, such as greeting (e.g., hello, goodbye), informing (e.g., I'm going to get a cookie), demanding (e.g., Give me a cookie), and requesting (e.g., Could I please have a cookie?);
2. **Changing** language according to the needs of a listener or situation, such as talking differently to a baby than to an adult, or speaking differently in a classroom than on a playground; and
3. **Following** rules for conversations, such as taking turns in a conversation, introducing topics of conversation, staying on topic, physical proximity to/from a speaker, and use of facial expressions and eye contact.

Collectively, the skills of language form, content, and use comprise our language competence.

LANGUAGE DEVELOPMENT

Knowledge of the normal, developmental features of language is important for determining the existence of a language disorder. The area of expressive language development, particularly the form of language, has been studied extensively over the past 50 years. Some of the most well established features of normal language are described next as they occur across the period of infancy to school-age development.

Infant/Toddler Language Development

The term, **infant** has its origins in Latin and means "without speech." So when referring to the period of infant development, we are considering a period during which the child has yet to utter a single word. That is not to say children remain silent during infancy. The development of language begins before a child says her first word.

Indeed, some may argue that language begins in the mother's womb. Before children begin talking, they communicate using a combination of vocal and gestural behaviors known as **prelinguistic** communication. One form of prelinguistic communication is that which occurs between mother and child. We know that as early as 3 months of age, infants take part in a conversational turn-taking with their mothers, called **gaze coupling**. Gaze coupling occurs when an infant turns toward the speaker and gains eye contact; it establishes a bond between mother and infant. The infant also produces a rich array of **vocalizations**. The production of vocalizations is not unique to human infants. To vocalize simply means to produce voice and many nonhuman species also vocalize. Among human infants, a distinct developmental pattern of vocalizations has been charted covering the first 12 months of life. The stages of vocal development are illustrated in Figure 4.2. A similar pattern of vocal development is found in infants throughout the world. The earliest vocalization produced by infants is **crying**. The infant quickly learns to produce cries for varying reasons such as when hungry, fussy, or experiencing discomfort. Between 2 and 4 months of age, the infant begins to use vowel-like sounds and consonant-like sounds similar to /k/ and /g/. These comfort sounds are referred to as **cooing** or **gooing**. Around 5 months of age and continuing to 11 months of age, infants produce a wide range of **babbling** sounds. These babbles consist of strings

---

FYI

It is often reported that a child's first words are either *mom* or *dad*. The reason for this is twofold. First, these are important people in a young child's daily life. Secondly the /m/ and /d/ sounds are the earliest and easiest sounds for young children to articulate, which helps pave the way for saying these two words.

FIGURE 4.2. The stages of early vocal development from the period of birth to 18 months of age.

FYI

Professor Ray Kent (1984) has theorized that the reason children produce repetitive strings of babbling is part of a larger human developmental process. During the first year of life, children demonstrate a number of rhythmic motoric behaviors such leg, arm, and finger movements. These rhythmic behaviors are thought to reflect a necessary activity in the development of motor control (skilled performance). Thus, babbling is just one of many rhythmic behaviors related to the development of physical coordination.

---

of syllable combinations that are either reduplicated (e.g., *ba-ba-ba-ba*) or non-reduplicated (*ma-ba-da-ba*) (i.e., variegated) that also have strong intonation patterns. Babbling represents a rich form of vocal behavior that reflects improvements in maturation and coordination of the speech musculature. The infant is truly on the cusp of talking during the babbling period.

By the time an infant reaches his first birthday, the child becomes a toddler. The period of toddlerhood covers the approximate ages of 1 to 2 years of life and reflects a period of rapid development in motor, cognitive, and linguistic abilities. The production of **single words** also marks the moment when the child is no longer just producing vocalizations, but rather, **verbalizations** (i.e., language-based). These verbalizations represent a distinct **sound-to-symbol** relationship. One of the earliest types of sound-symbol relationship is found in the production of **onomatopoeia**, whereby the toddler makes a sound to suggest a thing or action (cow says "*moo*," car goes "*beep*"). Children's vocabularies tend to include the names of important people in their environments and referents that they can interact with, manipulate, or change. For example, children are more likely to say something like *ball* rather than *tree* because a ball has movement and the

child is able to manipulate the object. A child's understanding (comprehension) of vocabulary normally is more advanced than his or her expressive vocabulary. Research has shown that children comprehend their first 50 words at about 13 months of age, but they cannot produce 50 words until they reach 20 months of age. Another language behavior that begins to surface by 18 to 24 months is "**fast mapping**." Fast mapping refers to the process by which children connect a word onto an underlying concept after minimal physical exposure (i.e., seeing the object and quickly linking a word to the object). By the time a child reaches the age of 2-years, the production of **two-word combinations** should be apparent (e.g., "*more juice*" or "*daddy go*"). Two-word combinations occur once a child achieves a single-word vocabulary in excess of 50 words. Examples of the first 50 words produced by children are shown in Table 4.1.

Preschool Language Development

The most well-charted areas of language development during the period from 2 to 5 years are morphology and semantics. During this time frame, the length of the child's expressive utterances

Table 4.1. Example of First 50 Single Words Produced by Three American Children

Daniel Age = 12-16 months		Will Age = 11-16 months		Sarah Age = 12-19 months	
1 light	26 nose	1 baby	26 apple	1 uh-oh	28 go
2 uh-oh	27 fire	2 mommy	27 nose	2 alldone	29 bump
3 wha that	28 hot	3 doggie	28 bird	3 light	30 pop-pop = fire
4 wow	29 yogurt	4 juice	29 all done	4 down	
5 banana	30 pee-pee	5 bye-bye	30 orange	5 shoes	31 out
6 kitty	31 juice	6 daddy	31 bottle	6 baby	32 hee-haw
7 baby	32 ball	7 milk	32 coat	7 don't throw	33 eat
8 moo	33 wack-wack	8 cracker	33 hot		34 neigh
9 quack		9 done	34 bib	8 moo	35 meow
10 cookie	34 frog	10 ball	35 hat	9 bite	36 sit
11 nice	35 hello	11 shoe	36 more	10 three	37 woof-woof
12 rock	36 yuk	12 teddy	37 ear	11 hi	
13 clock	37 aoole	13 book	38 nite-nite	12 cheese	38 bah
14 sock	38 Big Bird	14 kitty	39 paper	13 up	39 hoo-hoo = owl
15 woof-woof	39 walk	15 hi	40 toast	14 quack-quack	
16 daddy	40 Ernie	16 Alex	41 O'Toole	15 oink-oink	40 bee
17 bubble	41 horse	17 no (no)	42 bath		41 tree
18 hi	42 more	18 door	43 down	16 coat	42 mi-mi = ferry
19 shoe	43 mommy	19 dolly	44 duck	17 beep-beep	
20 up	44 bunny	20 wha tha	45 leaf	18 keys	43 ss = snake
21 bye-bye	45 my	21 cheese	46 cookie	19 cycle	44 ooh-ooh = monkey
22 bottle	46 nut	22 oh wow	47 lake	20 mama	
23 no	47 orange	23 oh	48 car	21 daddy	45 yack-yack = talk
24 rocky	48 block	24 button	49 rock	22 siren sound	
25 eye	49 nite-nite	25 eye	50 box	23 grr	46 hohoho = Santa
	50 milk			24 more	47 bye bye
				25 off	48 doll
				26 ticktock	49 kite
				27 ball	50 Muriel

From Stoel-Gammon, C., & Cooper, J. (1984). Patterns of early lexical and phonological development. *Journal of Child Language, 11*, 247–271. Reprinted by permission of Cambridge University Press.

begins to increase by leaps and bounds. This increase is accompanied by the acquisition and use of grammatical morphemes (see later discussion). As children gain mastery over language skills, they also become more sophisticated in their conversational abilities. Between the ages of 4 and 5 years they can follow complex directions and enthusiastically talk about things they do. They can make up stories, listen attentively to stories, and retell stories. At this age, children usually are able to understand that letters and numbers are symbols of real things and ideas. By the age of 5 years a child's expressive vocabulary is between 1,000 and 2,000 words and she is able to understand twice as many words spoken to her. They know gender and names of family members. They often play with words and make up silly words and stories. Toward the end of the preschool period, a child should have intelligible speech, although there may be some mild speech misarticulations. A summary of the language milestones covering the first 6 years of life is provided in Table 4.2.

School-Age Language Development

As children progress through the elementary school years, their language skills continue to develop. Growth in all aspects of language occurs with obvious changes seen in the areas of semantics (vocabulary) and pragmatics (language use). It is estimated that a 6-year-old child has a vocabulary of anywhere from 8,000 to 14,000 words. Beginning with the production of single words at 12 months of age, this means the child must (on average) acquire four to eight new words every day. By school age, a child should be able to speak in complete sentences with minor grammatical errors. The school-age period also marks the development of **metalinguistic awareness**. Metalinguistic awareness is the ability to reflect consciously on the nature and properties of language. Understanding that words and sentences can have more than one meaning is a form of metalinguistic awareness. Children begin to appreciate language in terms of humor, puns, poetry, and use in different situations. The knock-knock joke told by a 6-year-old captures metalinguistic awareness in the form of word play:

Knock knock.
Who's there?
Cargo.
Cargo who?
Cargo BEEP BEEP!

Written Language Development

Most of what is currently known about child language development is based on examining comprehension and pro-

---

FYI

A popular myth is that twin children, when learning to talk, develop their own form of communication known only to them. This has been termed **idioglossia**. However, the phenomenon is actually a case of one twin copying the immature or disordered speech pattern of their co-twin in their attempts to use language.

Table 4.2. Normal Language Development Across the First 6 Years of Life

Age	Language Level
Birth	Cries
2–3 months	Cries differently in different circumstances; cooing/gooing
3–4 months	Babbles randomly
5–6 months	Babbles rhythmically
6–11 months	Babbles in imitation of real speech, with expression
12 months	Produces jargonlike utterances and a small number of single words; recognizes name; imitates familiar sounds.
18 months	Single word vocabulary of 5–20 words, understands simple instructions.
2 years	Expressive utterances of 2 words; vocabulary is growing; waves goodbye; makes "sounds" of familiar animals; make wants known; understands "no."
2–3 years	Identifies body parts; combines nouns and verbs; has a 450 word vocabulary; uses short sentences; matches 3 to 4 colors, likes to hear the same story repeated; forms some plurals.
3–4 years	Can tell a story; expressive utterances of 4 to 5 words in length; vocabulary of about 1000 words; knows last name, name of street, several nursery rhymes.
4–5 years	Expressive utterances of 4 to 5 words in length; uses past tense; vocabulary of about 1500 words; identifies colors, shapes; asks many questions like "why?" and "who?"
5–6 years	Utterances of 5 to 6 words in length; vocabulary in excess of 2000 words; knows spatial relations (like "on top" and "far"); knows address; understands same-different; identifies simple currency, knows right and left hand; uses all types of sentences.

FYI

For years, scientists have argued that language is what sets humans apart from all nonhuman species. Although other animals can communicate, it seems that only humans are capable of using symbols (i.e., words) that have meaning. However, some researchers have suggested that apes are capable of learning sign language that provides evidence of their ability to use symbols that have meaning. The most famous of these apes was a gorilla called Koko who learned over 200 signs.

duction of spoken (oral) language. Less attention has been given to the relationship between oral language competency and written language. Yet, a child's written language skills begin to surface as early as 2 years of age and these abilities provide insight as to a child's overall knowledge of language (Table 4.3). Learning to write involves the ability to translate the sounds of a word to discrete letters (i.e., spelling). So a child's mastery in writing represents an achievement in generalizing language across modalities of communication (MacDon-

ald, 1997). As covered in Chapter 13, the analysis of a written language sample among individuals with deafness is thought to provide an indication of a person's oral language abilities, as well.

HISTORIC ASPECTS OF CHILD LANGUAGE DISORDERS

To speak about language is to speak about the development of the human

Table 4.3. Stages of Written Language Development

Stage	Age	Ability
I. Random Scribbling	2–3 years	Children make marks on paper randomly with little muscular control.
II. Controlled Scribbling	3 years	Children "write" across the paper in linear fashion, repeating patterns over again showing increased muscular control.
III. Letterlike Forms	3–4 years	Children make mock letters. These are written lines of letters that have letter characteristics but are misshapen and written randomly. They like to pretend they are writing, and are able to separate writing from drawing. They have purpose to their letterlike forms.
IV. Letter/Symbol Relationship	4 years	Children write letters to create words. They can write their name. They know the word that represents their name. They can copy words. Letter reversals are frequent.
V. Invented Spelling	4–5 years	Children make the transition from letter forms to invented spelling. They use a group of letters to form a word. Many of the letters will be consonants. They understand that letters relate to sounds. Some punctuation appears. They can copy words from their environment.
VI. Standard Spelling	5–7 years	Most of the words children use are written correctly. They organize their words in lines with spaces between the words; and, they move from left to right, and from the top of the page to the bottom.

race (Butler, 1986). There is evidence to suggest that language originated during the Ice Age, approximately 30,000 years ago. When language was created, it is likely that language disorders were soon to follow; frequently as a result of a physical accident or intellectual disability. One of the earliest detailed reports of a language disorder was by the French physician **Jean-Marc Gaspard Itard** (1774–1838) (Figure 4.3). The report was based on the case of the **wild boy of Aveyron**. Discovered in 1799, the boy (named Victor) had been lost or abandoned in childhood, apparently surviving on his own in the wild up to the age of approximately 11 years. The boy spoke no language and Itard undertook to educate Victor. Itard believed that two things separated humans from animals: empathy and language. He wanted to be the first person to fully civilize a wild child and attempted to teach Victor to speak and show human

emotion. Though initially successful in understanding language and reading simple words, Victor's abilities eventually plateaued to the point where Itard abandoned the experiment. The only words that Victor ever actually learned to speak were *lait* (milk) and *oh Dieu* (oh God). Victor died at the age of 40. This early study supported the theory that an enriching environment was vital to the acquisition of normal language.

In the early 1960s Roger Brown from Harvard University performed some pioneering research in the area of normal language development in a longitudinal study of three children, Adam, Eve, and Sarah (Brown, 1973). Brown recorded the conversations of these children with their parents at home every 2 weeks for the first 5 years of life. Brown calculated a measure called **mean length of utterance** (MLU) to assess the children's increasing ability to combine words and produce complex utterances. MLU is calculated by taking 100 utterances produced by a child (excluding all cases were the utterance is a repetition of a statement made by an adult) and then working out the average length in morphemes. The number of morphemes in an utterance often is the same as the number of words because, in children's early multiword speech, their words usually consist only of a single morpheme. For example, the utterance *"Daddy go"* consists of two morphemes. However, as a child's speech becomes more complex, she begins to modify words by the addition of morphemes, such as plural "s" or present progressive "ing," resulting in utterances such as *"Daddy going"* (3 morphemes).

A great deal of what is currently known about the development of expressive language during the preschool period is based on Brown's research. He identified five stages in language

FIGURE 4.3. Jean-Marc Gaspard Itard provided one of the earliest detailed reports of a language disorder based on the "wild boy of Aveyron."

development that were organized according to the child's MLU. There was an orderly development in 14 grammatical morphemes across the first 5 years of life that corresponded to the child's MLU (Table 4.4). The order of acquisition was similar for the three children. Brown argued that the order in which all children acquired various grammatical morphemes was identical with the progression from simple morphemes to more complex ones. However, more recent studies have shown that by the end of the preschool period, most children have acquired a full range of grammatical morphemes in their expressive

Table 4.4. Brown's (1973) Stages of Grammatical Morpheme Development and the Approximate Age at which Each Stage Should Be Attained

Stage	MLU	MLU Range	Age in Months	14 Grammatical Morphemes	Examples
I	1.75	1.5–2.0	15–30	combine basic words	more juice daddy go
II	2.25	2.0–2.5	28–36	(1) present progressive	daddy go*ing* fall*ing* down
				(2) preposition "in"	*in* house
				(3) preposition "on"	*on* top
				(4) -s plurals (regular)	my toy*s*
III	2.75	2.5–3.0	36–40	(5) irregular past tense	I *fell* down She *sat* on
				(6) -s possessives	Mommy*'s* house
				(7) uncontractible copula	*Are* they here?
IV	3.5	3.0–3.7	40–46	(8) articles	*a* ball *the* cat
				(9) regular past tense "ed"	He walk*ed* She danc*ed*
				(10) third-person regular present tense	He push*es* She *walks*
V	4.0	3.7–4.5	46–52+	(11) third-person irregular	Kathy *has* He *does*
				(12) uncontractible auxiliary	*Is* he going? What *are* you doing?
				(13) contractible copula	*Matt's* tall *I'm* short
				(14) contractible auxiliary	*They're* walking *He's* running

language; although the precise order in which they are acquired may not be identical.

TYPES OF CHILD LANGUAGE DISORDERS

Language disorders in children are characterized by deficiencies in the comprehension and/or production of spoken and written language (Figure 4.4). Deficiencies in language can have a profound impact on a child's academic, social, and emotional development. Roughly 7% of preschool and school-age children exhibit significant limitations in language ability. Some language disorders in children can result from organic factors, such as intellectual impairment, hearing loss, and head injury. Often, child language disorders are functional in nature, where a specific etiology for the disorder cannot be determined. Later chapters in this book address language disorders resulting from specific conditions such as genetic abnormalities (Chapter 11) and hearing impairment (Chapter 12). Some common conditions indicative of language impairment are provided below.

Specific Language Impairment

Specific language impairment (SLI) is characterized by difficulty with language that is not caused by known neurological, sensory, intellectual, or emotional deficit. SLI can affect the development of vocabulary, grammar, and conversation (discourse) skills. Children with SLI may be intelligent and healthy in all regards, with the exception of a specific difficulty with language. They may in fact be extraordinarily bright. Children with SLI usually learn to talk late. It is not unusual to first encounter a child with SLI at the age 3 or 4 years, with limited vocabulary and short utterances. As they mature and the problem goes undetected, they may be described by teachers as being smart but unmotivated. The incidence of SLI is approximately 8% among 5-year-old children. Although SLI is not a reading disability, 50% to 75% of children with SLI also experience problems in learning to read.

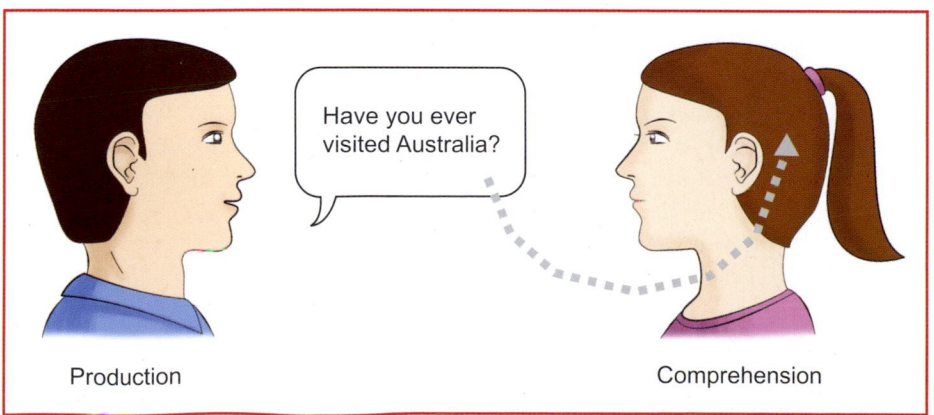

FIGURE 4.4. Conceptualization of the processes of language production and comprehension.

Intellectual Impairment

The acquisition of language is a remarkable human achievement. Within a few short years children make the transition from cooing and babbling to becoming fully communicative individuals. Generally, children acquire the essential components of language by the age of 3 or 4 years. However, this may not be true for children with an intellectual disability (i.e., mental retardation). Intellectual impairment is characterized by significantly subaverage intellectual functioning, which is determined on the basis of a mathematical ratio known as an **intelligence quotient** (IQ). A standard way of determining IQ is to note the discrepancy between an individual's true, chronological age (CA) and their mental age (MA), as derived from a test of intelligence. The formula for calculating IQ is *100 * MA/CA*. So two possible IQ examples would be:

- MA = 6 years / CA = 5 years
  (IQ = 120 which means gifted)
- MA = 6 years / CA = 9 years
  (IQ = 66 which means impaired)

In the late 1800s, intellectual disability used to be classified using descriptive terms such as idiot (IQ = 0–19), imbecile (IQ = 20–24), moron (IQ = 25–49), simpleton (IQ = 50–69), and dullard (IQ = 70–99) until these terms began to be abused by the rest of society. The terms have become obsolete and intellectual impairment is now defined by an IQ of approximately 70 or below. Four degrees of impairment severity can be specified: mild (IQ = 50–70), moderate (IQ = 35–49), severe (IQ = 20–34) and profound (IQ = 0–19). The prevalence of intellectual impairment in the noninstitutionalized population of the United States is 7.8 people per 1000. If institutionalized individuals are included in the prevalence rates, the number increases to 8.7 per 1000.

Intellectual impairment is associated with limitations in learning and can have a profound effect on a child's ability to talk. At one time it was believed that the language acquisition of all persons with an intellectual impairment represented a slow-motion version of normal language development. That is, children with an intellectual impairment demonstrated normal language behavior; however, it was behavior expected in younger, non-impaired children. We now know there is no consistent pattern of language behavior shown in children with an intellectual impairment due to differences in the type and severity of impairment. The overall picture of early language development in children with intellectual impairment is one of differences and similarities in comparison to normal children. Impaired children appear to follow the same set of universal principles in the acquisition of word meaning, although this is not always the case for profoundly impaired children. Intellectually impaired children are found to acquire syntactic and morphological knowledge in the same order as normally developing children. Children with intellectual impairments also are able to acquire basic pragmatic skills; yet more subtle aspects of conversational competence are less commonly displayed.

Autism

Autism was first identified in 1943 by **Leo Kanner** (1896–1981) who described 11 self-absorbed children who had "autistic disturbances of affect contact" (Figure 4.5). Autism originally was thought

FIGURE 4.5. Leo Kanner was the first person to identify distinct features of autism.

to reflect an attachment disorder resulting from poor parenting. The cause of autism is still unknown but most specialists believe it is a brain disorder that makes it difficult for the person to process and respond to the world. The term **autism spectrum disorders** (ASD) is now used to capture the wide range of autistic behaviors. Research has shown that many people who engage in autistic behaviors have related but distinct disorders. These include, Asperger syndrome, Fragile X syndrome, Williams syndrome, and Savant syndrome, to name a few. Details of Fragile X syndrome are covered in Chapter 11. ASD is also known as a type of **pervasive developmental disorder** (PDD), because it can cause a severe impairment in thinking, feeling, language, and the ability to relate to others.

Parents are usually the first to notice autisticlike behaviors in their child. In some cases, the baby seemed "different" from birth, unresponsive to people, or focusing intently on one item for long periods of time. The first signs of an ASD also can appear in children who had been developing normally. When an affectionate, verbal toddler suddenly becomes silent and withdrawn from social activities, something is wrong. Autism is one of the most common developmental disabilities of childhood. Individuals of all races, ethnicity, and socioeconomic backgrounds can show autism. The conservative estimate of the occurrence of ASD is about 2 per 1000 people, with about four times as many boys as girls affected. The number of people

FYI

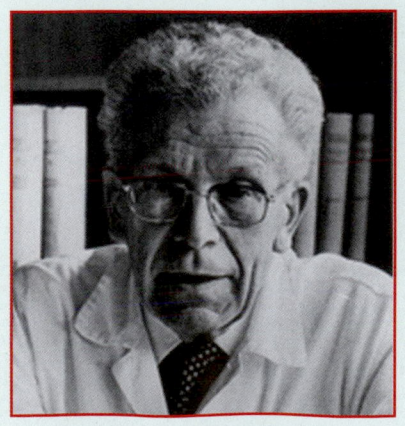

Asperger syndrome is considered a mild form of autism that is characterized by concrete thinking, obsession with certain topics, social isolation, excellent memory, and being 'eccentric.' Individuals have an average to above average IQ, are capable of holding a job and living independently. The cause of the condition is unknown. The condition is named after **Hans Asperger** (1906–1980), an Austrian physician who first described the syndrome in 1944.

known to have autism has increased dramatically since the 1980s, partly due to changes in diagnostic practice. Some research suggests that ASD can be as high as 10 per 1,000 people. Current estimates suggest that approximately 500,000 individuals in England and the United States have ASD and over 12,000 in Australia. Autism occurs in individuals of all levels of intelligence. Approximately 75% are of low intelligence whereas around 10% show **savant** skills such as extraordinary abilities in specific areas like music and mathematics.

Three crucial areas of development are affected by ASD: (1) verbal and nonverbal communication, (2) social interaction, and (3) creative or imaginative play. The communication problems of ASD vary, depending on the intellectual and social development of the individual. For many, speech and language develops to some degree, but not to a normal ability level. This development usually is uneven. For example, vocabulary development in areas of interest may be accelerated. Many have good memories for information just heard or seen. Some may be able to read words well before the age of five but cannot demonstrate understanding of what is read. Some may be unable to speak, whereas others might have rich vocabularies and are able to talk about topics of interest in great depth. Despite this variation, the majority of autistic individuals have little or no problem with speech articulation. Most have difficulty effectively using language. Their expressive language is likely to contain no content or information. For example, an autistic individual may repeatedly count from one to five. Others use **echolalia**, a repetition of something previously heard. One form, **immediate echolalia**, may occur when the individual repeats the question, "Do you want something to drink?" instead of replying with a "yes" or "no." In another form called **delayed echolalia**, an individual may say, "Do you want something to drink?" whenever he or she is asking for a drink. Other distinct features of autism are a lack of eye contact and poor attention duration. Individuals with ASD often are unresponsive to the speech of others and may not respond to their own names. As a result, some are mis-

---

FYI

Savant syndrome is a *juxtaposition* of severe intellectual disability and prodigious (narrow) mental ability. Individuals have an IQ generally below 70. The syndrome occurs more often in males. The most common savant skills are music (playing piano by ear), art (painting or drawing), lightning-quick mathematical calculating, calendar calculating, and mechanical/spatial skills. The condition was first identified by in 1887 by **John Langdon Down** (1828–1896), who used the term "idiot savant." The condition known as Down syndrome was first identified by Down.

takenly thought to have a hearing problem. Children with ASD fail to interact with others, which adversely effects communication. The simple act of communication involves two individuals, a speaker and a listener. The child with autism fails to engage in communication, resulting in a potentially severe communication disorder.

Late Talkers

The term **late talker** is used to describe a group of children who have an impoverished expressive vocabulary, usually within the age range of 16 to 30 months of life. These children are slow to acquire their first 50 words and also slow to combine two words. By 24 months of life most children have an expressive vocabulary of approximately 200 words, whereas late talkers may have a vocabulary of approximately 20 words. These children are developing typically in the areas of language comprehension, play, motor and cognitive/learning skills, with the sole exception being language expression. Children who are late talkers are thought to be at risk for subsequent language problems. The challenge presented to the SLP is determining which of these children will simply outgrow the delay and which will not.

> ### CURRENT THEORIES REGARDING CHILD LANGUAGE DEVELOPMENT AND DISORDERS

Theories regarding the cause of a child language disorder usually attribute the disorder to biological (nature) or environmental (nurture) factors. For exam-

ple, a biological cause would be seen in a child born with a profound hearing loss that interfered with his ability to hear and subsequently learn language. Alternatively, an environmental cause would be seen in a child deprived of human contact (e.g., wild boy of Aveyron), thus preventing him from experiencing the language of others. Either of these situations would have an effect on a child's subsequent language development. However, it is equally possible for the combined effects of nature and nurture to contribute to a language disorder. One possible scenario would be a situation where a child born with an intellectual disability (a biological condition) receives inadequate language stimulation in the home environment. Needless to say, there are a wide range of situations that can contribute to a language disorder. There are four major theories concerning normal language acquisition. These are the: (1) behavioral, (2) nativist, (3) interaction, and (4) statistical learning theories. Regardless of the theory one may ascribe to, a disruption in the normal process of language acquisition more than likely will lead to a language disorder.

The **behaviorist theory** is perhaps the oldest theory about language development. This theory assumes that children learn language the same way they learn everything else, namely, through imitation and reinforcement. The Swiss psychologist **Jean Piaget** (1896–1980) and American psychologist **Burrhus Frederic (B.F.) Skinner** (1904–1990) were strong advocates of a behavioral influence on language acquisition (Figure 4.6). The child's path to learning language involves a trial-and-error process. In other words, the child tries and fails to use correct language until he or she succeeds. The child's success with language is based on reinforcement and shaping provided

A

B

FIGURE 4.6. Famous behavioral psychologists: **A.** Jean Piaget and **B.** B. F. Skinner.

by the parent's gestures (smiles, attention and approval) which are pleasant to the child. Parents who ignore unfamiliar sounds produced by the young child and show increased attention to his production of word-like utterances further shape the child's language learning. Although research has shown that children who imitate the actions of those around them during their first year of life generally are those who also learn to talk more quickly, there is also evidence that imitation alone cannot explain how children become talkers.

The **nativist theory** of language stresses the contribution of the child's biological makeup to language acquisition. This theory was advocated in the early 1960s by the American linguist **Noam Chomsky** (b. 1928) (Figure 4.7). He suggested that humans are born with a special biological brain mechanism, called a **language acquisition device** (LAD). This theory supposes that the ability to learn language is inborn, that nature is more important than nurture, and that experience using language is only necessary to activate the LAD.

FIGURE 4.7. Noam Chomsky, American linguist.

Chomsky claims that it would be little short of a miracle if children were to learn their language strictly through the imitation of others. This is because children are exposed to very little correctly formed language. When people speak, they constantly interrupt themselves, change their minds, and make slips of the tongue. Yet children manage to learn their language all the same. Children do not simply copy the language that they hear around them. They deduce rules from it, which they can then use to produce sentences that they have never heard before. This also accounts for the common observation of young children inventing novel words such as "throwed." Because it is highly unlikely such a word was previously modeled to the child, it is doubtful this reflects imitation by the child.

An alternative to the behavioral and nativist theories of language acquisition is the **interactionist theory**. Interactionists consider language development to involve a combination of behavioral and nativist processes. According to this theory, language learning is influenced by the desire of children to communicate with others. Children are born with a powerful brain that matures slowly and predisposes them to acquire new understandings that they are motivated to share with others (Bates & Carnevale, 1993).

Some researchers believe that language acquisition is based primarily on general learning mechanisms, namely statistical learning (Saffran et al., 1996). Imagine that as an infant you are placed in an environment where you overhear an immense language system that contains thousands of unusual sounds. As an infant, you must discover the underlying structure of this system that consists of the individual sounds of language, and the larger pieces that are the words, which in turn combine to form sentences. Somehow you must rapidly figure out the structure of this system so that you can use it appropriately early in your childhood. The use of statistical cues may help young children discover some of the consistent patterns found in the language they overhear. This theory proposes that infants and toddlers learn statistical probabilities in speech, such as natural breaks between syllables, words,

and sentences. The **statistical learning theory** of language asserts that, with repeated exposure to many language examples, the statistical structure of the language is deciphered, which streamlines the process of language acquisition.

ASSESSMENT OF CHILD LANGUAGE DISORDERS

The classic diagram developed by Bloom and Lahey shows the relationship between the three components of language; form, content, and use (Figure 4.8). Communicative competence is achieved when a child is able to manage all of these components effectively. In the event of a communicative breakdown, the SLP identifies whether the problem is one of form, content, or use—or some combination of these components. Once the problem is isolated, an intervention plan can be developed to target the area that is hindering the acquisition of communicative competence. When a child has a suspected language disorder, he is usually brought to the speech-language clinic for an assessment. The assessment is a process of observation and measurement of the child's language behaviors to determine: (1) whether a language disorder exists and (2) the nature and severity of the disorder.

Does a Language Disorder Exist?

To answer this question, the SLP must examine and assess the child's comprehension and production of the various language components. Some features of a language assessment include: (1) a **case history**, (2) **standardized testing**, and

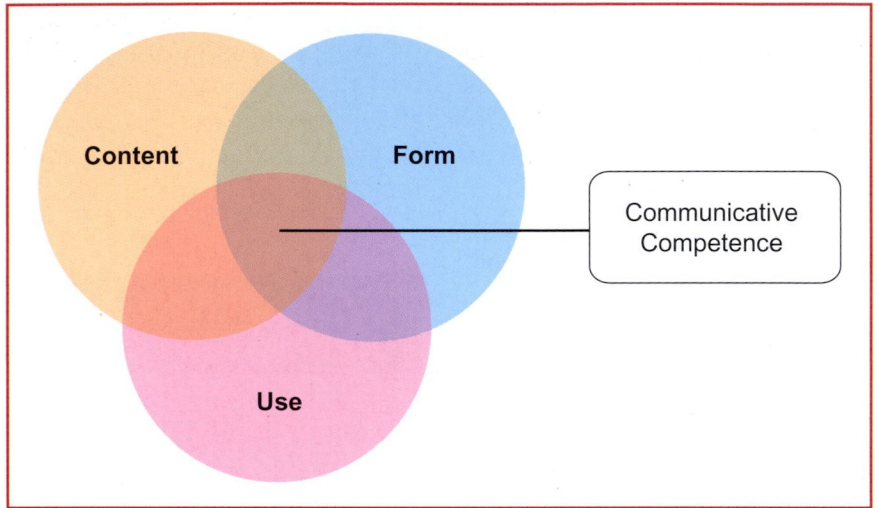

FIGURE 4.8. A Venn diagram showing the three components of language and their contribution to communicative competence.

(3) **language sampling** or **nonstandardized testing**. Each of these features is briefly defined.

Case History

The collection of a **case history** is vital to any assessment of communication disorders. The collection of this information typically is done via a questionnaire type format (Table 4.5) and can be completed by the parents prior to their visit to the clinic or can be completed as part of an interview with the parents at the beginning of the assessment session. The SLP uses the case history gathering as an opportunity to become acquainted with the parents and ascertain their understanding of their child's problem, and the concerns for the child. As part of the case history, the SLP gathers information about the child's general development, as well as communication behavior as reported by the parents. The SLP also learns about the possible coexistence of complicating conditions such as ear infections. The collection of information during the case history can

be crucial in situations where the child may be quite young and or severely disabled, where more emphasis is placed on the parent interview process rather than the child assessment process.

Standardized Testing

The use of **standardized testing** is a central feature to assessing a child's language abilities. There are many standardized measures of language ability. Some provide a comprehensive view of all language functioning; others measure specific features of language. Standardized tests are those that are sold by publishing companies. When using a standardized test, children are assessed in precisely the same fashion, with specific instructions provided by the tester. Every standardized test has a consistent, uniform way in which a child's language behavior is elicited and evaluated. Many standardized tests have **norms** that provide a way for the clinician to compare the child being tested with normally developing children of the same age and socioeconomic status. Standardized tests

Table 4.5. Abbreviated Example of a Case History Questionnaire

Identifying Information

Child's Name: _____ Sex: F   M

Date of Birth: _____ Age: _____

Statement of Problem

Describe your child's communication problem: _____

_____

When did you first notice the problem? _____

Has your child's communication problem changed since then? _____

_____

Is your child aware of her or his communication problem? _____

Is there a history of communication problems in your family? _____

Communication Development

At what age did your child begin to babble? _____

At what age did your child produce single words? _____

At what age did your child say two-word sentences? _____

Developmental History

Was the pregnancy normal? _____

When did your child sit upright? _____

When did you child begin to walk? _____ run? _____

Medical History

Has your child had any illnesses or accidents? _____

Has your child experienced any ear infections? _____ Frequency? _____

are the basis for many decisions in our culture. They are used for determining school placement, university entrance, and intelligence level. The score a child receives on a standardized test predicts a certain level of performance. A number of standardized tests are available to evaluate a wide range of language abilities. Two popular tests are the **Peabody Picture Vocabulary Test** (PPVT) (Dunn et al., 2006), which is designed to estimate vocabulary comprehension abilities, and the **Clinical Evaluation of Language Fundamentals** (CELF), (Semel et al., 2003), which involves a myriad of lan-guage comprehension and expression abilities (Table 4.6). Tests such as these examine a child's language abilities on the basis of picture-pointing tasks. The tester will present the child with a spe-

Table 4.6. Various Subtests Comprising the Clinical Evaluation of Language Functions Standardized Test (Semel et al., 2003)

Subtest/Scale	Description
Concepts and Following Directions	Measures auditory comprehension and recall of utterances of increasing length and complexity
Word Structure	Assesses morphology and pronoun use
Recalling Sentences	A sentence imitation task
Formulated Sentences	Child is given a word or words and must generate spoken sentences in reference to a picture cue
Word Classes (Receptive and Expressive)	These subtests measure the student's comprehension of relationships between words
Word Definitions	A measure of word meanings
Sentence Structure	A measure of auditory comprehension
Sentence Assembly	A measure of verbal expression
Semantic Relationships	Assesses comprehension of complex language relationships
Expressive Vocabulary	Vocabulary
Understanding Spoken Paragraphs	A measure of auditory comprehension, memory, and logic
Number Repetition—Forward	A measure of attention and memory
Number Repetition—Backward	A measure of attention and memory
Familiar Sequences (1 & 2)	Assess retrieval of well-learned information
Rapid Automatic Naming	Assesses naming speed
Word Associations	Assesses semantic knowledge
Phonological Awareness	Assesses phonological knowledge
Pragmatics Profile	Assesses comprehension of social rules
Observational Rating Scale	Assesses the impact of language functioning across situations

cific language model, and the child is required to match a specific picture to the language model. Figures 4.9 and 4.10 provide examples of picture stimuli that might be used in standardized testing.

Language Sampling

It is important to recognize that standardized tests generally are not sensitive to the subtleties of natural, spontaneous

A

B

C

D

FIGURE 4.9. Example of test pictures used for standardized testing of vocabulary comprehension. The clinician would prompt the child by stating, "Point to giraffe."

FIGURE 4.10. Example of test pictures used for standardized testing of language comprehension of sentences. The clinician would prompt the child by stating, "Point to, The girl pushes the boy."

communication. Therefore, in addition to standardized tests, a language assessment should include collection of a naturalistic sample of the child's language. The key to **language sampling** is to obtain a representative sample of the child's typical expressive language behavior. Language sampling is a form of **nonstandardized** (or informal) testing because there is no consistent or standardized manner in which the sample is collected. Language samples can be obtained through checklists or observational recording systems, or through casually conversing with the child. Language sampling is a four-step process. The first step involves eliciting and recording the language sample. Eliciting good language samples takes time, training, and practice. The sample is obtained by encouraging the child to speak while playing with toys, describing pictures, and answering open-ended questions. The sample is audio- and/or video-recorded for later analysis. The second step is transcribing the language sample. The child's utterances are transcribed verbatim. The third step in this process entails analyzing the language sample in a number of ways, including calculation of the child's size of vocabulary, MLU, syntactic structure, and sentence types. The fourth step in the language sampling analysis process requires interpretation of the analyses. The child's language abilities noted in the language sample can be compared to reference databases of typical children to provide an indication of his expressive language and whether he may exhibit a language disorder. Computer software known as **SALT** (Systematic Analysis of Language Transcripts) is in regular use for transcribing and analyzing language samples, as well as comparing them to reference databases of typical children. The SALT program was developed by Dr. Jon Miller and Dr. Robin Chapman at the University of Wisconsin-Madison. An example of MLU calculation is shown in Table 4.7.

What Is the Nature and Severity of the Disorder?

On the basis of the information collected from the child and parents, the SLP will make a number of decisions regarding

Table 4.7. Example of MLU Calculation. A typical MLU Calculation Is Based on a Sample of 100 Utterances.

Utterance Transcription	Number of Grammatical Morphemes
I see daddy.	3
More juice.	2
What man doing.	4
Mommy driving.	3
Ball in cup.	3
Baby pulled the wagon.	5
The girl likes eating.	6
He's falling down.	5
The bus is yellow.	4
Where mommy go?	3

Number of utterances = 10

Number of grammatical morphemes = 38

MLU = 38/10 utterances = 3.8

the child's language abilities. The most immediate decision is a determination as to whether the child exhibits a language disorder. The disorder could be in any area of language form, content, or use. If the child's language abilities are not equivalent to those found for same-aged normally developing peers, then the diagnosis of a language disorder is made. If a disorder is present, the SLP will next determine the nature of the disorder, by indicating whether the impairment is indicative of a **language delay** or **language deviance** (Figure 4.11). A language delay means that the child's language system is similar to younger, nondisordered children. The various components of the child's language system are not unusual. Rather, the child's

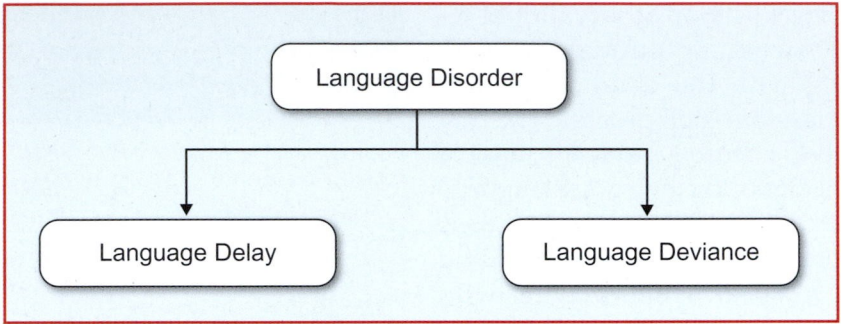

FIGURE 4.11. Classification of language disorders.

language is trailing behind in development compared to her peers. A child demonstrating a language deviance is exhibiting a linguistic system that is unlike that of younger nondisordered children. A language deviance often is found in situations where a child may exhibit a variety of physical and or cognitive impairments. Children exhibiting a language deviance are less common than those showing a language delay. The SLP also will make a decision concerning the severity of the language disorder that is based on determining the extent to which the child's language abilities are impaired. As a general rule, a language deviance is considered more severe than a language delay. However, a language delay also can be severe if a number of language abilities are impaired, such as vocabulary size, utterance length, and language syntax.

TREATMENT OF CHILD LANGUAGE DISORDERS

Treatment of child language disorders involves determining the best course of action to assist the child. There is no standard approach to treating child language disorders. Some approaches work better for some children than others. The particular approach and success of an approach is dependent on factors such as the child's age, attention span, and type and cause of language disorder. The set of goals and treatment strategies are unique to the child and his particular difficulties with language. An overarching theme in the treatment of child language disorders is to help the child improve his communication. Parents and teachers can contribute a great deal to the child's success in therapy. The child may only spend a few short hours each week receiving formal therapy from an SLP. The remainder of the time is spent outside the clinic in the home and school environment. So the SLP is likely to provide parents and teachers with activities that can be used in these settings to help facilitate the child's language abilities. Goals developed for helping children improve their language comprehension abilities might be to help the child increase receptive (listening) vocabulary, comprehension of directions, understanding of grammar, and recognition of the role of a listener in a conversation. Examples of expressive language goals would be to expand vocabulary development and the child's use of language (pragmatics) in various speaking contexts.

Once specific goals of treatment are identified, the SLP can opt to use either an adult-centered approach or child-centered approach in helping the child achieve these goals. Language therapy is characterized as **adult-centered** if the therapist takes a direct approach to teaching specific language skills to the child. This approach has been in widespread use for many years and involves giving the child frequent prompts to produce the desired utterances. The SLP may also use instructional materials such as charts that focus on the particular language skill being taught. The treatment goal of a session might be, for example, to get the child to correctly use verb forms such as "is walking," "is playing," and "is eating," or learning to follow directions. Adult-centered therapy is found to be most affective with school-age children.

In contrast, therapy that is **child-centered** uses a less directive path to improving the child's language abilities. This approach has been referred to as *speech on the run*, whereby the SLP provides therapy by following the child's lead and using a more conversational give-and-take rather than an instructional format. In these therapy sessions, an SLP will interact with a child by playing and talking. The therapist may use pictures, books, objects, or ongoing events to stimulate language learning. Four therapy techniques used in child centered therapy are: (1) self-talk, (2) parallel talk, (3) description, and (4) expansion. **Self-talk** involves the SLP (or parent) talking out loud about what they are doing as they engage with the child. As part of self-talk, the therapist provides a rich array of language models for the child in a noninvasive, natural fashion. For example, while playing with a doll, the SLP may say, *"Oh there's my doll; she is sitting on the chair."* **Parallel talk** involves the SLP describing out loud what the child is seeing, hearing, or thinking during the play activity. For example, if the child is playing with a train set, the SLP may comment, *"You put the train in the tunnel."* **Description** involves use of labeling or explanations by the SLP that call attention to the child about objects or happenings in the play setting. The SLP may say *"Here comes the train."* The use of **expansions** by the SLP requires a restatement of the child's utterance, however with a fuller and grammatically correct language model. For example, the child may say, *"train go,"* and the SLP responds with, *"Yes. The train is going."* The SLP adds the missing parts to the utterance and elaborates on the utterance, without overtly correcting the child or interfering with the flow of communication. The use of these child-centered techniques is particularly effective in providing language remediation to preschool-age children.

These two therapy approaches are not mutually exclusive. It is quite possible the SLP may develop some sort of hybrid therapy approach involving both adult- and child-centered techniques. One likely situation when a hybrid approach may be used is when the SLP wishes to implement a therapy program that involves both the home and school setting. The parents could be using *speech on the run* techniques to model general language skills for the child at home, and the SLP could use direct therapy techniques when the child is attending school.

CULTURAL CONSIDERATIONS AND CHILD LANGUAGE DISORDERS

Assessment

As the world becomes more globally connected, the diversity of cultural and language backgrounds represented among today's children is expanding. Most SLPs working in schools are likely to be confronted with children who differ in culture, dialect, as well as primary language compared to their own. Culturally and linguistically diverse children exhibit differences in behaviors, expectations, and belief systems. They use languages other than English and/or dialectical variations different from those used in the school setting. Special considerations must be taken to address the complex issues of these populations. The percentage of children living in the United States who are Hispanic doubled between 1980 and 2004 (from 9% to 19%) and is projected to increase to nearly 25% of the child population by 2020. Recent census statistics in England indicated that close to 4 million residents were of Asian/Indian and Black African/Caribbean background. Over 2 million Australians, or about 14% of those aged 5 years and over, speak a language other than English at home. Languages such as Italian and Greek, and to a lesser extent Chinese, German, and Arabic, are spoken in Australia as community languages.

Bilingualism is defined as the ability to communicate in two languages (Figure 4.12), but not necessarily at the same level of proficiency. There are two forms of bilingualism: (1) simultaneous, and (2) consecutive. **Simultaneous**

FIGURE 4.12. Bilingualism is becoming a part of our everyday world.

bilingualism also is referred to as spontaneous bilingualism. In this form of bilingualism, an individual has presumably spoken (or has been spoken to) two or more languages in the home since birth. In **consecutive bilingualism**, an individual learns one language after already knowing another. This is the situation for individuals who become bilingual as older children and adults. Consecutive bilingualism is by far the most common form of bilingualism. Most linguistically diverse children speak a form of English that varies from Standard English. These variations should not automatically be considered a language disorder.

The challenge for the SLP when confronted with a bilingual child is to distinguish between aspects of linguistic variation that represent regular patterns in the speaker's language or dialect and those that represent true disorders in language. This is known as the difference versus disorder paradox. A **language difference** is a situation in which the language features of a community differ from the majority language. The rules are normal for the smaller community. Consider the case of a child who is speaking Spanish-accented English. The child's first or dominant language (**L1**) is Spanish, and the second language (**L2**) is English. The SLP must determine if the child's differences with the English language are due to variation that is caused by normal linguistic processes, resulting from the competition between two languages, or a more basic problem, reflecting a language disorder. If the language of the child's L2 is found to be disordered, it is highly likely the L1 also is disordered. It is inappropriate to label a child as language disordered if his second language is in transition. It is also inappropriate to overlook a child who is speaking L2 when the L1 may be disordered.

Great care must be taken to ensure that language assessment of bilingual children is culture-free and dialect-sensitive. Problems may arise when the language tester (the SLP) and the child being assessed come from different linguistic or cultural backgrounds. In addition, there are few language tests that have been adapted to the bilingual population. Most tests are developed using speakers of Standard English. So, in addition to the mismatch between the SLP and the child in regard to cultural and linguistic differences, there is also a mismatch in the tools available to evaluate the child's language abilities. If the SLP is monolingual and is not fully aware of the possible factors influencing a child's L1 on the L2, the therapist should recruit the services of an interpreter or family member as part of the assessment protocols. It is crucial that SLPs exercise diligence in distinguishing between a language difference and a language disorder.

Intervention

The traditional role of the SLP has been to provide therapy services to individuals with diagnosed communication disorders. It is also within the scope of practice for SLPs to provide what is termed, **elective therapy**. Given that a standard form of English is often required to be successful in business, economic, and educational sectors, speakers of nonstandard English may be at a disadvantage. In these cases, the role of the SLP is to help the client acquire the desired competency in speaking a standard form of English and reducing the affects of the accent resulting from the individual's L1 or primary dialect. Normally, the services of the SLP would not be required because the language demonstrated by the client technically is not disordered. In these cases, the client chooses to receive therapy on an elective basis.

CURRENT RESEARCH IN CHILD LANGUAGE DISORDERS

The Genetics of Child Language Disorders

Children with unexplained difficulties with learning and using language have puzzled researchers for many decades. The term SLI is used as the umbrella term for language disorders that cannot be attributed to retardation, autism, deafness, or other general causes. Today, research is actively taking place to identify a genetic cause for SLI. Evidence is available to show that language impairment can run in families, transferring down from one generation to the next. The gene, called *FOXP2*, was identified in a detailed study of a severe speech and language disorder that affected almost half the members of a large family, identified only as "KE" (Lai et al., 2000). Based on examination of the genetic makeup of each member of the KE family, researchers narrowed the location of the *FOXP2* gene to a region of chromosome 7 that contained about 70 genes. The discovery of this gene was the first to be linked to the normal development of speech and language. At present, it seems that disruption in this gene accounts for severe language disorders but it is unlikely to account for less severe language disorders such as SLI (see also Chapter 11).

Social Communication

Successful communication involves social interaction. A person needs to have the necessary language abilities and social skills to engage in day-to-day communication. This interaction occurs most often among one's peers. Challenges in social communication are a defining characteristic among children with SLI or ASD. The requirements for successful social communication are complex. Children must be aware of their own intentions and perspectives, as well as those of their peers. Ultimately, social communication is successful when children have both the motivation and desire to interact with others, as well as an understanding of the explicit and subtle social rules for communicating in a particular environment. Increasing emphasis is now being placed on identifying the skills necessary for children to be successful in social communication, and

how these skills can be addressed in treatment of children with language disorders (Timler, 2008).

CHILD LANGUAGE DISORDERS ON THE WORLD WIDE WEB

Listed below are Web sites that provide further information on the topic of child language disorders. At the time of publication, each Web site was freely accessible.

Autism Speaks Video Series
http://www.autismspeaks.org/video/index.php

Language Development Video
http://www.learner.org/discovering psychology/06/e06expand.html

Specific Language Impairment
http://www.ldonline.org/spears werling/Specific_Language_ Impairment

Speech and Language Delay Video
http://www.webmd.com/video/conquering-speech-struggles

Speech and Language Disorders Resources
http://www.angelfire.com/nj/speechlanguage/index.html

REFERENCES

Bates, E., & Carnevale, G. F. (1993). New directions in research on language development. *Developmental Review, 13,* 436–470.

Brown, R. (1973). *A first language.* Cambridge, MA: Harvard University Press.

Butler, K. (1986). *Language disorders in children.* Austin, TX: Pro-Ed.

Dunn, L. M., Dunn, L. L., & Dunn, D. M. (2006). *Peabody Picture Vocabulary Test* (4th ed.). Upper Saddle River, NJ: Pearson Education.

Kent, R. D. (1984). Psychobiology of speech development: Coemergence of language and a movement system. *American Journal of Regulatory Integrative and Comparative Physiology, 246,* R888–R894.

Lai, C., Fisher, S., Hurst, J., Levy, E., Hodgson, S., Fox, M., & Monaco, A. (2000). The SPCH1 region on human 7q31: Genomic characterization of the critical interval and localization of translocations associated with speech and language disorder. *American Journal of Human Genetics, 67,* 357–368.

MacDonald, S. (1997). *The portfolio and its use: A road map for assessment.* Little Rock, AR: Southern Early Childhood Association.

Saffran, J., Aslin, R., & Newport, E. (1996). Statistical learning by 8-month-old infants. *Science 274,* 1926–1928.

Semel, E., Wiig, E., & Secord, W. (2003). *Clinical Evaluation of Language Fundamentals* (4th ed.). Upper Saddle River, NJ: Pearson Education.

Stoel-Gammon, C., & Cooper, J. (1984). Patterns of early lexical and phonological development. *Journal Child Language, 11,* 247–272.

Timler, G. (2008). Social communication: A framework for assessment and intervention. *The Asha Leader, 13*(15), 10–13.

CHILD PHONOLOGICAL DISORDERS

OBJECTIVES

After reading this chapter, the student should be able to:

- Describe consonants and vowels according to categories of articulation.
- Describe theories regarding phonological development and disorders.
- Identify individuals who have made historic contributions to the area of phonological disorders.
- Compare, contrast, and discuss typical and atypical phonological development
- Compare, contrast, and discuss articulation versus phonological assessment.
- Compare, contrast, and discuss articulation versus phonological treatment.
- Describe phonological awareness.
- Describe cultural considerations in phonological disorders.

INTRODUCTION

As children learn to speak, they begin producing single words. The words typically are only one or two syllables in length and are created using a small number of consonants and vowels. Advances in a child's age are accompanied by advances in the length of spoken utterances, as well as increases in the number and variety of consonants and vowels. Children progress through phases of speech sound acquisition so that, by no later than 6 to 7 years of age, they should be overheard producing the entire repertoire of speech sounds. For a variety of reasons, children may be unable to accurately produce certain consonants and vowels by the age at which they are expected. Such children are described as having a **phonological disorder**. The severity of a phonological disorder can range from speech that is completely incomprehensible, even to a child's immediate family members, to speech that can be understood by everyone but with a few slightly mispronounced sounds. A phonological disorder has long been recognized as the most common type of communication disorder. In the following chapter, the nature of phonological disorders is described.

TERMINOLOGY AND DEFINITIONS

The consonant and vowel sounds comprising a language are known as **phonemes**. The term **phonology** refers to the study of how sounds are organized and used in a language. Diagonal marks (/) known as **virgules** are used to signify the individual phonemes of a language (e.g., /m/, /b/, /z/, etc.). The symbols of the English alphabetic system serve as a poor example of depicting the **sound-symbol relationship** of the English language. The English alphabet consists of 26 letters (5 vowels and 21 consonants), yet these individual letters or combinations of these letters can represent the same or different sounds. For example, the /s/ sound is depicted differently in the words _bass_, _base_, and _face_. In the word _scissors_, the /s/ sound is written as "sc," while the remaining /s/ symbols are produced more like a /z/ sound. This rather fuzzy sound-symbol relationship is not unique to English—this situation prompted a group of French and English linguists to gather in 1886 and develop a symbol system called the **International Phonetic Alphabet** (IPA), which has become the standard notation system used worldwide to describe the sound patterns of various languages. The basic idea behind developing the IPA was to create an alphabet in which each symbol would have a distinctive sound. According to the IPA system, the English language consists of 42 symbols (18 vowels and 24 consonants). A portion of the IPA symbol system is shown in Figures 5.1 and 5.2. The figures depict the various ways in which consonant and vowels sounds can be classified. This classification relates to the pattern of articulation within the vocal tract.

Consonant Classification

When a consonant is articulated there is almost always some form of obstruction or at least a narrowing of the vocal tract

Place of Articulation

Manner of Articulation		Bilabial	Labiodental	Lingua-Dental	Lingua-Alveolar	Lingua-Palatal	Lingua-Velar	Glottal	Examples
Stops	Voiceless	/p/			/t/		/k/		pin tin kin
	Voiced	/b/			/d/		/g/		bust dust gust
Fricatives	Voiceless		/f/	/θ/	/s/	/ʃ/		/h/	fin thin sin shin hit
	Voiced		/v/	/ð/	/z/	/ʒ/			van the zoo treasure
Affricates	Voiceless					/tʃ/			cheap
	Voiced					/dʒ/			jeep
Nasals	Voiced	/m/			/n/		/ŋ/		seem scene sing
Liquids	Voiced				/l/	/r/			late rate
Glides	Voiced	/w/				/y/			well yell

FIGURE 5.1. Categorization of consonants according to place, manner, and voicing features of articulation. Where there are voiced and voiceless consonants within the same manner of articulation, the voiceless consonant is listed in the top of the box.

FIGURE 5.2. Categorization of vowels according to tongue elevation and tongue advancement categories.

that causes a disruption in the air flowing upward from the lungs. The three major ways of classifying the pattern of consonant articulation are according to: (1) place of articulation, (2) manner of articulation, and (3) consonant voicing.

Place of Articulation

Place of articulation refers to the location where the constriction or obstruction of the vocal tract occurs. An illustration of the various places of consonant articulation is shown in Figure 5.3. Beginning at the front of the mouth and working toward the back of the throat, the places of consonant articulation include:

Bilabial. As the name implies, a bilabial articulation is carried out by using both lips for consonant articulation. The bilabial consonants are /p/, /b/, and /m/.

Labiodental. In labiodental articulation, the lower lip and the upper teeth act together to produce the consonant sound. The labiodental consonants are /f/ and /v/.

Linguadental. Articulation of these consonants involves placement of the tongue between (or just behind) the teeth. The sounds /θ/ and /ð/ are included in this category.

Lingua-Alveolar. The alveolar ridge, situated just behind the upper teeth, is a common place of articulation for English consonants. No less than six sounds are produced there, including /t/, /d/, /n/, /s/, /z/, and /l/.

Linguapalatal. In linguapalatal sounds, the tongue makes direct (or close) contact to the region of the hard plate. Similar to lingua-alveolar consonants, this is a popular place of articulation for English consonants, and includes /ʃ/, /ʒ/, /tʃ/, /dʒ/, /j/, and /r/.

FIGURE 5.3. Cross-sectional view of the vocal tract depicting consonant places of articulation. 1 = bilabial, 2 = labiodental, 3 = linguadental, 4 = lingua-alveolar, 5 = lingua-palatal, 6 = linguavelar, and 7 = glottal.

Linguavelar. The linguavelar place of articulation is limited to the /k/, /g/, and /ŋ/ sounds.

Glottal. The glottal place of articulation is located at the back of the throat at the lower end of the pharynx (i.e., near the glottis). The primary glottal consonant is /h/, although there is another, less frequently produced consonant known as a glottal stop /ʔ/.

Manner of Articulation

The term **manner of articulation** refers to the way in which the obstruction inside the oral cavity is made. There are six distinct manners of articulation including:

Stops. For the production of stops a solid obstruction is built up somewhere within the oral cavity, initially completely blocking the airstream coming up from the lungs. This blockage is then abruptly released so the air that was compressed behind the obstruction can escape with a kind of explosive movement. The stop consonants are /p/, /b/, /t/, /d/, /k/, and /g/.

Nasals. For the production of nasal consonants, the velum is lowered, allowing air to escape through the nasal cavity rather than the oral cavity. Nasal consonants in English are fairly limited in number. There are only three: /m/, /n/, and /ŋ/.

Fricatives. Where stops are produced with complete obstruction in the oral cavity, fricatives are produced by creating a partial obstruction of the airstream. This makes turbulence arise at or near the point of obstruction, where the airstream is forced through a greatly narrowed channel. Fricatives comprise the largest class of English consonants according to manner of articulation, including /f/, /v/, /θ/, /ð/, /s/, /z/, /ʃ/, /ʒ/, and /h/.

Affricates. Affricates are a combination of a stop and a following fricative, where the quality of the stop remains largely the same, but the fricative part tends to be shorter than a "pure" fricative. The affricates are /tʃ/ and /dʒ/.

Liquids and Glides. These consonants differ from the other consonants by the fact they are produced with far less obstruction in the vocal tract. Instead, there is a subtle narrowing of the vocal tract. These consonants are sometimes referred to as **approximates** because their manner of articulation seem to lie between true consonants and pure vowels. The liquid consonants are /l/ and /r/. The glide consonants are /w/ and /j/.

Consonant Voicing

The **voiced consonants** are those that require vocal fold vibration to be produced correctly. These include /b/, /d/, /g/, /v/, /ð/, /z/, /ʒ/, /dʒ/, /w/, /j/,

/l/, /r/, /m/, /n/, and /ŋ/. Not all consonants involve vocal fold vibration. These are referred to as **voiceless consonants** and include /p/, /t/, /k/, /f/, /θ/, /s/, /ʃ/, /tʃ/, and /h/. Collectively, all consonants can be described using the categories of voicing, place, and manner of articulation. The phoneme /b/ is an example of a voiced bilabial stop. The phoneme /ʃ/ is an example of a voiceless palatal fricative (see Figure 5.1).

Vowel Classification

As noted above, consonants are characterized by an obstruction of the vocal tract, which causes a disruption in airflow. The opposite is true of vowels. Here, the characteristic feature is the absence of closure of the vocal tract, so that air can flow in a relatively unimpeded fashion. There are two major ways of classifying vowels according to the positioning of the tongue body within the oral cavity: tongue elevation and tongue advancement (Figure 5.4).

Tongue Elevation

As implied, **tongue elevation** (or tongue height) refers to the distance that the tongue is moved from the base of the mouth toward the roof of the mouth for the production of vowels (see Figure 5.4).

FYI

The ability to articulate an innumerable number of speech sounds in an oral cavity that is less than 3 inches in length is considered the most sophisticated and coordinated activity performed by the human body.

FYI

American English uses a vowel that is found in less than 1% of the world's languages. The vowel is found in words such as *fur*, *stir*, and *her*.

A

B

C

FIGURE 5.4. The articulation of vowels according to tongue elevation. The three panels depict tongue articulation (**A** to **C**) ranging from high, mid, and low, respectively.

There are three general locations of vowels according to tongue elevation: high /i, ɪ, u, ʊ/, mid /ɛ, ɛ, ə, ʌ, o/, and low /æ, ɔ, ɑ/.

Tongue Advancement

The classification of vowels according to **tongue advancement** (or tongue carriage) refers to the movement of the tongue body from the back of the oral cavity towards the front (Figure 5.5). There are three locations of vowels according to tongue advancement: front /i, ɪ, ɛ, e, æ/, central /ə, ʌ/, and back /u, ʊ, o, ɔ, ɑ/. Collectively, all vowels can be described using the categories of tongue elevation and advancement. The phoneme /u/ is an example of a high-back vowel. The phoneme /æ/ is an example of a low-front (see Figure 5.1).

Children do not acquire all the sounds of their language at once; the process is gradual and covers the approximate age range of 1 year to around 6 years of age. Although some variability

A

B

C

FIGURE 5.5. The articulation of vowels according to tongue advancement. The panels depict tongue articulation (**A** to **C**) according to front, central, and back, respectively.

is naturally expected between children, most tend to acquire the sounds of speech in an orderly fashion. As a general rule, vowels of the English language are acquired by children slightly earlier than consonants. The 24 consonants of English can be loosely organized into three phases of development (Table 5.1). The first phase contains the **early eight** consonant sounds such as "m," "b," and "w." The next phase involves acquisition of the **middle eight** consonants such as "t," "k," and "f." The last phase includes the **late eight** consonants such

as "sh," "th," and "z." The latter sounds generally involve more precise articulatory movements compared to early developing sounds, so it is not unusual for children to require more time to master these articulations. Some children may not acquire the late eight until they reach 6 years of age. So it is important to emphasize that these phases are not set in stone. Children are known to show variability in the order and pace at which they acquire speech sounds, especially the middle eight consonants. If a child's speech does not consistently contain

Table 5.1. Acquisition of 24 English Consonants Organized According to the Early, Middle, and Late periods of Acquisition. The phonetic symbol is listed on the left and a word example in standard orthography is provided on the right.

Early Eight (1;5 to 2 years of age)	Word Examples
Nasals m n	movie, north
Stops b p d	boy, pea, do
Fricatives h	hat
Glides w j	wind, yell
Middle Eight (3 to 4 years of age)	
Nasals ŋ	wing
Stops t k g	toy, cat, go
Fricatives f v	food, vine
Affricates tʃ dʒ	church, jump
Late Eight (5 to 6 years of age)	
Fricatives θ ð s z ʃ ʒ	thick, these, sew, zoo, ship, beige
Liquids l r	lamp, ramp

these various consonants by a particular age range, suspicion is raised about the possibility of a phonological disorder.

Any deviation, great or small, in the articulation of phonemes can lead to **misarticulations**, or what is simply referred to as a **speech sound disorder** (or **phonological disorder**). Phonological disorders affect 15% of preschool children. In a majority of cases, the type of phonological disorder demonstrated by children results from inaccurate production of consonants. This is not always the case, especially among children with severe phonological disorders who demonstrate impaired consonant and vowel production. By the time children enter school, approximately 6% continue to exhibit a phonological disorder ranging from mild to severe. For 80% of children with a phonological disorder, the condition is sufficiently severe that they will require the services of an SLP to help them improve the quality of their speech. As noted in other chapters, many medical conditions found to occur during the childhood period seem to affect boys more often than girls. Phonological disorders are no exception. Estimates suggest that two to four times as many boys as girls exhibit the disorder. As of 2006, approximately 90% of SLPs working in the United States reported that their caseloads included individuals with a phonological disorder. Children who have a phonological disorder are more likely to have additional difficulties with their communication such as language problems and academic difficulties. A relationship can be observed between early phonological disorders and subsequent reading, writing, spelling, and mathematical abilities.

HISTORIC ASPECTS OF CHILD PHONOLOGICAL DISORDERS

A great deal of research has occurred over the past 100 years examining phonological disorders, and a large body of this historical research has centered on approaches to correcting the disorder. In the early 20th century, **E. W. Scripture** (1864–1945), who was a professor of psychology at Yale University (Figure 5.6), recommended specific treatment approaches for a speech condition he called "negligent lisping." In current times, we would refer to this phonological disorder

FIGURE 5.6. E. W. Scripture. Early 20th century psychologist who recommended specific treatment approaches for speech sound disorders.

as *stopping of fricatives*, where "s" might be produced with a "t" ("soup" is produced as "toup"). Scripture attributed the condition to mental carelessness and his cure for the condition consisted of teaching the individual to carefully correct his faults. To elicit correct articulation for /s/, for example, Scripture wrote:

> One cure consists [of] inserting a probe, an applicator, a toothpick, or a pencil just over the middle of the tongue and pressing it down as the person begins to speak a word beginning with "s" . . . He cannot close the passage completely and instead of saying "t" he is forced to say "s." This catches his ear, and he notices the difference in sound. Constant repetition enables him to train his tongue in the new way. (Scripture, 1912, pp. 132–133)

Lee Edward Travis (1896–1987) made contributions to a number of areas in communication disorders; including phonological disorders (see also Chapter 2). He developed treatment programs that differed depending on whether the disorder was organic (anatomical) or functional (nonanatomic) in nature. Travis wrote:

> The articulatory case frequently shows inferior ability in controlling the lips, tongue, jaw and diaphragm in voluntary rhythmical movements not involved in speech. This would imply, as does the speech defect itself, that he possesses poor control of these structures in speech. (Travis, 1931, p. 223)

Grant Fairbanks (1910–1964) was a well-respected speech scientist at the University of Illinois who wrote a therapy manual known as the *Voice and Articulation Drillbook*, published in 1940 (Figure 5.7). The book was filled with a number of word- and sentence-naming

FIGURE 5.7. Grant Fairbanks. American speech scientist who wrote a manual for treating voice and speech sound disorders.

FIGURE 5.8. Charles Van Riper. Established what is now known as the **traditional approach** to treating speech sound disorders. (Reprinted with permission from Van Riper, C. [1981]. An early history of ASHA. *ASHA Magazine, 23*[11], 855–858.)

activities for correcting the speech misarticulations of children and adults. Fairbanks firmly believed that good listening skills, in addition to repeated practice in producing specific misarticulated speech sounds, were essential for the correction of any phonological disorder. He wrote:

> When articulating a sound in isolation it is valuable to start with prolonged examples, since you can listen carefully, make the necessary adjustments and perceive the position of your articulators. (Fairbanks, 1940, p. xxi)

Charles Van Riper (1905–1994), a contemporary of Fairbanks, was undoubtedly one of the leading researchers in child phonological disorders and stuttering during the mid-20th century (Figure 5.8). Van Riper was a skilled SLP who also happened to stutter. He devoted his career to developing effective treatment approaches. In his seminal publication, *Speech Correction* (Van Riper, 1947), he recommended a series of procedural steps for the treatment of phonological disorders. The steps begin with helping to establish a new sound (that is misarticulated) in a person's speech and working through increasingly complicated speaking situations, with the end goal of producing the new sound in natural conversational speech. This management program has since been referred to as the **traditional approach** and is still used today. Additional details regarding the traditional approach are provided later in this chapter.

There was a short period during the 1950s where a group of researchers attempted to link phonological disorders to a larger emotionally based disorder

(Rousey, 1957). With the exception of obvious physical impairments of the speech anatomy, the assumption was that a functional phonological disorder was indicative of a **psychological disturbance**. The treatment for phonological disorders was thus focused on psychotherapy. This view was prompted by existing research at the time which indicated that children showed considerable variability in acquiring speech sounds. This variability was attributed to developmental differences between children in their social and emotional development. A number of theories were proposed concerning the psychological underpinnings of specific consonant and vowel misarticulations. For example, substitution of the /d/ for the /th/ sound ("the" is produced as "duh") was assumed to be related to an oral expression of aggression. That is, a pattern of speech utilized by "tough guys." The resultant therapy focused on reducing aggression as a means of improving speech clarity. This perspective on phonological disorders was short lived. Large scale studies examining the acquisition of speech have since confirmed there is considerable similarity across children in achieving normal milestones. Furthermore, we now have a much clearer understanding of the patterns of speech sound misarticulations that are produced by children, which attribute the problem to either motor or language-based difficulties, as opposed to psychological difficulties.

Finally, no history of phonological disorders would be complete without mentioning the contributions of **Mildred Templin** (1913–2008) (Figure 5.9). Templin earned her PhD in child development from the University of Minnesota in 1947. She conducted a series of longitudinal and cross-sectional studies of spelling, vocabulary, and cognitive be-

FIGURE 5.9. Mildred Templin. Expert in the communication disorders of children. (Printed with permission of the Trustees for the Estate of Mildred Templin.)

havior of children with hearing disabilities and normally developing children. Her work led to the publication of *Certain Language Skills in Children* (1957). At the time, this was a definitive work in the field. Together with her colleague Dr. Frederick Darley in 1969, she created the Templin-Darley Tests of Articulation, which are still used today to evaluate speech sound production skills in children.

TYPES OF PHONOLOGICAL DISORDERS

The types of phonological disorders can be organized into three categories based on the presumed cause of the disorder: (1) **structural**, (2) **neurological**, and (3) **functional**. Structural and neurological disorders are sometimes referred to as **articulation disorders** rather than phonological disorders, the reason being that the cause of the disorder is related to problems in the motor movements required to produce clear speech. Functional disorders are simply referred to as phonological disorders because there are no clearly identifiable motor problems. Instead, the difficulty observed in producing speech sounds appears to be related to a problem in learning to organize the sounds of the language.

Structural Cause

Structural problems involve abnormalities of the mouth that are necessary for speech sound production, such as the teeth, tongue, or palate. These abnormalities make it difficult for children or adults to produce certain sounds, and in some cases make it impossible to produce the sounds at all. The structural problem causing the phonological disorder generally needs to be surgically or medically treated before the child receives any sort of speech therapy. Correction of the structural problem is likely to greatly assist in correction of the speech sound difficulties. One such example is a **cleft lip and palate**. Chapter 8 is specifically dedicated to this condition. A cleft lip and palate is one of the most common and obvious phonological disorders that has a structural cause. Another structural problem contributing to a phonological disorder is **dentition**. It is not unusual for children to develop temporary speech articulation difficulties during the time when primary teeth are being replaced by permanent teeth. This condition is found in nearly all first graders (see Chapter 2, Figure 2.3). Indeed, the child who loses her front two teeth experiences considerable difficulty pro-

ducing consonants that require articulation between the tongue tip and central incisors (e.g., "s" and "t').

More permanent forms of dental-related articulation problems concern the alignment of the upper and lower teeth, which is referred to as **occlusion**. An uneven alignment between the upper and lower teeth is called a **malocclusion**. This situation occurs in approximately 90% of the population. There are three types of malocclusion patterns that help to create the overall appearance of our faces (Figure 5.10). A **Class I** malocclusion involves normal alignment of the upper and lower teeth with only one or two teeth slightly misaligned. A **Class II** malocclusion (or distocclusion) is an overbite. This pattern can result from one of two conditions, the first being a small **maxilla** (upper jaw) with a normal sized **mandible** (lower jaw). The second condition is a result of a normal sized maxilla but a large mandible. The third type of malocclusion is referred to as a **Class III** condition resulting in an underbite (or mesiocclusion). In this condition, the maxilla may be unusually small with a normal-sized mandible or the mandible may be unusually large with a normal-sized maxilla. In extreme instances of either a Class II or Class III malocclusion, oral surgery may be required to correct the alignment pattern. However this situation usually is prompted by other medical conditions, aside from speech problems. Most notable is a condition in which the **temporomandibular joint** (TMJ) works abnormally. This joint serves as the socket location where the mandible fits into the side of the skull (temporal bone). When the TMJ fails to function normally, an individual may experience severe headaches. There also are extreme instances of TMJ dysfunction when the jaw may open and stay locked (i.e., lockjaw).

A   **B**   **C**

FIGURE 5.10. Dental and jaw alignment (occlusion) patterns. The patterns represent Class I, Class II, and Class III occlusions (from **A** to **C**).

FYI

Some famous people who have a Class III malocclusion (underbite) include the U.S. First Lady Michelle Obama; TV personality Jay Leno; former Prime Minister of Canada, Brian Mulroney; and film actors Casey Affleck, Keira Knightley, and Quentin Tarantino.

Two conditions concerning *tongue mobility* contribute to a structurally based phonological disorder: **ankyloglossia** and **reverse swallow**. The first condition involves the **lingual frenulum**, which is the tendon that extends from the floor of the mouth to the underside of the tongue. A child may be born with a condition where the length of the tendon is abnormally short. The short length of the tendon restricts tongue mobility and possibly, tongue-related speech sounds. In the past, there were suggestions that clipping the tendon would help to improve speech clarity. There is little evidence to indicate that undergoing this rather drastic surgical procedure serves to correct a phonological disorder, and it should only be considered when the tendon is so short that it impairs more basic biological functions such as swallowing. Another term for ankyloglossia is "tongue tie." An illustration of a lingual frenulum is provided in Figure 5.11.

The condition of reverse swallow also is called **tongue thrust**. The condition is reflective of an orofacial muscular imbalance. A reverse swallow normally is seen during the early infancy and tod-

A   **B**

FIGURE 5.11. Illustration of a normal lingual frenulum (**A**), and an abnormally short frenulum (ankyloglossia) (**B**).

dler periods of normal development. During this time period, swallowing is achieved by pushing the tongue forward, rather than backward, to assist with the digestion of food and liquid (Figure 5.12). By the time children reach the age of 6 years, most have automatically changed to a normal swallowing pattern, which involves squeezing the tongue against the roof of the mouth instead of pushing it forward against the teeth. Research suggests that hereditary factors, learned behavior such as thumb sucking, and/ or medical conditions may be responsible for tongue thrust. For whatever reason, a child may experience a delay or interruption in the oral maturational process and fail to progress to an adult swallowing pattern. This delay may also affect motor skills required for speech sound production.

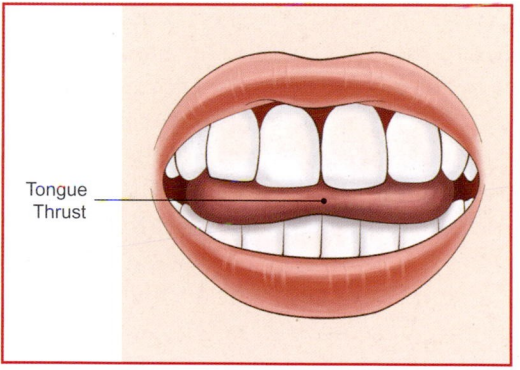

FIGURE 5.12. Illustration of tongue thrust during moments of swallowing.

Neurologic Cause

The second category of phonological disorders reflects problems attributed to

the nervous system. The nervous system is responsible for activating and controlling the various structures and muscles needed for producing speech sounds. Depending on the location of the nervous system impairment, an individual could show excessive speed or stiffness in the execution of speech. It is equally possible for the nervous system impairment to result in slow or labored speech production. Some neurologic conditions that are known to cause a phonological disorder are **Parkinson disease** and **amyotrophic lateral sclerosis**. A portion of Chapter 9 is dedicated to phonological disorders of this particular neurologic origin. One type of neurologically based phonological disorder that has been discussed for over 25 years is **childhood apraxia of speech** (CAS). CAS is thought to be a disorder of the nervous system that affects a child's ability to organize and sequence the sounds of speech when producing words. This difficulty occurs in the absence of any muscle weakness or paralysis. The problem lies with the inability to plan movements of the speech articulators for the purpose of volitional (i.e., on command) speech. The child has difficulty making speech movements when he is consciously aware of trying to do so or in instances when he is requested to do so by others. The same speech movements are produced correctly when the child is producing natural, conversational speech. A key feature of CAS is that the child's misarticulations are inconsistent. CAS is a relatively rare, poorly understood phonological disorder that continues to be a topic of debate among researchers. There are varying opinions regarding the existence, cause, symptoms, and treatment of CAS. There is no clearly defined set of speaking behaviors that identify the presence of CAS, rather it is a spectrum of characteristics and consequently no two children with CAS are alike.

Functional Cause

The third category of phonological disorder is considered functional because the precise cause of the disorder is unknown. In this condition, the phonological disorder results from impairments in the organization of phonemes and/or their application in speech. A child may be able to say a sound correctly but not use it appropriately in all words containing the sound. The child may also display a reduction in the total number of consonant and vowels sounds in his or her speech repertoire. In either case, the speech patterns displayed by the child are different from those of same-age peers. Phonological disorders of a functional nature make up the largest percentage of child-based phonological disorders. A functional phonological disorder can be further divided into disorders that reflect a **speech delay** or those that reflect **residual errors**. A delay is characterized by speech that is unclear (or unintelligible) and contains many consonant misarticulations. Children with a speech delay also are found to be at an increased risk for broader communication and academic difficulties. Children with a speech delay represent the most severe form of functional phonological disorder. Children with a phonological disorder who show residual errors are those who may only have one or two speech sounds that are misarticulated. The speech sound in error is usually a fricative (e.g., thumb is produced as *fumb*) or liquid consonant (e.g., radio is produced as *wadio*). This category represents a less severe form of functional phonological disorder.

CURRENT THEORIES REGARDING CHILD PHONOLOGICAL DISORDERS

A number of theories have attempted to explain the fashion in which children normally learn the sounds of their language. The same theories have been used as a backdrop for the assessment and treatment of phonological disorders.

Three of these theories are the: (1) behaviorist theory, (2) natural phonology theory, and (3) optimality theory.

Behaviorist Theory

The **behaviorist theory**, developed by Mower (1960), suggests that a child's acquisition of consonants and vowels has its roots in early babbling behavior. The child's babbling is shaped and directed toward the adult pronunciation of words through selective reinforcement of sounds that approximate the target language. The child is a passive learner in acquiring the sounds of the language. According to this theory, children may not acquire speech sounds in an identical fashion. Instead, their speech development is based on the environment in which they are reared. In the case of a phonologically disordered child, a faulty environment would be viewed as contributing to the child's speech difficulties.

Distinctive Features and Natural Phonology Theory

Chomsky and Halle (1968) proposed that the unique sound systems of all the world's languages could be described according to a specific number of phonological patterns, which they termed **distinctive features**. By simply noting the presence or absence of these features, the phonology of a particular language could be captured. Examples of distinctive features include nasality, consonantal, vocalic, and lip rounding. This approach to describing phonology according to patterns represented a dramatic shift in the way theorists viewed a child's acquisition of speech sounds.

The early work of Chomsky and Halle was a turning point in phonological theory and led to the development of other theories examining patterns of speech sound development. Notable among these theories was the **natural theory** proposed by David Stampe (Donegan & Stampe, 1979). In this theory, a child's speech development is thought to be affected by naturally occurring phonological patterns (or "processes"), some of which remain active and others that are suppressed (or disappear) as the child learns his or her language. The child's task is to either "allow" or deliberately "suppress" various sound patterns that match those of the native language. The phonological system of a particular language is based on retaining some of these patterns while suppressing others. An example of a phonological pattern would be *final consonant deletion* (i.e., producing words that do not end with a final consonant—only vowels). A child acquiring English would learn to deliberately suppress this pattern because many of the words of English contain final consonants. On the other hand, a young child learning Mandarin would naturally accept this phonological pattern as part of the language because the words of Mandarin do not contain final consonants. The notion of phonological patterns has received widespread attention over the past 20 years as a framework to evaluate and treat the speech of children with severe phonological disorders. The theory provides an approach to treating entire classes of misarticulated speech sounds rather than individual phonemes.

Optimality Theory

Optimality theory is a general model of how grammars are structured. The theory was originally developed in the field of linguistics but has since been applied to phonological disorders. In its approach to the acquisition of phonology, optimality theory focuses on two important aspects of any phonological system: (1) the patterns that are impossible for a language and (2) the patterns that are possible. It is distinguished from other theories of phonological development in the role that is assigned to **constraints** (Geruit & Morrisette, 2005). A constraint is a limit on what constitutes a possible pronunciation of a word. The child's role in learning the sounds of the language is to learn these constraints. For example, in English some of the various phonological constraints are:

- No word may end in /tp/, although /pt/ is possible.
- No word may start with /tl/ or /dl/, but /pl/, /bl/, /tr/, and /dr/ are possible.
- No word may start with /mr/ or /nr/, though /br/ and /fr/ are possible.

ASSESSMENT OF CHILD PHONOLOGICAL DISORDERS

The goal of assessment is to obtain and establish an accurate profile of the child's articulation of vowels and consonants. The diagnosis of a phonological disorder depends greatly on the age of the child in question. Children who are 3 years old may show mispronunciation of words but these mispronunciations are expected (normal) for their age. On the other hand, an 8-year-old child who makes the same mispronunciations may have a phonological disorder. Listed below are some of the fundamental steps in performing a phonological assessment. These steps include: (1) speech sampling, (2) collection of a phonetic inventory, (3) describing speech patterns, (4) estimation of age expectancy, (5) severity estimation, and (6) performing an oral-facial examination.

Speech Sampling

The first step in determining whether a phonological disorder exists is to collect a sample of the child's speaking behavior. There are numerous ways of collecting the sample that vary according to **speech spontaneity** and **structure**. Spontaneity refers to whether the child is asked to speak freely or whether he is required to name specific words or sounds. Structure refers to the particular environment in which the speech sample is being collected. At one end of the continuum, the sample could involve collection of spontaneous speech in a typical environment such as the child's home. The advantage of this approach is that the sample is natural and reflects normal speaking behavior. A particular disadvantage to this approach is that it is time-consuming and may not elicit a broad sample of speech from the child containing all possible consonants and vowels. On the other end of the continuum, the speech sample may be based on having the child name specific pictures that result in a one-word response. This type of activity usually occurs in a clinic setting. The advantage of this approach is that the child is required to deliberately produce specific consonants and vowels, although a disadvantage is that this is not a typical, natural setting of free speaking. In spite of this unnaturalness, picture-naming is the preferred approach to speech sampling. A number of commercially available tests exist that are designed to sample a child's phonology using a **picture-naming** task. The pictures comprising the test have been chosen because they contain consonants and vowels in various locations within a word (initial, medial, and final). There is no universally accepted picture- naming test used across English-speaking countries. A depiction of a picture-naming task and the associated scoring sheet is shown in Figure 5.13.

A

FIGURE 5.13. (**A**) Example of a picture inventory test *continues*

Picture-Naming Test

Word	Phoneme	Initial	Medial	Final
Mouse	/m/	x		
Hammer	/m/		x	
Lamb	/m/			x
Goat	/g/	x		
Dragon	/g/		x	
Frog	/g/			x
Fence	/f/	x		
Elephant	/f/		x	
Leaf	/f/			x

B

FIGURE 5.13. *continued* **(B)** Corresponding test form

Phonetic Inventory

Once the speech sample is collected, the SLP next transcribes the sample using symbols of the IPA. Based on the transcribed sample, a **phonetic inventory** is created. A phonetic inventory is a list of the consonants and vowels noted in the speech sample. The list can be organized in a number of ways, such as noting those sounds that occurred at the initial, medial, or final position of a word. The inventory provides useful information regarding a child's ability to produce the consonant and vowel sounds of the language. Sounds absent from the inventory may be indicative of a phonological disorder.

Description of Speech Patterns

On the basis of the phonetic transcription, the SLP then compares the child's pronunciation of each word to the intended pronunciation of the word. Based on this comparative analysis, the SLP is able to describe the pattern of the child's pronunciations. There are two notational systems for the description of disordered speech patterns. The first notational system is the **SODA** system. This system considers four general types of misarticulations: (1) **s**ubstitutions, (2) **o**missions, (3) **d**istortions, and (4) **a**dditions (SODA). Examples of these patterns are provided in Table 5.2. The speech sound misarticulations demonstrated by children with a functional phonological that are of a residual nature are often described using the SODA system. The second notational system is used in instances when a child exhibits a severe functional phonological disorder (i.e., speech delay). The system describes the speech pattern according to large classes of sounds that may be misarticulated; these patterns are referred to as **phonological processes** (or patterns). Examples of common phonological processes are shown in Table 5.2.

Age Expectancy Estimation

Once the speech patterns demonstrated by the child are determined, the SLP must make a determination whether these patterns are acceptable or disordered. The child's age is an important factor when determining whether a phonological disorder exists. Normative data are available to the SLP to guide in the decision. The normative data are presented in two ways: (1) age of mastery and (2) age of suppression. Using **age of mastery** norms involves examining each misarticulated sound produced by the child in regard to the age at which the sound should be acquired.

Table 5.2. The SODA Patterns of Speech Misarticulations and Some of the More Commonly Occurring Phonological Processes

Error Patterns	Example	
SODA Patterns		
Substitution	rabbit → wabbit	cat → tat
Omission	hat → at	blue → bue
Distortion[1]	soup → *oup	ladder → *adder
Additions	green → gareen	swim → sawim
Phonological Process		
Final Consonant Deletion	hat → ha	leaf → lea
Stopping of Fricatives	fish → pish	zoo → doo
Cluster Reduction	spoon → poon	broom → boom
Gliding of Liquids	lazy → wazy	broom → bwoom

[1]Distortions involve the substitution of a phoneme with an undecipherable sound. The * is used to denote an undecipherable sound.

If a child is unable to produce a sound after the age at which it should normally be acquired, the child is assumed to be disordered in regard to the production of the sound. For example, the "g" sound is normally acquired by the age of 4 years (see Table 5.1). If a 6-year-old child was to demonstrate misarticulations of "g" there would be cause for concern. **Age of suppression** norms refer to the age at which specific phonological processes should no longer be apparent in a child's speech. If a child still demonstrates a particular process after the age at which it should have disappeared, the child would be exhibiting a phonological disorder. For example, the phonological pattern of final consonant deletion ("hat" is produced as "ha") should disappear by the age of 3;6 years. If a 4-year-old child is observed deleting final consonants, there would be cause for concern. Some age of disappearance (suppression) norms for phonological processes are listed in Table 5.3.

Severity Estimation

If a child is found to demonstrate a phonological disorder, the SLP must determine the severity of the phonolog-ical disorder. Severity refers to the affect of the phonological disorder on the **intelligibility** of speech. Intelligibility is defined as a listener's ability to understand a speaker's words. This judgment can be based on **qualitative** and **quantitative** criteria. Qualitative criteria involves an impressionistic judgment as to the impact of the disorder on the clarity of the child's communication. This may simply involve a judgment by the SLP using a continuum of good-fair-poor. This estimation is generally influenced by the characteristics of the phonological disorder. For example, a pattern involving a high number of consonant omissions is likely to result in a severity judgment of "poor" compared to a pattern involving a simple substitution of one sound for another such as "f" used in place of "th" (thumb is pronounced as "fumb"). Another qualitative scale of speech severity involves judgments by the child's parents or teachers in regard to how well the child communicates. For example, a teacher might be asked to rate how well they understand the child on a 10-point scale, with 1 meaning *all the time* and 10 meaning *never*.

A quantitative estimate of severity is based on more objective criteria such as: (1) the exact number of misarticulated

Table 5.3. Age of Suppression for Some of the More Commonly Occurring Phonological Processes

Phonological Process	Example	Age of Suppression
Velar fronting	gun → dun	3 years
Final consonant deletion	bat → ba	3;6 years
Unstressed syllable deletion	balloon → loon	4 years
Gliding of liquids	rabbit → wabbit	4 years
Vowelization	flower → flowa	4 years

phonemes, (2) the length of time the disorder has existed, and (3) the age of the child. A popular measure of severity is known as the **percentage of consonants correct** (PCC) (Shriberg, 2003). The PCC is calculated from the phonetic inventory by tabulating the total number of consonants produced in a speech sample and dividing this into the total number of consonants that were produced correctly. The formula is as follows:

$$\frac{\text{Number of correct consonants}}{\text{Total number of consonants}} \times 100 = \text{PCC}$$

On the basis of PCC calculation, the severity of the disorder is categorized as normal to mild (85%–100%), mild to moderate (65%–84%), moderate to severe (50%–64%), or severe (below 50%).

Oral-Facial Examination

The phonological assessment continues with an examination of the child's oral-facial patterns. Assessment of the oral-facial mechanism is divided into two key areas: (1) **structure** and (2) **function**. Some individuals with a phonological disorder may show structural and/or functional peculiarities that affect speech sound production, including dental malocclusion, cleft palate, and tongue abnormalities. Structural assessment includes examination of the lips, teeth, tongue, hard palate, and soft palate. The functional assessment involves examination of the same structures in a variety of speaking and nonspeaking tasks. These tasks are designed to evaluate the **range of motion**, **strength**, and **rate of movement**. The information derived from this examination helps to guide the SLP in determining the nature of the phonological disorder. The information also can shed light on the client's general oral-motor skills, which can be useful when developing a treatment program. A simple checklist of features considered in an oral-facial examination is provided in Table 5.4.

TREATMENT OF CHILD PHONOLOGICAL DISORDERS

Decisions about whether to treat and how often the child should be seen are based primarily on the severity of the disorder. Treatment for a phonological disorder is important not only for the child to be able to form speech sounds, but for other reasons, as well. Children who have problems creating speech sounds may have academic difficulties in subject areas such as spelling or reading. Also, children whose speech sounds different than their peers can find themselves frustrated and ridiculed, and may become less willing to participate in play or classroom activities. The prognosis for children with a phonological disorder generally is good. For many children, the problem resolves spontaneously. It is reported that in 75% of children with mild or moderate forms of the disorder, and whose problems do not stem from a medical condition, the disorder is resolved by the age of 6 years. In many other cases, children who receive treatment eventually develop normal or close to normal speech. In some instances, there may be mild misarticulations that last until adulthood, but speech is completely understandable. For children with a phonological disorder due to a structural or neurologic cause, the outcome generally is dependent on how well the underlying cause of the problem is treated.

Table 5.4. Example of a Typical Oral-Facial Examination

Oral Facial Examination

	Structure	**Function**
Lips	Symmetry: _____	Purse: _____
	Scarring: _____	Retract: _____
		Purse and Retract: _____
Teeth	Alignment: _____	
	Gap or missing teeth: _____	
	Facial pattern: _____	
Tongue	Scarring: _____	Moves side to side: _____
		Moves up and down: _____
		Moves in and out: _____
Hard Palate	Vault height: _____	
	Vault width: _____	
	Scarring: _____	
Soft Palate	Symmetry: _____	Lifts on sustained "ah": _____
	Scarring: _____	Lifts on repeated "ah": _____
		Symmetry of movement: _____

The treatment approaches to resolving a phonological disorder can be categorized into two primary approaches: (1) the **articulation approach** and (2) the **phonological approach**. Within each of these approaches, there are variations in management techniques.

Articulation Approach

The articulation approach focuses on motoric aspects of producing individual consonants and vowels. Techniques include the use of mirrors, tongue depres-sors, oral-motor exercises, and sensory motor training. Repetition of the misarticulated sounds is an integral part of treatment. Two well-known techniques that use a motor-oriented framework of speech treatment are the traditional approach and maximal contrast approach.

Traditional Approach

The **traditional approach** was first developed by Charles Van Riper. This style of treatment emphasizes correct articulation of individual speech sounds. Through a series of graduated steps, the child is

FYI

Children with a phonological disorder typically receive individualized treatment from an SLP on a twice weekly basis. The duration of each therapy session lasts between 30 minutes to 1 hour, depending on the age of the child and the severity of the disorder.

taught to consciously learn to produce the sound. The child has to be successful at each step before proceeding to the next level of speaking complexity. The first step involves sensoriperceptual (ear) training, whereby the child must first be able to correctly perceive the misarticulated speech sound as spoken by others before attempting to produce the sound himself. The ensuing steps entail teaching the child to articulate the sound in short syllables, followed by words, then sentences, and eventually, in a conversational speaking context. The sounds targeted for treatment are those that should have been mastered earliest by the child but, as yet, are not articulated correctly (see Table 5.1).

Maximal Contrast Approach

There is debate over the way children with more severe forms of a phonological disorder should be treated. Some SLPs believe sounds that are learned later in development should be addressed first in therapy, even if the child has not yet learned to produce some of the earlier developing sounds. Research has shown that earlier developing sounds are likely to improve on their own, so it may not be necessary to target them in therapy. The focus of the **maximal contrast** approach is to enact widespread change

in children with a severe phonological disorder. Rather than targeting early developing sounds, later developing sounds are the focus of therapy. Presumably, by targeting these more difficult sounds, they assist in "filling the gap" for less difficult sounds.

Phonological Approach

Whereas traditional and maximal contrast approaches focus on teaching the child to articulate specific sounds correctly, the phonological approach focuses on having the child change his or her phonological system, using cognitive techniques such as semantic images. The phonological approach is used in cases where children have multiple misarticulations (speech delay) and highly unintelligible speech. Using a phonological treatment approach with severely unintelligible children shortens the length of time necessary to improve their sound systems. Two phonological treatment approaches are the cycles approach and minimal pairs approach.

Cycles Approach

This **cycles approach** was developed by Hodson and Paden (1991). The general idea behind the approach is to facilitate the emergence of speech sound patterns rather than attempting to work on mastery of individual speech sounds. For example, if a child is showing the phonological patterns of final consonant deletion (e.g., "hat" is produced as "ha"), cluster reduction (e.g., "blue" is produced as "bue"), and stopping of fricatives (e.g., "see" is produced as "tee"), the treatment program would involve working on each of these patterns in a staggered fashion. A typical treatment cycle might involve working on final

---

FYI

The **electropalatograph** is a recording device that provides a form of biofeedback to a client with speech articulation difficulties. A specifically designed acrylic palate is created that contains touch-sensitive sensors spaced along the surface of the palate. The device is attached to the roof of a person's mouth and is capable of detecting the location and amount of contact between the tongue and palate during the articulation of speech. A visual display of the location of tongue-palate contact is provided on a computer monitor. The device is used primarily for research but is gaining popularity as an alternative approach to the treatment of some speech disorders (McAuliffe et al., 2003).

---

consonant deletion for 2 weeks, and then switching to cluster reduction for 2 weeks, followed by stopping of fricatives for 2 weeks. At the conclusion of this "cycle" the SLP probes to determine whether the child's overall pattern of speech sound production is improving. If not, another cycle of therapy would commence with possible changes to the particular sounds targeted during a treatment session.

Minimal Pairs Approach

A **minimal pair** refers to a situation where two words differ in pronunciation by only one sound, and the change in sound results in a change in word meaning. For instance, the words "sea" and "seat" differ only by the absence or presence of the last consonant [t] and this difference signals a change in meaning. For a phonologically disordered child who deletes final consonants, it is likely the child would produce "seat" as "sea." A minimal pair treatment approach might involve the SLP presenting pictures of "sea" and "seat" simultaneously to the child. In a game format, the child would be instructed to name one of the pictures, with the SLP guessing which picture was named. Because the child is likely to produce

both words as "sea," the SLP would deliberately point to the picture of "sea" even when the child had intended the alternate "seat." Thus, to resolve this confusion the child must learn to revise his productions until his SLP is no longer confused between the two words.

Phonological Awareness

As an adjunct to both articulation and phonological approaches to the management of phonological disorders, it is important to consider the child's understanding of his speech sound system. Treatment programs often rely on the repeated production of speech sounds and may fail to link the child's awareness with production. **Phonological awareness** refers to the ability to think about and manipulate the sound system apart from meaning. Children with impaired phonology may have incomplete (or inaccurate) awareness of their speech sound system. Training in the types of skills that deliberately involve phonological awareness has shown to help children change their disordered phonological system, as well as help children with literacy (reading) problems (Gillon, 2004). A simple phonological awareness task involves the child's recognition of words that rhyme (e.g., asking the child, "Do the words *cat* and *hat* sound alike?"). A more complicated phonological awareness task involves the child's ability to segment sounds and words (e.g., asking the child, "How many words do you hear in the sentence, '*I have a blue pen*'?"). Examples of phonological awareness tasks, ranging in level of complexity are provided in Figure 5.14.

CULTURAL CONSIDERATIONS AND CHILD PHONOLOGICAL DISORDERS

English is spoken throughout the world. While the English of England might be construed as the true mother tongue of the language, there are enormous varieties in spoken English. Each particular variety of English is often described in reference to the geographic region where the language is spoken. English is spoken around the world, resulting in geographically rich varieties of the language. We find English varieties such as British English, Irish English, Australian English, American English, New Zealand English, South African English, Indian English, and Singapore English, to name a few. Each variety is characterized by particular dialectical features, including unique vocabulary and specific phonological patterns. **Dialect** refers to a regional variety of a particular language. Dialects are distinguished by variations in vocabulary (word choice), grammar, and pronunciation. They are based on geography or socioeconomic level. **Geographic dialects** are the most common form of dialect. They are thought to be related to the immigration of certain ethnicities to specific regions of a country. The dialect reflects the vestiges (i.e., roots) of the original language. Examples of geographic dialects found in England and the United States are shown in Figure 5.15.

FIGURE 5.14. Examples of phonological awareness tasks according to increasing levels of complexity.

A

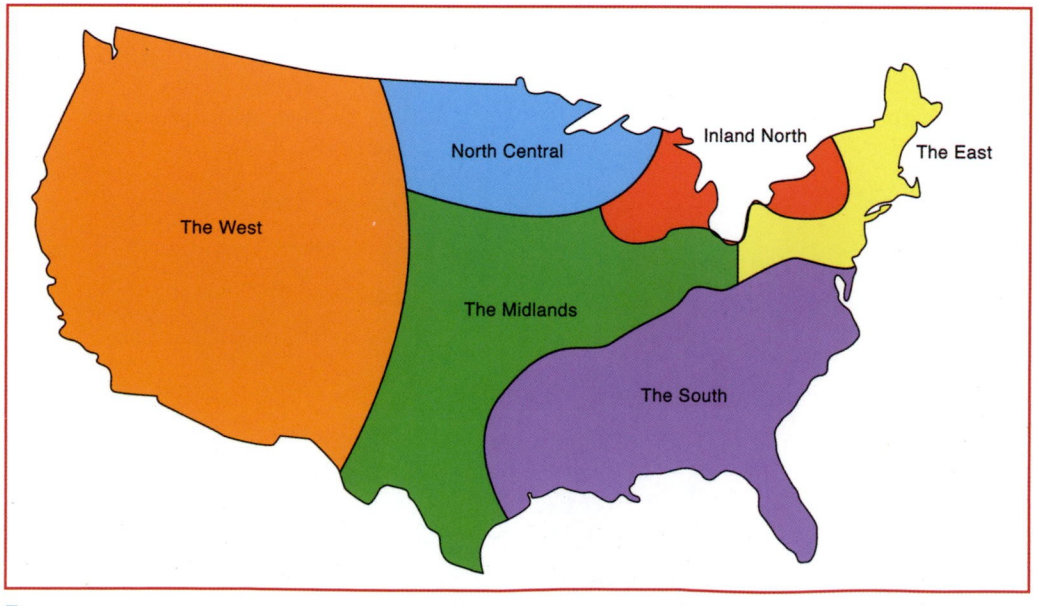

B

FIGURE 5.15. The approximate geographic boundaries for various accents of English spoken in England (**A**) and the United States (**B**).

Socioeconomic dialects are less common, with word choice being one of the more obvious features. Individuals who vary in income level, educational level, and occupation may be found to speak differently than individuals residing within the same geographic region. For example, consider the term used in England to describe pieces of candy. Individuals from high economic levels often used the term "sweets," whereas someone from a lower economic class is likely to use the term "lollies."

The term **accent** refers to the manner of pronunciation of a language. Accents are found in all varieties of English. For example, a common feature of New Zealand English is the "vowelization" of postvocalic /r/ ('bear" → "bea-ah), that is produced throughout most of the country. Yet, in the most southern region of the same country, the postvocalic /r/ is clearly produced. This peculiar variation in pronunciation is attributed to a large Scottish immigrant population in the southern part of New Zealand, which is known to produce a distinct /r/. A wide range of variation is also found in American English production, including New England English, Appalachian English, and African American English (AAE). There is a popular misconception that AAE is incorrect, lazy, defective, ungrammatical, and broken English. On the contrary, evidence from many years of linguistic investigation establishes that AAE is a legitimate, rule-governed, socially constructed variety of American English (Payne, 2000). Some of the phonological patterns that are unique to AAE are shown in Table 5.5.

Bilingualism refers to the ability to communicate in two languages. This ability can found in four modalities: (1) speaking, (2) understanding, (3) reading, and (4) writing. **Multilingualism** is

Table 5.5. Some Phonological Rules of African American English (AAE)

AAE Rule	Examples
Final Consonant Reduction	old → ole
	missed → miss
	tests → tesses
Devoicing of Voiced Sounds	they → dey
	feather → feavuh
	bathe → bave
	eating → eatin
Modification of Voiceless Sounds	nothing → nufin
	liked → lik-ted
	ask → aks
	asked → ast

the ability to communicate in more than two languages. An individual who is multilingual can also be referred to as a polyglot (i.e., multiple tongues). Approximately 50% of the world's population is bilingual. Indeed, individuals who speak only one language (i.e., monolingual) are becoming the exception rather than the norm. The learning of two or more languages can occur simultaneously or consecutively. A **spontaneous bilingual** is one who has learned two or more languages at precisely the same time and continues to use multiple languages. Spontaneous bilinguals will not exhibit an accent when speaking various languages. A **consecutive bilingual** is one whose second language was learned sometime after learning a first language. In this case, the first language is referred to as **L1** and the second language is **L2**. The majority of the world's bilinguals is consecutive and will exhibit an accent in their L2 speech. When the L2 spoken is English, the term **English as a second language** (**ESL**) is used.

When we encounter a foreign language, our natural tendency is to hear it in terms of the sounds of our own language. We actually perceive it differently from the way native speakers do. Equally, when we speak a foreign language we tend to attempt to do so using the familiar sounds and sound patterns of our mother tongue. This is the well-documented phenomenon known as **phonological interference**. Our L1 (mother tongue) interferes with our attempts to produce the L2 (target language). Phonological interference can occur in many ways. Perhaps the most common interference concerns sounds in the L2 that are not found in L1. In these cases, the speaker of the L2 may either replace the foreign sound with one found in the L1 or completely delete the sound. Some aspects of accented speech are generally attributed to differences in the phonemic inventories of a speaker's native language and their second language. Some examples for French, Spanish, and Mandarin are provided below, all of which pertain to production of the phoneme /ð/ (the first sound in the English word "this). In each of these languages, this particular phoneme is not found in the native L1.

French. In French-accented English, the French phoneme /z/ is often produced as a substitute for the English phoneme /ð/. For example, the word "thee" is likely to be produced as "zee."

Spanish. In Spanish-accented English, the Spanish phoneme /d/ is often produced as a substitute for the English phoneme /ð/. So, instead of saying "this" the speaker is likely to say "dis."

Mandarin. In Mandarin-accented English, the English phoneme /ð/ frequently sounds like a soft "d," produced with the tongue either immediately behind the front teeth or protruding slightly from the mouth.

An issue that confronts the SLP when evaluating the speech of an ESL speaker is determining whether the speech pattern demonstrated is indicative of a phonological difference or a phonological disorder. A **phonological difference** is a pattern where the sound productions are within the norms for the community but different from the standard. For instance, a person who produces Mandarin accented English (MAE) is likely to pronounce English in the same way as other speakers of MAE (Chen, 1999). Speech therapy is not warranted for an ESL speaker showing a phonological difference. Rather, the speech pattern is considered normal

---

FYI

Click sounds serve as phonemes in some South African languages. Clicks are produced on ingressive (inward) airflow compared to all other phonemes, which are produced on egressive (outward) airflow. However, click sounds are sometimes found in languages when we least expect them, including English. For example, consider the ingressive sound sometimes used to express regret or disapproval, written as *tsk-tsk*.

and serves a communicative function, as well as a social solidarity function. Sometimes, an accent or dialect may be a problem if it interferes with a person's goals in life. For example, an ESL speaker may choose to receive therapy to help reduce their accent, such as a Japanese executive who wishes to do business with American companies. Another situation might be where an aspiring actor from a European country wishes to "lose" his foreign accent by learning the standard form of the L2. This type of therapy would be considered "elective" as opposed to mandatory and could be provided by the SLP.

It is possible that a bilingual speaker might show a phonological disorder. In this condition, the sound productions of the speaker fall outside the norms of the community. Referring back to an MAE speaker, this would be a situation in which the individual's speech productions of English differ from those of other MAE speakers. As is often the case, if the person's L2 is found to be phonologically disordered, the L1 is most likely phonologically disordered as well. In order for the SLP to make this diagnosis, she would need to be aware of the phonological rules of the accent.

CURRENT RESEARCH IN CHILD PHONOLOGICAL DISORDERS

Genetic Factors

Searching for the cause of phonological disorders has typically not been of primary interest to SLPs. Rather, the research focus has been to develop effective treatment programs. This has certainly been the case for functional phonological disorders. However, recent advances in behavioral molecular genetics over the past decade have made it possible to investigate genetic factors that may contribute to phonological disorders. We typically assume that functional phonological disorders have a cause that is unknown or perhaps may even reflect learned behavior. Yet, mounting evidence suggests that at least some functional phonological disorders may actually have a genetic (i.e., organic) origin. Work in this area is still quite limited (Shriberg, 2003).

Treatment Efficacy

Minimal research has been undertaken that directly compares the effect of treatment procedures in facilitating improved speech sound production. Research is now underway to more critically examine the effectiveness of various treatment approaches for children with phonological disorders. The aim of this research is to determine whether the intervention has the desired outcome and which treatment(s) is/are most effective, as well as determining the impact that a phonological disorder has on the lives of children (Baker & McLeod, 2004).

Childhood Apraxia of Speech (CAS)

Although there is agreement that CAS is a unique form of phonological disorder, we still do not know what causes CAS. Research is desperately needed in this area. At present, there are several theories about the cause of CAS. One view is that children with CAS have problems producing speech because of auditory deficits, although they may show normal hearing sensitivity. The belief is that these deficits adversely affect the child's ability to detect and/or encode speech sounds from conversational speech. Another theory is that CAS may be caused by a child's difficulty in learning and building an adultlike language system. Yet another viewpoint is that CAS is caused by problems in a child's organization and sequencing of speech components such as sounds, syllables, and melody. The belief is that the child has mentally stored these speech components, but does not possess the skills to consistently organize and sequence the movements of the articulators into words and sentences.

CHILD PHONOLOGICAL DISORDERS ON THE WORLD WIDE WEB

Listed below are Web sites that provide further information on the topic of phonological disorders. At the time of publication each Web site was freely accessible.

Child Speech Sound Disorders Q&A
http://members.tripod.com/ Caroline_Bowen/phonol-and-artic.htm

Childhood Apraxia of Speech Association of North America (CASANA)
http://www.apraxia-kids.org/

Expert Information on Speech and Language Delays
http://www.speechdelay.com/

Phonological Disorders
http://www.speechpathology.com

Speech Sound Disorders Information
http://www.brighttots.com/Speech _and_Language_disorders/Speech_ Sound_Disorders.html

REFERENCES

Baker, E., & McLeod, S. (2004). Evidence-based management of phonological impairment in children. *Child Language Teaching and Therapy, 20,* 261–285

Chen, Y. (1999). *Acoustic characteristics of American English produced by native speakers of Mandarin.* Unpublished doctoral dissertation, University of Connecticut, Storrs, CT.

Chomsky, N., & Halle, M. (1968). *The sound pattern of English.* New York: Harper and Row.

Donegan, P., & Stampe, D. (1979). The study of natural phonology. In D. A. Dinnsen (Ed.), *Current Approaches to phonological theory* (pp. 126–173). Bloomington: IN: University Press.

Fairbanks, G. (1940). *Voice and articulation drillbook.* New York: Harper & Brothers.

Geruit, J., & Morrisette, M. (2005). The clinical significance of optimality theory for phonological disorders. *Topics in Language Disorders, 25,* 266–280.

Gillon, G. (2004). *Phonological awareness: From research to practice.* New York: Guilford Press.

Hodson, B. W., & Paden, E. P. (1991). *Targeting intelligible speech.* San Diego, CA: College-Hill Press.

McAuliffe, M. J., Ward, E. C., & Murdoch, B. E. (2003). Variation in articulatory timing of three English consonants: An electropalatographic investigation. *Clinical Linguistics and Phonetics, 17,* 43–62.

Mowrer, O. H. (1960). *Learning theory and behavior.* New York: Wiley.

Payne, K. (2005). African American English: Nature, origin, and implications for clinicians. *ECHO, 1*(2), 95.

Rousey, C. (1957). The psychopathology of articulation and voice deviations. In L. E. Travis (Ed.), *Handbook of speech pathology and audiology.* Englewood Cliffs, NJ: Prentice-Hall.

Scripture, E. W. (1912). *Stuttering and lisping.* New York: MacMillan.

Shriberg, L. (2003). Diagnostic markers for child speech-sound disorders: Introductory comments. *Clinical Linguistics and Phonetics, 17,* 501–505.

Travis, L. E. (1931). *Speech pathology: A dynamic neurological treatment of normal speech and speech deviations.* New York: Appleton-Century.

Van Riper, C. (1947). *Speech correction: Principles and methods.* Englewood Cliffs, NJ: Prentice-Hall.

Van Riper, C. (1981). An early history of ASHA. *ASHA Magazine, 23*(11), 855–858.

FLUENCY DISORDERS

OBJECTIVES

After reading this chapter, the student should be able to:

- Define and describe speech fluency and factors that interfere with fluency.
- Understand the cross-cultural and cross-linguistic differences that may impact communication.
- Understand the etiologies of various types of fluency disorders, including stuttering, neurogenic and psychogenic fluency disorders, and cluttering.
- Understand the nature, characteristics, and onset of stuttering.
- Understand past and present theoretical models concerning the etiology of stuttering.
- Describe methods for evaluating and measuring disfluent speech.
- Describe the role of family involvement in the prevention and intervention strategies for young children and adolescents.
- Describe procedures for the treatment of stuttering.
- Understand the role of age and culture in the management and treatment of stuttering.
- Understand the diagnostic and treatment principles for clients who demonstrate cluttering, neurogenic disfluency, and psychogenic disfluency.

INTRODUCTION

Most of us have met someone with a **fluency disorder** or know of someone who has a fluency disorder (Figure 6.1). The peculiarity of the disorder is undeniable and is one of the most identifiable communication disorders by both trained and untrained listeners. When an SLP is asked to provide a general description of their occupation to a layperson, mentioning the treatment of individuals with a fluency disorder is readily recognizable. After holding a conversation with a person who has a fluency disorder one may wonder: (1) What caused the disorder? (2) Can the disorder be cured?, and (3) What can I, as a listener, do to best communicate with a person who has a fluency disorder? The answers to these questions are still unknown but we do know a great deal about fluency disorders and have developed treatment approaches that help improve a person's ability to produce speech fluently. Interestingly, some of the world's leading experts in the area of fluency disorders were drawn to the field because they themselves have a fluency disorder. Who would be a better expert then someone who has first-hand experience with the disorder? There is a documented history of research on fluency disorders that has led to a wealth of information on the topic. The information presented in the following chapter is an introduction to the fascinating area of fluency disorders.

TERMINOLOGY AND DEFINITIONS

The term **fluency** refers to the effortless flow of speech. Fluency encompasses many features that contribute to this

FIGURE 6.1. Pictures drawn by children in response to instructions, "Draw a picture of what it feels like to stutter." Permission granted by Andriana DiGrande, New England Fluency Program, USA. From http://www.mnsu.edu/comdis/kuster/stutter.html .

effortless flow, such as: (1) the rate or quickness of a person's speech, (2) the silent periods or pauses that may occur within or between words, (3) the stress or emphasis placed on various syllables or words, and (4) the inflection or intonation used by the speaker during the production of an utterance. Collectively, we think of fluent speech as the pleasant sing-song pattern of talking. Fluency encompasses qualities that make speech sound natural and normal. This definition is specific to the spoken word; however, fluency can also apply to other areas of communication such as written language.

The term **disfluency** is the opposite condition, whereby a disruption or breakdown in the flow of speech occurs. A change in any single feature, or combination of features, that contribute to fluent speech, can result in disfluent speech. For example, excessively fast speaking can interfere with the correct articulation of vowels and consonants, thereby affecting the naturalness of speech. Unusually long pauses between the syllables of words can likewise affect speech naturalness. It is important to keep in mind that we all produce speech disfluencies, although this does not necessary mean we have a fluency disorder. The simple interjection of "um" between words, or changing our choice of words in mid-conversation would classify as forms of disfluency. The job of the SLP is to distinguish between what is considered normal, natural speech disfluencies and unnatural speech disfluencies. When speech disfluencies fall outside the boundary of what is considered natural, they are deemed to represent a fluency disorder. The two fluency disorders profiled in this chapter are **stuttering** and **cluttering**.

There is a bit of confusion in the terminology surrounding fluency disorders. Students frequently ask whether the terms *disfluency* and *dysfluency* are interchangeable. The answer is no, although the terms have been used interchangeably as recently as the 1990s. The prefix *dis* has its origins in Latin and is used to form words that are the opposite of the core word, such as *honor* versus *dishonor*, and *able* versus *disable*. Alternatively, the prefix *dys* has its origins in Greek and refers to something bad, harsh, or wrong, such as *function* versus *dysfunction*. We all demonstrate disruptions in fluency. To ascribe the prefix *dys* to this condition would be too strong a description. Rather, the disruption in fluency simply reflects the opposite state. Therefore, the term disfluency is preferred for the disruptions in speech that occur normally in the majority of speakers.

HISTORIC ASPECTS OF FLUENCY DISORDERS

Observations regarding fluency disorders, specifically stuttering, can be traced back centuries. A list of notable

---

FYI

The origins of the word "stuttering" are unclear but there are a few possibilities as to its derivation. The word *stue* is from a Greek word that means to strike. There is a Nordic word *stytta*, which means "to stop." There is also an old German word *stutten* that means "to make a series of repeated sounds."

individuals (past and present) known (or thought) to have a fluency disorder is provided in Table 6.1. Some of the earliest documented reports of individuals who stutter include **Moses**. There is a report in the Old Testament that Moses stuttered as depicted in the passage, *"O Lord, I have never been a man of ready speech, never in my life, not even now that thou has spoken to me; I am slow and hesitant of speech"* (Exodus 4:10). The Roman emperor Claudius (10 BC to 54 AD) was assumed to produce stuttered speech and showed signs of deafness. **King Louis II** of France (843–879) was also known to produce a stutter. He was called "le Begue" or "the Stammerer" (Figure 6.2).

Because of the unusual pattern of speaking associated with stuttering, the disorder has been of high scientific and medical curiosity. The interest has centered on determining either the cause of stuttering or how to cure stuttering. During the late 1700s and early 1800s the root cause of stuttering was thought to be related to faulty functioning of the tongue and/or larynx. **Jean-Marc Gaspard Itard** (1774–1838), a physician at the Institute of Deaf Mutes in Paris (see also Chapter 4), was the first to view stuttering as a pathological condition. In his opinion, stuttering was caused by a spasm induced by a weakness of the motor organs of the larynx and tongue. The Swiss scientist **Rudolf Schulthess** (1802-1833) also believed stuttering was due to spasms of the larynx and suggested using the terms *phonophobia* or *lalophobia* to describe the condition.

Table 6.1. Famous People Known to Have Displayed Stuttering

Rowan Atkinson	British Actor
Lewis Carroll	Author of *Alice in Wonderland*
Winston Churchill	Former Prime Minister of England
Cameron Daddo	Australian Actor
Charles Darwin	British Naturalist
King George VI	Former King of England
Marilyn Monroe	American Actor
Sam Neill	New Zealand Actor
Isaac Newton	Scientist
Gareth Gates	British singer
James Earl Jones	American actor
Porky Pig	Cartoon character from Looney Tunes series
Jimmy Volmer	Cartoon character on the TV series South Park
George Washington	American President
Bruce Willis	American Actor

FIGURE 6.2. King Louis II of France. Was called "le Begue" or "the Stammerer."

Toward the middle of the 19th century there was a shift from viewing the tongue and larynx as causal factors of stuttering toward viewing stuttering as a disturbance in the breathing patterns for speech. For example, the German scholar **A. Thome** (1867) held the opinion that stuttering was a result of spasms of the respiratory organs that were linked to an individual's emotional state. The disturbance of stuttering was triggered by emotionally based disruptions in the nervous system. Two types of emotional conditions were assumed to contribute to moments of stuttering: (1) embarrassment or lack of confidence and (2) excessive rapidity of thought.

During the 1800s, approaches to the treatment of stuttering also varied widely. Believing the tongue was responsible for stuttering led Itard to develop a small forked golden plate that was placed under the tongue to provide support while speaking. More drastic treatment of the tongue was proposed by German surgeon **Johann Friedrich Dieffenbach** (1792–1847) who recommended cutting the tongue with scissors and removing a triangular wedge from the back of the tongue (Figure 6.3). **James Yearsley** (1805–1869) was a British surgeon who advocated removal of the tonsils as a form of treatment for stuttering. All of these invasive procedures were ultimately abandoned for two reasons. First, performing surgery in this region of the body carries a level of danger because the speech organs receive heavy blood supply (i.e., they are highly vascular). Therefore, surgery performed in this part of the body was risky. A surgical error could lead to considerable blood loss and subsequent death. The second reason for abandoning invasive techniques was that the various surgical

FIGURE 6.3. Johann Friedrich Dieffenbach. German surgeon who recommended cutting out portions of the tongue to treat stuttering.

procedures were not found to be successful in curing stuttering.

During the first half of the 20th century, there was continued interest in isolating the cause and cure of stuttering. Although research undertaken during this time period was less invasive than earlier years, the approaches were no less unusual. **Lee Edward Travis** (1896–1987), who is considered a founding father of the speech-language pathology profession (Figure 6.4), devoted a majority of his career to understanding the cause of stuttering. Travis held the view that people who stutter have speech centers in both cerebral hemispheres of their brain instead of just the left hemisphere. Stuttering resulted from a lack of brain dominance when it came to producing speech. As a result of this condition,

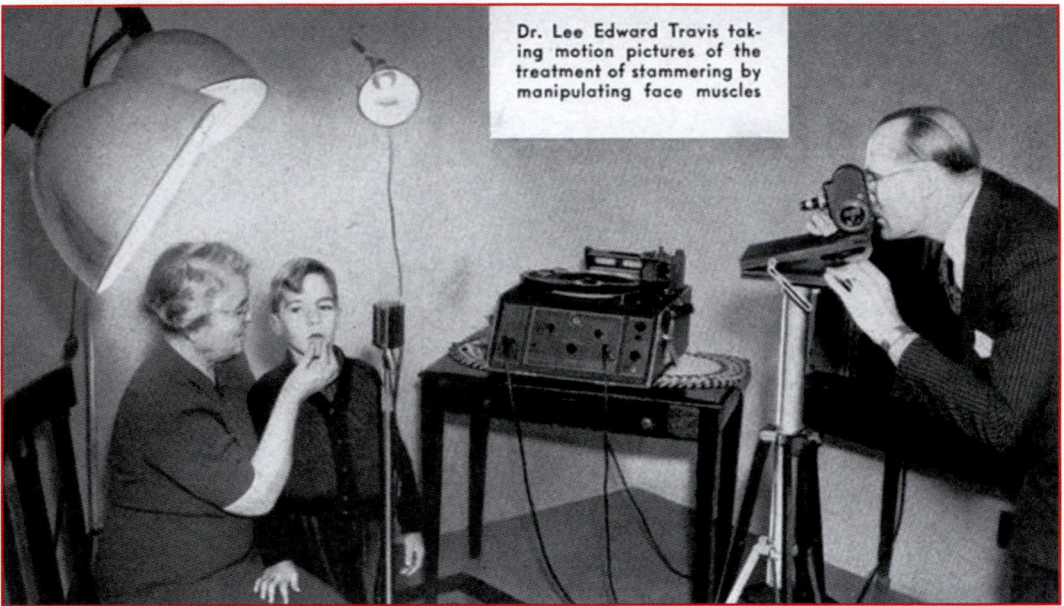

Dr. Lee Edward Travis taking motion pictures of the treatment of stammering by manipulating face muscles

FIGURE 6.4. Lee Travis in 1940. Known as the father of speech-language pathology, he had a strong research interest in stuttering.

when an individual began to organize the act of speech in their brain, the two sides of the brain were "competing" for control of the speech muscles. This competition led to a breakdown in the forward flow of speech and resulted in a stutter. This theory was based on Travis' observation that people who were left-handed or "forced" right-handers were more likely to stutter than pure right-handers. In the early 1930s, Travis took left-handed stutterers and forced them to write with their right hand. Two of these research participants later became eminent scholars in the field of stuttering, **Charles Van Riper** (1905–1994) and **Wendell Johnson** (1906–1965). Van Riper is quoted as saying, *"Both of us* [Van Riper & Johnson] *wore plaster casts upon our right arms to enforce left-handedness and again I found myself doing the interminable pages of talking and writing each day."* The activity did little to alleviate the production of stuttered speech.

Bryng Bryngelson (1892–1979) received his Ph.D. from the University of Iowa and went on to have a successful career at the University of Minnesota (Figure 6.5). Bryngelson is remembered for his research on the relationship between stuttering and left-handedness. However, after spending nearly 30 years on the topic, there was little evidence to suggest that shifting handedness would alleviate the production of stuttered speech. One of Bryngelson's important contributions to the field of stuttering therapy was his concept of voluntary stuttering. By having an individual who stutters do so deliberately in public settings helped to lower the anxiety associated with speaking situations. Gradually, deliberate stuttering was decreased with the aim of producing stutter-free speech at all times.

The area of stuttering in the early 1900s was also influenced by **Sigmund Freud's** (1856–1939) psychoanalytic the-

FIGURE 6.5. Bryng Bryngelson. Believed that a person's handedness was linked to stuttering. Reprinted with permission from Van Riper, C. (1981). "An early history of ASHA." *ASHA Magazine, 23*(11), 855–858.

FIGURE 6.6. Wendell Johnson. Believed the development of stuttering had a strong environmental influence. Reprinted with permission from Van Riper, C. (1981). "An early history of ASHA." *ASHA Magazine, 23*(11), 855–858.

ory. The cause of stuttering was felt to be a result of a deep-seeded psychological disturbance and that family relationships, especially parent-child relationships, lay at the root of the problem. An adaptation of this perspective was proposed by Wendell Johnson who felt stuttering was caused by the parents' misinterpretations of their child's speech (Figure 6.6). Parents confused the child's normal disfluency for stuttering. According to Johnson, *"Stuttering begins not in the child's mouth but in the parent's ear."* In doing so, parents' required from the child a level of speaking performance that the child could not attain. The subsequent reactions of both child and parents resulted in a worsening of the child's speech, leading to stuttering. In 1939, Johnson tested this theory, in what is now known as the Iowa Stuttering Study. In this study, 12 nonstuttering children who were residents in an orphanage were induced to stutter. Of these 12 children, half were told that they had symptoms of stuttering and their caregivers were instructed to correct their speech disfluencies whenever they occurred. These six children eventually developed symptoms of stuttering. The other six children were part of a control group and received no instructions to correct their speech disfluencies. These children never developed stuttering. The research would nowadays be considered unethical because of the lack of protection for the participants. The University of Iowa made a public apology in 2001 and subsequently agreed to pay approximately $1,000,000 to the six children and their heirs (ASHA, 2007).

Lena Rustin (1928–2004) was an inspirational pioneer in the treatment of stuttering (Figure 6.7). Born in England,

FIGURE 6.7. Lena Rustin. Inspirational pioneer in the treatment of stuttering. Photo courtesy of the British Stammering Association (www.stammering.org).

Dr. Rustin was a dedicated clinician who spent her career helping children who stutter and their families. She founded the Association for Research into Stammering in Childhood (ARSC) in 1991. She also was the cofounder of the Michael Palin Centre for Stammering Children in London.

TYPES OF FLUENCY DISORDERS

Stuttering

The World Health Organization (WHO) (1977) defines stuttering as, *"Disorders in the rhythm of speech in which the individual knows precisely what s/he wishes to say but at the same time is unable to say because of an involuntary repetition, prolongation, or cessation of a sound."* Speech-language pathology associations worldwide such as the American Speech-Language-Hearing Association (ASHA), Royal College of Speech-Language Therapists (RCSLT), and Speech Pathology Australia (SPA) have developed their own definitions of stuttering that vary slightly from the WHO definition but the general tenets of the definition are the same. Stuttering is a disruption in the flow of speech. Stuttering is also viewed as a **developmental disorder**. A child who eventually develops a stutter is considered to have been born with the condition; however, the condition is not perceptually apparent until the child begins using connected speech. The term **stammering** is synonymous with stuttering and is used often in the United Kingdom. Either term is appropriate and acceptable.

Stuttering is found to occur in all languages of the world, although precise

Speaking to the rhythmic beats of a metronome has been shown to help reduce stuttering. Although speaking in such a fashion sounds highly unnatural, the device has been used at the beginning of a therapy program to help gain control over severely disfluent speech.

Table 6.2. Words From Around the World Used to Refer to Stuttering

Language	*Word*
Afrikaans	hakkel
Arabic	rattat
Cherokee	a-da-nv-te-hi-lo-squi
Chinese (Cantonese)	hau hick
Chinese (Mandarin)	kou chi
Dutch	stotteren
Egyptian	tuhuhtuhuh
English	stuttering
Fijiian	kaka
French	begaiement
German	stottern
Hawaiian	uu uus
Hebrew	gimgum
Hindi	hakalaanaa
Hungarian	dadogo
Icelandic	stama
Italian	balbuzie
Japanese	domori; kitsuon
Korean	maldeodum
Maori	kikiki
Nigerian	nsu
Punjabi	totalaanaa
Russian	zaikatsia; zaikanie
Spanish	tartamudez
Swedish	stamning

estimates of its prevalence are unknown. Evidence of its occurrence around the world is provided by noting whether a word for stuttering exists in the vocabulary of the language. Table 6.2 provides some examples of various words for stuttering in languages around the world. Languages that do not have a word for stuttering does not necessarily mean the disorder is absent from the population. Rather, the condition may not be viewed as a disorder. As a general rule, stuttering is thought to occur in 1 out of every 100 individuals, or approximately 1% of the population.

The percentage of stuttering in preschool children is somewhat higher with approximately 3% of children showing early signs of stuttering behavior. However, this number is reduced to 1% once children enter school. Stuttering is three times more likely to occur in boys compared to girls (3:1 ratio). There are also reports of stuttering occurring more often among **twins** and for the disorder to run in families across generations, suggesting a **genetic** (hereditary) predisposition for the disorder among some individuals.

The development of stuttering is not sudden. The appearance of the disorder is often equated with phases of the moon, whereby the condition waxes and wanes. There will be periods in the child's daily/weekly speaking behavior when it seems like nearly every word produced is disfluent. The same child may then show long periods of time when nearly every word is produced fluently. The **onset** of stuttering typically occurs at 3 years of age but may vary in children anywhere from 2 years to 5 years of age. We also know that some situations can serve to raise or lower moments of stuttering in children and adults alike. Situations that tend to require high communicative demand such as answering questions, speaking to a stranger, or speaking on the telephone are likely to increase moments of disfluent speech. On the other hand, speaking one-on-one with a familiar individual (or even to a pet) is likely to be a situation of low communicative demand, resulting in more fluent speech.

Stuttering involves both **overt** (observable) and **covert** (nonobservable) behaviors. The combination of these behaviors has been likened to the shape of an iceberg. The tip of the iceberg that rises from the water reflects the overt behaviors, which are the audible and visible signs of stuttering (Figure 6.8). Van Riper (1982) refers to overt behaviors as the **primary characteristics** of stuttering. Yet, far greater and perhaps more detrimental is the portion of the iceberg that is submerged. This portion reflects covert behaviors, which comprise feelings of fear, shame, guilt, anxiety, hopelessness, isolation, and denial. Van Riper refers to covert behaviors as the **secondary characteristics** of stuttering.

Primary Characteristics of Stuttering

A popular approach to describing overt stuttering is to differentiate and label the various types of disfluencies. The premise for identifying disfluency types is that some sorts of disfluencies are most often associated with chronic stuttering. Therefore, differentiating disfluency types should aid in the assessment and diagnosis of stuttering. Johnson (1961) identified eight disfluency types

---

FYI

As the development of stuttering progresses from young children to adults, the earliest types of disfluencies tend to be repetitions of phrases and single words. Later, the types of disfluencies include blocks and prolongations, in addition to repetitions.

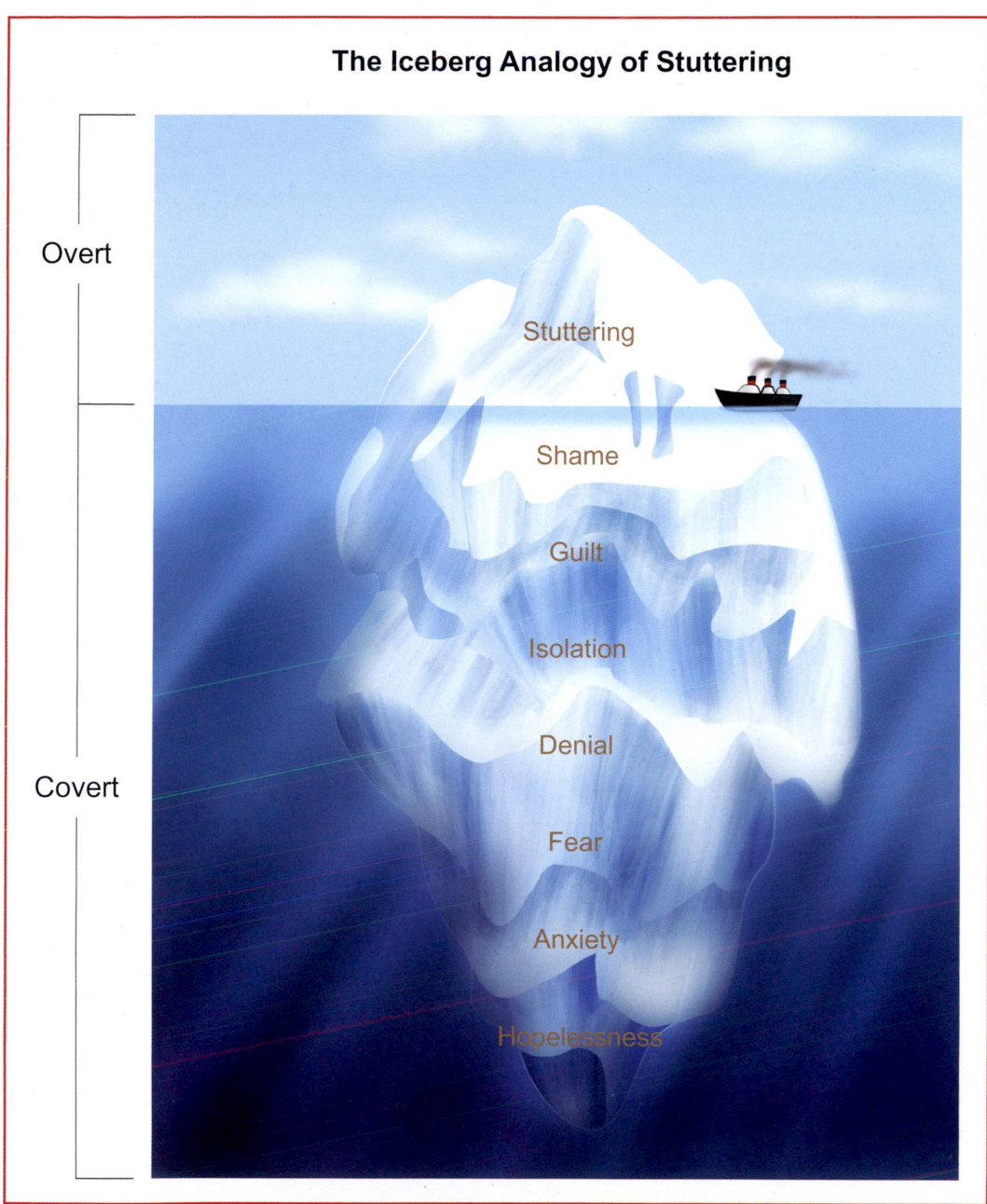

The Iceberg Analogy of Stuttering

Overt

Covert

Stuttering

Shame

Guilt

Isolation

Denial

Fear

Anxiety

Hopelessness

FIGURE 6.8. Classic depiction of the many facets of stuttering as analogous to the shape of an iceberg.

(Table 6.3). One thing to note with these various disfluency types is that some disfluencies occur within a specific word, while other disfluencies occur between (or across) words. Johnson suggested that the production of **between-word**

Johnson System	**Yairi & Ambrose System**
1. Part-Word Repetition For example, *"My t-t-t-tooth hurts"*	SLD
2. Single-Syllable Word Repetition For example, *"I-I-I-I want to go home"*	SLD
3. Multisyllabic Word Repetition For example, *"The ba-ba-ba-baby is crying"*	SLD
4. Dis-rhythmic Phonation (sound prolongation) For example, *"MMMMMMy tooth hurts"*	SLD
5. Tense Pause (silent prolongation or "block") For example, *" . . . The baby is crying"*	SLD
6. Phrase Repetition For example, *"I want- I want- I want to go home"*	OD
7. Interjection For example, *"I um, well, um, want to go home"*	OD
8. Revision-Incomplete Phrase For example, *"My too . . . my molar hurts"*	OD

Table 6.3. Disfluency Notation Systems*

*The Johnson (1961) system is based on the consideration of 8 disfluency types. Types 1–5 are considered within-word disfluencies. Types 6–8 are considered between-word disfluencies. The Yairi and Ambrose system (1992) is based on the original Johnson system but simplified to consider two major types of disfluencies, stutter-like disfluencies (SLD) and other disfluencies (OD).

disfluencies was a common feature in the speech of people who do not stutter. The production of **within-word disfluencies** (in addition to producing between-word disfluencies) most often was associated with stuttering behavior. The typology developed by Johnson is still used in research and clinical settings; however, it has since been simplified to two broad categories of disfluencies: **stuttering-like disfluencies (SLD)** and **other disfluencies (OD)** (Yairi & Ambrose, 1992). SLDs are those disfluencies indicative of chronic stuttering (i.e., part-word repetition, single-syllable word repetition, disrhythmic phonation, tense pause) and ODs are reflective of normal nonfluent speech (i.e., multisyllabic word repetition, phrase repetition, interjection, and revision-incomplete phrase). The reason for reducing the types of disfluencies to only two categories was to simplify the identification process for researchers and clinicians while still being able to capture the essence of stuttering behavior. An illustration of two common types of SLD, sound repetitions and sound prolongations, is shown in Figure 6.9.

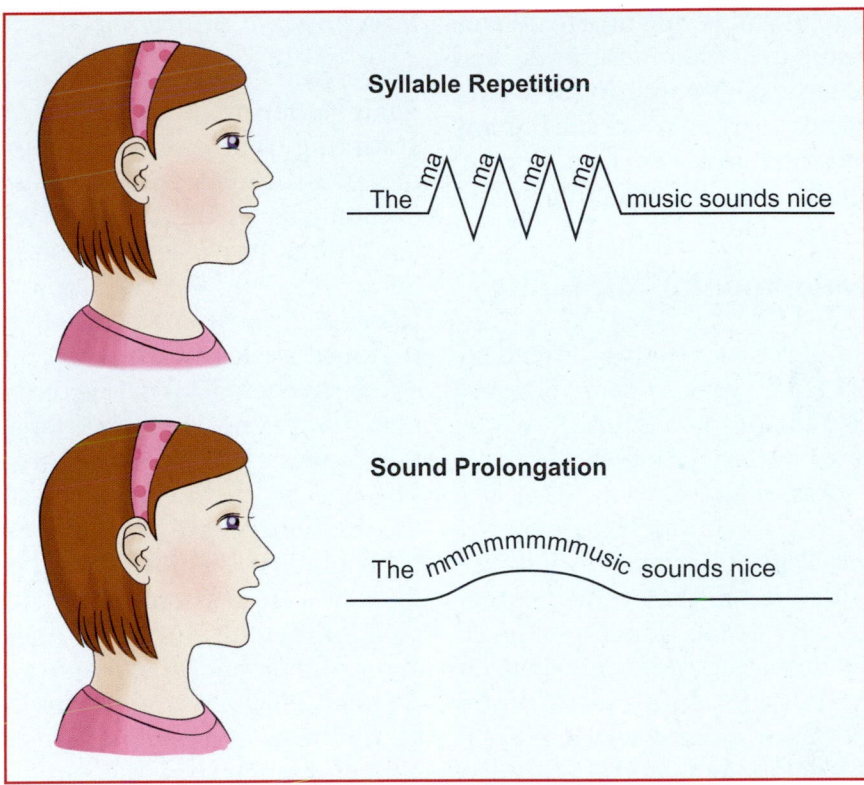

FIGURE 6.9. Illustration of a sound repetition and sound prolongation during production of the sentence: *the music sounds nice.*

Secondary Characteristics of Stuttering

The secondary characteristics of stuttering are more difficult to classify than primary characteristics. These features of stuttering seem to develop gradually over time. Many of these behaviors may be absent among young children during the earlier years of stuttering and only begin to develop as the child grows older and stuttering becomes more fixated. These secondary characteristics can be organized into two categories: **bodily movements** and **psychosocial behaviors**. Bodily movements typically are related to facial activity that accompanies a moment of stuttering. These might include eye blinks, facial grimaces, head movements, and loss of eye contact. In more extreme cases, there also might be torso and limb movements. Some theorists believe these body movements reflect a coping strategy by the individual, whereby the behavior was used successfully at some point in time to aid the individual in speaking fluently. However, over time, these behaviors were less successful in preventing moments of stuttering. Consequently, stuttering continued and the coping strategy (i.e., bodily movements) became uncontrollably linked to moments of stuttering. Psychosocial behaviors are the feelings experienced by the individual who stutters. A person's feelings can be as much a part of the disorder of stuttering as the speech behaviors. These feelings, which are usually negative, include fear, frustration, embarrassment, sadness, and anger. As a person's stuttering worsens, these psychosocial behaviors can become more enhanced and may lead to complete withdrawal from speaking.

Nondevelopmental Stuttering

The definition of stuttering offered by the WHO (1977) makes clear reference to fluency disorders (plural), which implies that stuttering does not occur as a single form of speech but rather in a variety of ways. Although the majority of instances of stuttering are developmental, there are forms of the disorder that arise later in life. These nondevelopmental forms of stuttering occur far less often but this does not minimize their importance on the caseload of a SLP. Two nondevelopmental forms of stuttering are neurogenic and psychogenic.

Neurogenic Stuttering

Conditions affecting various areas of the brain, including the cortex, cerebellum, and brainstem can cause **neurogenic stuttering**. The disfluency pattern in neurogenic stuttering is characterized by a high number of involuntary repetitions or prolongations of speech that do not seem to be a result of poor (hesitant) language formulation difficulties or as a result of psychiatric problems. Secondary behaviors may not be present, and if they do exist they are not associated with moments of disfluency. One example of neurogenic stuttering can be found among individuals with Parkinson disease. Goberman and Blomgren (2003) suggested that stuttering in Parkinson disease is related to impairment in the amount (i.e., reduction) of the neurotransmitter, dopamine in the brain.

Psychogenic Stuttering

There are far fewer reports of **psychogenic stuttering** compared to neurogenic stuttering. Whereas neurogenic stuttering is associated with various known pathologies in the brain, psychogenic conditions are less obvious. Psychogenic stuttering is a condition referring to people in whom a psychological distrubance is clearly diagnosed. Because of the psychological nature of this disorder, the diagnosis of psychopathology falls outside the expertise of the SLP. The speech disfluencies produced by the individual are strongly linked to psychological distress. The types of disfluencies are less consistent than both developmental stuttering and neurogenic stuttering. An example would be a situation where the person's speech disfluencies may change noticeably, either for better or worse. A reduction in stuttering during a person's disclosure of emotionally sensitive information is a strong indicator of a psychogenic stutter. Further evidence of a psychogenic basis for stuttering is related to response to treatment. If a person's speech fluency returns to normal or near normal, it is likely there was a psychological basis because this level of improvement is not found in developmental stuttering.

Cluttering

A third type of nondevelopmental stuttering that is considered a separate type of fluency disorder is known as cluttering. **Cluttering** is a disorder of speaking rate. In a person who shows cluttering, their speaking rate can be either abnormally fast, irregular, or both. Among normally fluent adult speakers, the typical rate of speaking is approximately 240 syllables per minute (spm). Individuals with cluttering will often demonstrate a speaking rate in excess of

300 spm. In cluttered speech, the rapid rate of speaking contributes to: (1) higher than normal speech disfluency, (2) the types of disfluencies are not like those found in stuttering, and (3) slurred speech misarticulations, such as consonant deletions and consonant substitutions during spurts of rapid speech. The general impression when listening to the speech of an individual with cluttering is that they are speaking so fast that their speech fluency deteriorates. A comparison of cluttered and stuttered speech is illustrated in Figure 6.10. Treatment for individuals with cluttering tends to focus on reducing speaking rate, which results in marked improvement in the overall fluency and clarity of their speech.

FYI

A peculiar pattern of stuttering is the production of a **disfluency cluster**, which is the production of two or more disfluencies on the same word and/or adjacent words. An example of a disfluency cluster would be the production of a sound repetition followed by a prolongation such as, *The b-b-boy wwwent*. Disfluency clusters seem to only occur in the speech of people with a diagnosed stuttering disorder.

A   B

FIGURE 6.10. The pattern of speaking found in a person who stutters (**A**) compared to an individual who clutters (**B**).

CURRENT THEORIES REGARDING STUTTERING

Modern theories about stuttering have been shaped over many years of research. Most attempt to explain why a moment of stuttering occurs—although stuttering is the most researched communication disorder, the actual cause of stuttering remains controversial. There is no unified theory of stuttering. The general consensus is that stuttering has a **multidimensional** etiology. The various theories include a number of factors that may contribute to the disorder including genetics, the environment, language complexity, motor coordination, and psychological influences. In essence, modern theories suggest both nature and nurture influences on stuttering. Some of the most popular theories to date include the demands and capacities theory, covert repair theory, and the neuropsycholinguistic theory.

Demands and Capacities Theory

This theory was proposed by Starkweather (1997) and views stuttering as occurring when the demands for fluency from the child's social environment exceed the child's cognitive, linguistic, motor, or emotional capacities for fluent speech. Children who eventually develop stuttering have a genetic predisposition for the disorder and will encounter a mismatch between their speaking capabilities and self-imposed or environmental demands.

Covert Repair Theory

This theory was proposed by Postma and Kolk (1993) and links together the production of language and moments of stuttering. This theory assumes that people who stutter have an internally disordered phonological system. During the internal planning for speech, we naturally form (i.e., encode) the necessary sounds for words and sentences before physically producing speech. For people who stutter, they experience frequent planning errors that need to be "repaired" before the words leave the speaker's mouth. Speech disfluencies occur when a speaker interrupts ongoing speech to repair these errors. This is why we often observe the frequent production of repetitions and pauses in people who stutter. These repairs do not occur at a conscious level.

Neuropsycholinguistic Theory

This theory was proposed by Perkins, Kent, and Curlee (1991) and is based on the assumption that producing fluent speech involves sophisticated timing between the formulation of language and the actual motor execution of speech movement. Stuttering results in a situation where there is a disruption in the timing (integration) of linguistic formulation and speech movement. People who stutter will often report experiencing a "loss of control" in producing speech, which is enhanced when there is time pressure to produce speech.

ASSESSMENT OF FLUENCY DISORDERS

The aim of fluency assessment is to determine whether the disfluency behavior demonstrated by an individual is typical or atypical of what we might expect of most people speaking on an

FYI

Stuttering disappears once a person begins to sing. The reason for this is twofold. First, the strings of words being sung are familiar and well rehearsed, which helps to reduce stuttering. Second, singing involves the natural blending together of sounds and words in a melodic fashion with the vocal folds in a constant state of vibration. This is a form of continuous phonation that likewise helps to reduce stuttering.

everyday basis. Two questions to be addressed in a fluency assessment include: (1) *Are speech disfluencies present in the person's speaking behavior?* and (2) *What is the nature of the speech disfluencies?* The SLP answers these questions according to the age of the individual being assessed as they differ between children and adults because **parent input** is vital to the diagnosis of the condition in young children.

Are Speech Disfluencies Present?

To answer the first question, a large sample of conversational speech is collected from the person. The sample needs to be large enough so a representation of natural speaking behavior is obtained. The generally accepted minimum amount of speech is 300 words of conversation. Once this sample is collected (usually audio-recorded), the SLP re-listens to the sample and identifies and tallies moments of speech disfluency occurring across the 300-word sample. This tally is then converted to a percentage of occurrence. For example, if 21 moments of disfluency were identified across the

300-word sample, the percentage of disfluency would be 7%. Conversational speech that is **3% disfluent** or higher is usually a rough indication of a fluency disorder. Alternatively, 2% disfluency or lower would be considered within normal limits for people speaking on an everyday basis.

What Is the Nature of the Speech Disfluencies?

The answer to the second question involves further analysis of the specific moments of disfluency. The stuttering typology systems developed by Johnson (1961) and Yairii and Ambrose (1992) can be used to assess the nature and severity of the fluency disorder. As a general rule, the greater the occurrence of within-word (or SLD) disfluencies, the greater the severity of the stuttering disorder. The **Iowa Scale for Rating the Severity of Stuttering** was developed by Johnson et al. (1963) over 40 years ago and remains quite popular. To use the scale, the SLP must first calculate the average percentage of disfluency produced by an individual. Based on the percentage of disfluency, a corresponding severity ranking is assigned ranging from 0 (no stuttering) to 7 (very severe stuttering) (Table 6.4).

A popular test used to determine the nature of speech disfluencies is the **Stuttering Severity Instrument** for children and adults (Riley, 1994). This test considers the frequency of disfluencies, the duration of disfluencies, and the physical concomitants of speaking to formulate a diagnosis. The use of a perceptual scale can also be used to determine the nature of speech disfluencies. Perceptual scales bypass any formal measurement of disfluent speech. The philosophy behind using a perceptual scale is that one simply needs to hear a moment of stuttering to make a judgment as to the existence and severity of the disorder. One such scale is a 9-point **severity scale** that requires a listener to assign a value ranging from 1 (not stuttering) to 9 (extremely severe stuttering) (Figure 6.11).

Other variables that are considered when describing the nature of disfluencies are the presence or absence of **secondary behaviors**. These can be ascertained by visually examining the person during moments of disfluency, as well as to simply ask the person how they feel about their speech. The calculation of **speaking rate** can also aid in the diagnosis of a fluency disorder, particularly in regard to cluttering. This calculation can be made using the same 300-word conversational sample that was collected for noting the frequency and type of disfluencies. It is equally important to examine a person's fluency behavior in the context of over-

Table 6.4. Iowa Scale for Rating the Severity of Stuttering*	
Severity Ranking	**Descriptions**
0	*No Stuttering*
1	*Very Mild*—Stuttering on less than 1% of words
2	*Mild*—Stuttering on 1% to 2% of words
3	*Mild to Moderate*—Stuttering on 2% to 5% of words
4	*Moderate*—Stuttering on 5% to 8% of words
5	*Moderate to Severe*—Stuttering on 8% to 12% of words
6	*Severe*—Stuttering on 12% to 25% of words
7	*Very Severe*—Stuttering on more than 25% of words

*The table is a condensed version of the overall scale.

FIGURE 6.11. Example of a 9-point scale for perceptually rating the severity of stuttering.

all communication abilities. So, assessment of the person's phonology and language abilities is also performed.

Once a diagnosis of a fluency disorder is made, the next step is to enroll the individual in a treatment program. There are instances when the SLP may recommend monitoring the client rather than direct therapy. This may be the case for young children who are on the "cusp" of developing a fluency disorder or if a child appears to be at low risk for persistent stuttering.

TREATMENT OF FLUENCY DISORDERS

There is no 100% cure for stuttering. Because we still do not know what causes stuttering, it is not surprising to find that we also do not know the best way to treat stuttering. Although there is general agreement that stuttering cannot be completely remedied, a great deal can be done to help reduce the frequency of disfluent speech. Regardless of the treatment approach, there are three general goals to therapy: (1) to change the speaking behavior of the person, (2) to change the way the person feels about their speech, and (3) to change the way the person interacts with their speaking environment. Most treatment approaches fall into one of two categories, **traditional** and **nontraditional**.

Traditional Treatment Approaches

The traditional approaches to treating fluency disorders can be broadly organized into two types: (1) fluency shaping and (2) stuttering modification (Zeb-rowski & Kelly, 2002). Both approaches use principles of behavior modification to change the existing pattern of speaking. Often times, the SLP may try one or the other approach with the client to determine which seems to work best. The SLP may also develop a hybrid approach that incorporates features of both types of therapy. Ultimately, the client's response to a particular approach serves as the best gauge to the preferred treatment approach.

The **fluency shaping** approach is designed to modify all aspects of the client's speaking behavior. That is, every syllable, word, and sentence uttered by the client is modified into an overall new pattern of speaking. This modification is made by instructing the client to: (1) speak at a reduced rate, (2) prolong the vowel portions of words, and (3) use slow and smooth speech initiation. A term associated with this pattern of speaking is **continuous phonation**, where the client attempts to maintain constant vocal fold vibration during the production of entire utterances of speaking. The **stuttering modification** approach is designed to address individual moments of stuttering, as opposed to changing the entire pattern of speaking behavior. This modification is made by teaching the client to: (1) stutter with less tension, (2) use light articulatory contacts during speaking, and (3) reduce situational fears and negative attitudes of stuttering.

One treatment approach to working with preschool children during the earliest years of stuttering is **parent-directed therapy** (Zebrowski & Kelly, 2002). As indicated, parents are taught to play a key role in the remediation of their child's stuttering behavior. Receiving treatment in a clinical setting may typically involve only one or two (1-hour) sessions per week, which accounts for only a fraction of a child's weekly speaking activity. Therefore, by involving parents, they are taught to reinforce goals established in the clinic setting. This form of therapy places emphasis on increasing *desirable* speaking behavior instead of *undesirable* behavior. Attention is directed away from the perception of what is happening to the child, toward those things he is doing to both facilitate and interfere with talking. Emphasis is also placed on increasing the child's awareness of physical aspects of speaking that contribute to fluent speech, such as articulatory tension and breathing patterns. A popular form of parent-directed therapy is the **Lidcombe Program** of early stuttering intervention (Onslow et al., 2003).

Nontraditional Treatment Approaches

Nontraditional approaches generally are not used by SLPs to manage a person's stuttering. These approaches are also typically not applicable to the majority of individuals who may stutter, or show a related fluency disorder. Nontraditional approaches to treating stuttering include hypnotherapy, drug therapy, and electronic devices. **Hypnotherapy** is a psychologically based approach to the treatment of stuttering. Psychological techniques emphasizing anxiety reduction and building self-confidence are presented under hypnosis to help the individual speak confidently. By reducing anxiety and increasing self-confidence, the person's severity of stuttering presumably will lessen. Use of this technique remains controversial but there is evidence to suggest the approach may be particularly effective for individuals with a mild stuttering disorder.

The use of **drug therapy** to manage stuttering focuses on an individual's anxiety that is often greatly heightened when anticipating moments of speaking. A number of antianxiety drugs have been shown to reduce moments of stuttering; however, only a small number of individuals tend to show a long-lasting reduction in stuttering once under the drug's influence. Those who do respond usually show only a modest reduction in stuttering (see also Current Research).

Electronic devices closely resemble hearing aids that are inserted into one ear. These "fluency aids" serve to alter the individual's overall speaking behavior (i.e., a form of fluency shaping). Some devices use a technology called **altered auditory feedback** or AAF. When fitted with the device, an illusion is created where the client hears his or her own voice with either a delay or slight shift in pitch. The client needs to reduce their speaking rate and prolong vowels in order to minimize the effect of the alteration, which subsequently results in fluent speech. Some devices transmit **white noise**, which is acoustically similar to the sound of a waterfall. By introducing noise into the speaker's ear, they are unable to hear their own voice. This form of distraction has shown to decrease moments of stuttering in some, but not all, individuals.

The use of electronic devices is often considered at two points in the continuum of therapy. Based on consultation with an SLP, a client may use such a device when first entering treatment to assist with gaining initial control over severe stuttering. Once control is established, the device is no longer used and the person transitions into a traditional treatment program. Alternatively, an

electronic device also might be used when other forms of treatment have proved unsuccessful. The device is used on an everyday basis.

CULTURAL CONSIDERATIONS AND FLUENCY DISORDERS

Careful considerations are required in the diagnosis and management of fluency disorders among individuals from diverse cultural backgrounds. The multicultural perspectives of the client can (and should) influence clinical practice. For example, in some cultures, such as Chinese, stuttering is not considered to be a prevalent communication disorder and thus there is less emphasis placed on correcting the disorder. In some African nations the cause of this speech problem and its treatment are deeply rooted in "folk" ideas. Some of the reported causes of stuttering include tickling a baby too much, or leaving a newborn child out in the rain. Corresponding treatments include praying or applying ointments to the throat. Therefore, an SLP should not assume there is a universally agreed upon approach to the management of fluency disorders.

To illustrate this point, consider the two common traditional approaches to treating stuttering, fluency shaping, and stuttering modification. Stuttering modification therapies utilize a counseling based methodology with a primary aim of developing positive attitudes toward communication. Although this goal may seem to hold wide universal appeal, the structuring of this form of therapy requires cultural sensitivity. Counseling has its roots in psychology and there-

fore it is important to consider features such as race, language, economic class, and differing worldviews as potential barriers to the counseling process (Hickson & Christie, 1994). The stuttering modification treatment approach has the potential to become a complex and multidimensional process, especially in a context of varying multicultural perspectives and beliefs.

There are reports that fluency shaping therapies appear to have better acceptance compared to stuttering modification therapy by clients of diverse backgrounds (Cooper & Cooper, 2001). Fluency shaping approaches, at least in the earliest phases of treatment, tend to focus exclusively on gaining control of speech fluency with less emphasis on counseling. Fluency shaping has its roots in behavioral conditioning and programmed instruction, so this approach tends to bypass matters concerning cultural sensitivity. Regardless of the treatment approach selected, those that are currently available to the SLP will likely need to be modified to make them applicable in a multicultural context.

Another multicultural consideration when dealing with fluency disorders is the influence of **bilingualism**. Over 50% of the world's population is bilingual. Thus, the trend is that most people are able to speak more than one language, and people who only speak one language are becoming far less the norm. Also consider that roughly 1% of the population stutters. So, in the context of bilingualism, it would seem that at some point in the career of an SLP, they will be confronted with a bilingual speaker who stutters. There are mixed views concerning the characteristics of stuttering in bilingual speakers. Although it would seem obvious that a bilingual person who stutters in one language will show the same pattern in another language, the research to date does not support this view. Individuals are likely to stutter in both languages; however, the less dominant or least proficient language will show a higher percentage of stuttering (Van Borsel et al., 2001). Therefore, the bilingual person who stutters poses unique concerns in regard to diagnosis and management of the disorder. For example, can the SLP make an accurate diagnosis of a fluency disorder when listening to a language that is foreign? Is it possible to differentiate stuttering from cluttering? Should the treatment of fluency disorders focus on only one language or both? These are important questions that still await answers.

CURRENT RESEARCH IN FLUENCY DISORDERS

Research in the area of fluency disorders has been broad and extensive over the past century. The current trends are diverse and likely to change in years ahead. At present, there is exciting research occurring in four particular areas: (1) **pharmacology**, (2) **treatment efficacy**, (3) the **brain**, and (4) **temperament**.

Pharmacology

As mentioned earlier in this chapter, a wide range of drugs have been tested on individuals who stutter to determine whether symptoms of the disorder can be extinguished. Most of these drugs fall within the class of drugs known as benzodiazepines, which serve to decrease anxiety. Many have proven to be either ineffective or have side effects that hin-

der its application. The most promising research to date has come from the antianxiety drug known as **Pagoclone**. This drug is one of a class of medications known as non-benzodiazepines, which have similar effects to the benzodiazepine group, but with quite different chemical structures. Currently, there is a large multisite study occurring in the United States testing its effectiveness as a treatment for stuttering (Maguire et al., in press).

Treatment Efficacy

Although past clinical research related to the treatment of fluency disorders is large and offers a number of approaches to reducing stuttering, there is limited research looking at the effectiveness (i.e., efficacy) of the various approaches. It is not uncommon for drug companies to first test their product in a controlled clinical trial before distributing the drug for public use. A controlled trial is perhaps the ideal approach to validating the efficacy of treatment. Yet, this form of validation is nearly absent when considering various treatments for fluency disorders, or most communication disorders for that matter. To date, only one treatment program, the Lidcombe pro-

---

FYI

SLPs typically advise that when speaking with a person who stutters, it is appropriate to allow the person to complete their utterances. It is important to maintain good eye contact and refrain from interrupting or finishing a stuttered utterance for the person.

gram, has been evaluated along a clinical trials format. The results concerning the effectiveness of the program are promising (Jones et al., 2005).

The Brain

Dating back to the work of Lee Travis in the 1920s, there has been evidence to suggest that stuttering results from either a lack of brain dominance or competing hemispheres when it comes to producing speech. This contention has received a resurgence of interest, motivated in large part by new technologies available to directly visualize the brain, such as functional magnetic resonance imaging (fMRI) and positron emission tomography (PET) scanning. Results from recent research tend to support the earlier views of Travis that individuals who stutter may indeed show different brain organization and functioning compared to individuals who do not stutter (Ingham, 2007).

Temperament

Temperament is a personality trait associated with childhood and refers to how a child reacts to a situation. Although research in the mid-half of the 20th century focused a great deal on emotional factors related to stuttering, interest in the topic gradually faded. There now is renewed interest in the exploration of personality traits (e.g., temperament) in young children who stutter and how these traits might be linked to the persistence of stuttering in some children. Guitar (2006) hypothesized that a sensitive (i.e., reactive) temperament contributes to a child being vulnerable to the development of a stuttering problem.

FLUENCY DISORDERS ON THE WORLD WIDE WEB

Listed below are Web sites that provide further information on the topic of fluency disorders. At the time of publication each Web site was freely accessible.

Developmental Stuttering Video
http://www.webmd.com/video/stuttering-study

SpeechEasy
http://www.speecheasy.com/press-releases.html

Stuttering Foundation Videos
http://www.stutteringhelp.org/

International Stuttering Association
http://www.stutterisa.org/

Stigma of Stuttering Video
http://www.cbsnews.com/stories/2008/12/25/eveningnews/main4686616.shtml

REFERENCES

ASHA. (2007, Nov 6). Iowa stuttering study settlement. *ASHA Leader*, p. 8.

Cooper, E. B., & Cooper, C. S. (2001). Fluency disorders. In D. Battle (Ed.), *Communication disorders in multicultural populations* (3rd ed.). Oxford: Butterworth-Heinemann Medical.

Goberman, A., & Blomgren, M. (2003). Parkinsonian speech disfluencies: Effects of L-Dopa-related fluctuations. *Journal of Fluency Disorders*, 28, 55–70.

Guitar, B. (2006). *Stuttering: An integrated approach to its nature and treatment* (3rd ed.). Baltimore: Williams & Wilkins.

Hickson, J., & Christie, G. M. (1989). Research on cross-cultural counselling and psychotherapy: Implications for the South African context. *South African Journal of Psychology, 19*, 162–169.

Ingham, R. J. (2007) *Neuroimaging in communication sciences and disorders.* San Diego, CA: Plural.

Johnson, W. (1961). *Stuttering and what you can do about it.* Minneapolis: University of Minnesota Press.

Johnson, W., Darley, F., & Spriestersbach, D. (1963). *Diagnostic methods in speech pathology.* New York: Harper & Row.

Jones, M., Onslow, M., Packman, A., Williams, S., Ormond, T., Schwarz, T., & Gebski, V. (2005). A randomised controlled trial of the Lidcombe Program for early stuttering intervention. *British Medical Journal, 331,* 659–661.

Maguire, G., Franklin, D., Vatakis, N., Morgenshtern, E., Denko, T., Yaruss, S., . . . Riley, G. (in press). *Exploratory randomized clinical study of Pagoclone in persistent developmental stuttering: The EXPRESS Trial.* Journal of Clinical Pharmacology.

Onslow, M., Packman, A., & Harrison, E. (2003). The Lidcombe program of early stuttering intervention. *Overview of the Lidcombe program* (pp. 3–15). Austin, TX: Pro-Ed.

Perkins,W. H., Kent, R. D., & Curlee, R. R. (1991). A theory of neuropsycholinguistic function in stuttering. *Journal of Speech, Language, and Hearing Research, 34,* 734–752.

Postma, A., & Kolk, H. (1993). The covert repair hypothesis: Prearticulatory repair processes in normal and stuttered disfluencies. *Journal of Speech and Hearing Research, 36,* 472–487.

Riley, G. (1994). *Stuttering Severity Instrument-3.* Austin, TX: Pro-Ed.

Starkweather, C.W. (1997). Therapy for younger children. In R. F. Curlee & G. M. Siegel (Eds.), *Nature and treatment of stuttering* (2nd ed., pp. 257–279). Boston: Allyn and Bacon.

Van Borsel, J., Maes, E., & Foulon, S. (2001). Stuttering and bilingualism: A review. *Journal of Fluency Disorders, 26,* 179–205.

Van Riper, C. (1981). An early history of ASHA. *ASHA Magazine, 23*(11), 855–858.

Van Riper, C. (1982). *The nature of stuttering* (2nd ed.). Englewood Cliffs, NJ: Prentice-Hall.

Yairi, E., & Ambrose, N. (1992). A longitudinal study of stuttering in children: A preliminary report. *Journal of Speech, Language, and Hearing Research, 35,* 755–760.

Zebrowski, P., & Kelly, E. (2002). *Manual of stuttering intervention.* San Diego, CA: Singular.

CLEFT LIP AND PALATE

OBJECTIVES

After reading this chapter, the student should be able to:

- Demonstrate knowledge of the biological aspects of embryonic development that impact the process of developing a cleft.

- Understand the differences between normal lip/palate and cleft lip/palate anatomy and physiology.

- Describe the characteristics of different types of cleft lips and palates.

- Identify the impact of cleft lip and palate on speech and language development.

- Demonstrate knowledge regarding the fundamental aspects of assessing clients and students with cleft lip and palate.

- Have a basic knowledge of the surgical and nonsurgical management techniques for cleft lip and palate.

- Demonstrate basic knowledge of and be able to accurately identify the articulation, voice, and resonance characteristics which are typical of clients with cleft lip and palate.

- Demonstrate basic knowledge of the team concept in the habilitation of individuals (and families) who have cleft lip and palate.

- Identify cultural issues impacting individuals with cleft lip and palate.

- Identify current research issues in the area of cleft lip and palate.

INTRODUCTION

The birth of a child is one of the most joyous experiences in a parent's life. However, it is not uncommon for expectant parents to alternate between visions of a healthy baby and worries that the baby will be born with health problems. A **birth defect** is a problem that happens while a baby is developing in the mother's body. Birth defects are defined as abnormalities of structure, function, or body metabolism that are present at birth. Most birth defects happen during the first 3 months of pregnancy. The majority of babies with birth defects are born to two parents with no obvious health problems or risk factors; a woman can do everything her doctor recommends to deliver a healthy child and still have a baby with a birth defect. A cleft of the lip and/or palate is a birth defect that affects an estimated 6800 infants annually in the United States, according to the Centers for Disease Control and Prevention. Among the various types of communication disorders to be covered in this text, cleft lip and palate is by far the most physically obvious type of communication disorder.

TERMINOLOGY AND DEFINITIONS

A cleft of the lip or palate (CL/P) is defined as an elongated opening, resulting from failure of parts of the mouth to fuse or merge. A CL/P is an organic, developmental communication disorder. A CL/P is also a type of **craniofacial abnormality**, reflecting involvement of the bony features of the skull, as well as tissue features of the face. CL/P is the most common congenital abnormality. Because it is present at birth, the developmental disruptions that result in CL/P occur during the prenatal period of growth.

The study of prenatal growth and the developing process of an individual is

---

FYI

Some well-known people who were born with a CL/P include Wendy Harmer (comedian), Jesse Jackson (politician), Stacy Keach (actor), Nikki Payne (comedian), Joaquin Phoenix (actor), Peyton Manning (professional football player), and Cheech Marin (comedian). According to diagnostic imaging of the Egyptian Pharaoh Tutankhamun (1341–1323 BC), he too may have had a CL/P. (Image of Joaquin Phoenix. From H. Cauldfield at Wikimedia Commons. Released under the GNU Free Documentation License, CC-BY-SA-2.5.)

called the science of **embryology**. Human pregnancy is approximately 9 months (40 weeks) in duration. This time period starts immediately after conception, when the ovum is fertilized by sperm. The prenatal period is divided into three phases of pregnancy: the first phase is **zygote**, which is the period of conception through the first 2 weeks of pregnancy; the second phase is **embryo**, which is the period of 2 weeks through the eighth week; and the third phase of pregnancy is **fetus**, which is the period of 9 weeks through birth.

Physical formation of the face occurs during the period of embryonic development and early fetal development. A visual timeline of facial development is provided in Figure 7.1. Late in the first month of pregnancy, the baby's developing face and mouth is effectively split into two halves with the eyes and nose spread out toward the sides. The two sides gradually begin growing closer

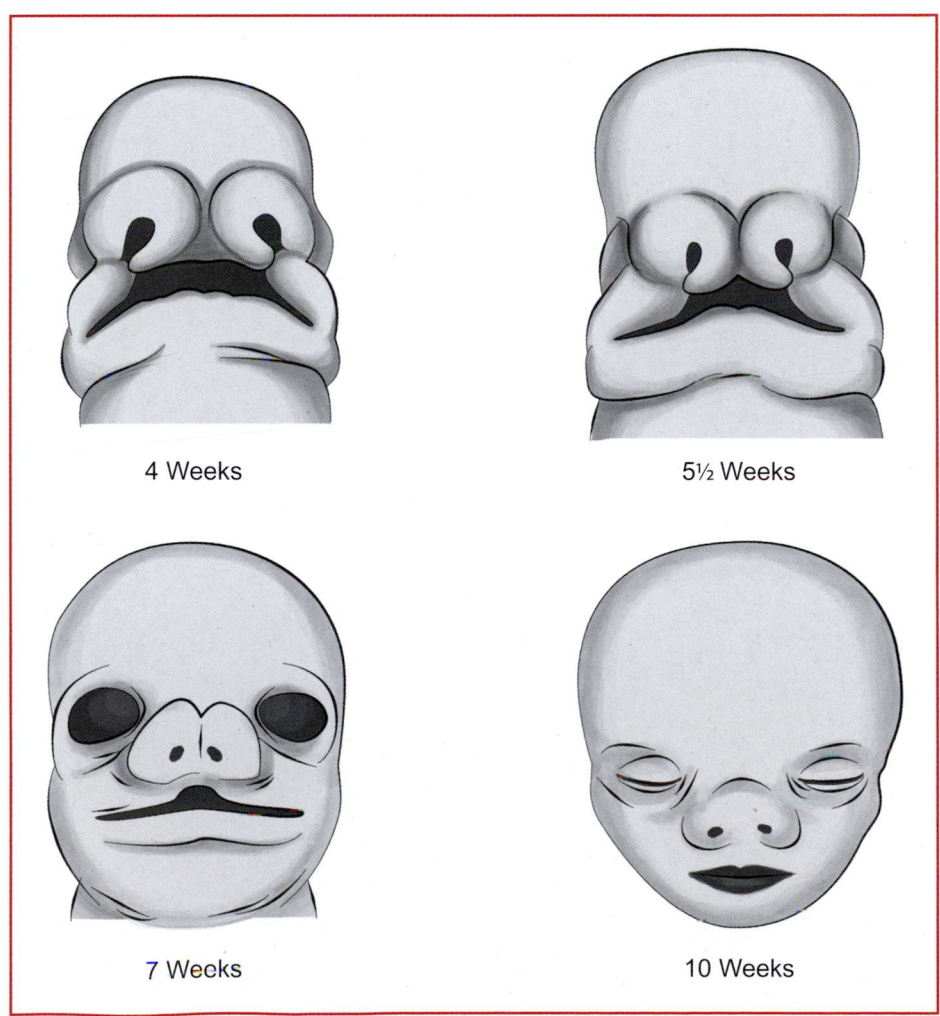

4 Weeks   5½ Weeks

7 Weeks   10 Weeks

FIGURE 7.1. Prenatal development of the face.

together beginning around the fourth week of prenatal development. First to fuse are the lips. The face continues developing and changing shape considerably. The eyes move forward, the nose comes together, and the face appears much narrower. Following fusion of the lips, the **alveolar** ridge is formed, which is the boney gum ridge that serves as sockets for our teeth. Next, the fusing seam travels backward to form the hard palate and then the soft palate (i.e., **velum**). The tip of the soft palate is called the **uvula**, and is recognized as the teardrop-shaped tissue that hangs at

the back of the throat. By the 12th week of pregnancy, the mouth is fully formed (Bzoch & Williams, 1979). An illustration in the timeline of palate development is provided in Figure 7.2.

Various landmarks on the face (Figure 7.3) that can be affected by a CL/P include the **columella**, which is the fleshy strip underneath the nose that separates the right and left nostrils (also called **nares**). The **philtrum** is the midline groove in the upper lip that runs from the top of the lip to the nose. The slight curve in the upper lip directly below the philtrum is called **Cupid's**

8th Week

9th Week

10th Week

12th Week

FIGURE 7.2. Major stages of hard and soft palate development during the 12 weeks of prenatal development.

FIGURE 7.3. Some anatomic landmarks of the face.

bow, said to resemble the bow of Cupid, the Roman god of love and beauty. The **vermilion border** is the edge of red pigment around the upper and lower lips of the mouth.

HISTORIC ASPECTS OF CLEFT LIP AND PALATE

For centuries, research and interest in CL/P was lacking because the deformity was thought to occur as a result of syphilis. Many children born with CL/P were unable to nurse, and subsequently failed to survive because of malnutrition. Others were simply left to die either because the birth defect was too hideous for society, or as a result of superstition. One of earliest reports of CL/P was by a French surgeon **Ambroise Pare** (1510–1590) who is considered the greatest surgeon of the 16th century (Figure 7.4). When discussing a patient with a cleft, Pare first coined the phrase, *le bec-de-lièvre* with an English transition of, "lip of the hare." He was merely observing that

FIGURE 7.4. Ambroise Pare, considered one of the greatest surgeons of the 16th century.

the lip was split, as is the lip of a rabbit (and several other animals). Among these animals, the split lip is used like forceps in picking up food (Figure 7.5).

A

B

FIGURE 7.5. Example of two animals that have a split lip used for grasping food during eating.

Unfortunately, this terminology led to the development of superstitions as to the cause of the disorder. For example, it was once believed that children with cleft lips were born to women who, when pregnant, were frightened by the devil, who had assumed the shape of a hare. In 1887, a passage was published in the journal of *Lancet* stating that one of the laws of heredity is that hideous physical impressions on the mind of a mother are capable of producing deformity and monstrosity in the offspring. Support of this notion was based on report at the time of a pregnant woman attending a carnival. One of the attractions she observed involved a trained horse pulling the trigger of a pistol, pretending to shoot a rabbit. Upon shooting, the rabbit was replaced with a stuffed (toy) rabbit that appeared to have had its head shot off. This greatly distressed the pregnant woman who later gave birth to a child resembling a rabbit. Fortunately, the term harelip is no longer in use and is considered demeaning. However, as a society, we have not yet moved beyond using names of animals

FYI

The occurrence of a CL/P is not unique to humans. They also are found in the animal world, including dogs and cats. Purebred dogs and cats are at the highest risk for CL/P, and they are most common in Boston terriers, Pekingese, bulldogs, beagles, cocker spaniels, dachshunds, and Siamese cats. Heredity is considered the primary cause of CL/P in animals.

to describe human conditions. For example, the phrase "pigeon-toed" is used to refer to the turning in of feet while walking, and "crow's feet," is a phrase used to refer to small wrinkles around the outer corners of the eyes.

Cosmetic surgery began in the ancient world. The Romans performed simple techniques such as repairing damaged ears. Physicians in ancient India used skin grafts for reconstructive work as early as 800 BC. The first report of surgical cleft lip repair came from China in 390 AD when an 18-year-old named Wei Yang Chi received the surgery. Chi subsequently became the Governor General of six Chinese Provinces (Rogers, 1971). The treatment consisted of cutting and stitching the edges of the cleft lip together, followed by 100 days of complete bed rest, when the patient could eat only thin gruel and was not allowed to smile or talk.

Jehan Yperman (1260–1331) was a medieval Belgian surgeon who is believed to have been the first person to provide a detailed description of cleft lip repair. Yperman published a treatise on surgery that so meticulously described the details of needle-and-suture surgery that some of his advice is still considered in modern surgical procedures (Figure 7.6).

The Swiss surgeon **Pierre Franco** (1506–1580) is known as the "Father of Cleft Palate Surgery." In 1556 he described in detail the principles and techniques for repairing a cleft of the palate. Because of the dangers associated with surgery in any form, especially that involving the head or face, the repair of CL/P was almost nonexistent until the 19th century. Besides, in the absence of anesthesia the operation was extremely painful. It was not until the 19th and 20th centuries that such surgeries became commonplace.

FIGURE 7.6. Example of the 13th–14th century surgical treatise written by medieval surgeon Jehan Yperman. Techniques related to cleft lip repair were included in the treatise.

Some of the well known CL/P surgeons during the 1800s included the Germans **Karl Ferdinand von Graefe** (1787–1840) (Figure 7.7), **Johann Friedrich Dieffenbach** (1792–1847), **Bernard von Langenbeck** (1810–1887) (Figure 7.8), and **Philip Gustav Passavant** (1815–1893). Von Graefe was a pioneer of plastic and reconstructive surgery. Dieffenbach applied his surgical talents to the correction of CL/P, as well as other communicative disorders such as stuttering (see also Chapter 6). Von Langenbeck was a skilled surgeon who developed a procedure for the closure of the hard palate. Passavant was a dedicated surgeon who was interested in developing surgical techniques to help improve speech production. In particular, he recommended reconstruction of the velar muscles and lengthening of the soft palate as important steps to helping individuals develop normal speech.

During the time of CL/P repairs in the mid-1800s, infants and children were rarely operated on and most patients were mature adults with speech defects that were nearly impossible to correct. However, as improvements were introduced in surgical techniques and anesthesia, the age of the patients receiving surgery gradually became younger. One of the first surgeons to recognize the importance of speech therapy was **Carl Casper von Siebold** (1736–1807) (Figure 7.9). He conducted detailed studies of the speech difficulties of a 3-year-old boy with a CL/P and noted that he had difficulty pronouncing the letters b, s, z, and r. Siebold expressed deep regret at the "impossibility" of correcting this defect surgically.

The effect of CL/P on speech was also studied in the United States by **Matthew Wilson** (1734–1802). Wilson was an American Revolutionary War minister and physician who wrote a compendium of medicine called the *Therapeutic Alphabet* that contained an alphabetical listing of diseases, symptoms, and their cures. Among the various listings was a reference to CL/P and the poor speech pronunciation that accompanied the affliction.

FIGURE 7.7. Karl Ferdinand von Graefe, a cleft lip and palate surgeon of the 1800s.

FIGURE 7.8. Bernard von Langenbeck was a skilled surgeon who developed a procedure for the closure of the hard palate.

FIGURE 7.9. Carl Casper von Siebold. One of the first cleft lip and palate surgeons to recognize the importance of speech therapy for his patients.

Herbert K. Cooper (1897–1978) established the first CL/P clinic in the United States when his recognition of the need for multidisciplinary involvement resulted in the formation of a unique clinic in 1939. It was the first of its kind, having all the necessary dental and surgical specialists in one location. The team concept Cooper created is still the accepted standard of care for children with CL/P. The clinic remains in existence in Pennsylvania and has been renamed the Herbert Cooper-Lancaster Cleft Palate Institute.

DISORDERS OF CLEFT LIP AND PALATE

Clefts of the lip and palate can be categorized according to the affected structures and location of the cleft. The degree of clefting is related to the amount of embryonic damage to the lip and palate.

Cleft Lip

If the cleft does not affect the palate structure of the mouth, it is referred to as cleft lip. When the cleft occurs on only one side of the upper lip, it is called a **unilateral cleft lip**. When it occurs on both sides of the upper lip, it is called a **bilateral cleft lip**. When the cleft results in a gap that goes all the way from the lip and mouth into the nostril, it is referred to as a **complete cleft lip**. When the gap does not extend from the mouth all the way into the nostril, it is an **incomplete cleft**. When the incomplete cleft lip is very minor (a groove or a notch), it is called a **microform cleft**. A microform cleft can appear as small as a slight indentation in the vermilion border of the lip or look like a scar from the lip up to the nostril. Examples of the various types of cleft lip are shown in Figure 7.10.

Cleft Palate

A cleft palate can be either complete or incomplete. A **complete cleft palate** involves an opening between the hard and soft palates that extends through to the uvula. In most cases, a cleft lip is also present in conditions of a complete cleft of the hard palate. An **incomplete cleft palate** is a condition in which the hard palate may be fully developed with a cleft only found for the soft palate. In these cases, it is likely there is no cleft of the lip. Another less common and minor form of cleft palate is known as a **submucous cleft**. In this condition there is a cleft of the muscular layer of the soft palate with an intact layer of mucosa lying over the defect. A telltale sign of a submucous cleft is a bifid (or notched) uvula. In most cases, a submucous cleft does not adversely affect swallowing and speech production. Examples of

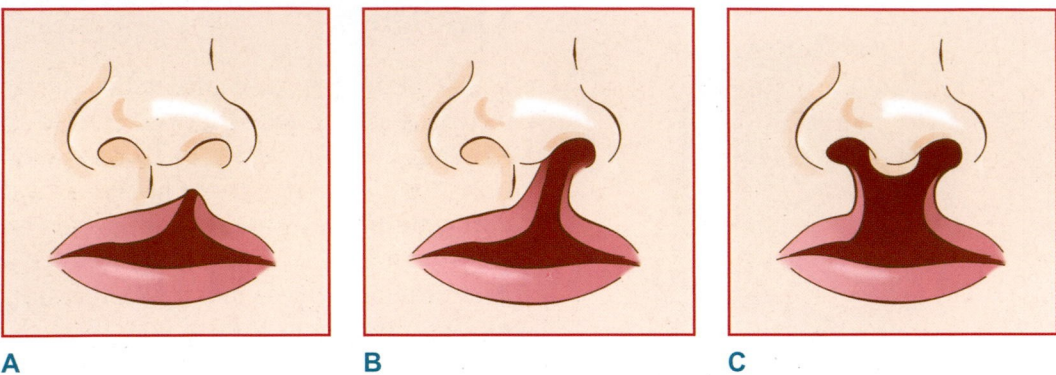

A   B   C

FIGURE 7.10. Types of cleft lip: unilateral incomplete cleft lip (**A**), unilateral complete cleft lip (**B**), and a bilateral complete cleft lip (**C**).

A   B   C

FIGURE 7.11. Types of cleft palate: incomplete cleft of the soft palate only (**A**), unilateral complete cleft of lip and palate (**B**), and a bilateral complete cleft of lip and palate (**C**).

various types of clefts to the hard palate are shown in Figure 7.11.

Characteristics of Cleft Lip and Palate

Approximately 50% of all clefts involve a cleft of both lip and palate. A cleft of the lip alone, or the palate alone, each account for 25% of all clefts, respectively. Instances when there are isolated clefts of the lip or palate alone are most often associated with birth defects affecting other parts of the body and/or brain. Ten percent of cleft lips are incomplete. Approximately 85% of cases of bilateral cleft lip and 70% of unilateral cleft lip

also involve a cleft of the palate. Cleft lip and palate is more common on the left side, less common on the right, and least common bilaterally. There are sex differences in the occurrence of various types of clefts: males are twice as likely to have a cleft lip and palate or an isolated cleft of the lip compared to females; females are twice as likely to have an isolated cleft of the palate compared to males. So across the various types of clefts, males are far more likely to be born with a cleft compared to females.

The occurrence of CL/P varies considerably according to race. In the United States, American Indians show the highest occurrence of clefting with 7 per 10,000 live births, followed by Latinos with a prevalence of 5 per 10,000 live births. Among the Japanese population, the occurrence of CL/P is 4.5 per 10,000, and among the Chinese, the occurrence is 3.4 per 10,000 live births. Among Caucasians, the occurrence of CL/P is approximately 2 per 10,000 births. The lowest occurrence of CL/P is found among African American births with only 0.6 per 10,000 births.

The prevalence of CL/P also differs among various countries around the world. The prevalence of children born with CL/P in the United Kingdom is around 3 per 10,000 live births, similar to what is found in Arab countries. In Australia, Canada, and New Zealand the prevalence is approximately 7 per 10,000 births. At the extreme ends of the continuum, Cuba and South Africa show fewer than 2 children with CL/P per 10,000 births, whereas Finland and Malta have more than 14 CL/P births per 10,000.

CURRENT THEORIES OF CLEFT LIP AND PALATE

The exact cause of CL/P is not completely understood. Cleft lip and/or cleft palate are caused by multiple genes inherited from both parents, as well as environmental factors that scientists do not yet fully understand. About 25% of occurrences of CL/P can be attributed solely to genetic inheritance. If either parent has a cleft, the relative risks become about 5%t higher for having a baby with a cleft compared to nonclefted parents. If both parents have clefts, the risks are much greater. When a combination of genes and environmental factors cause a condition, the inheritance is called **multifactorial** (i.e., many factors contribute to the cause). By far, the majority of children born with a CL/P acquire the condition as a result of combined genetic and environmental factors. There are a number of environmental conditions that interact with one or more genes to increase the risk of CL/P. These include: (1) lack of a balanced diet, (2) maternal illness, (3) cigarette smoking, (4) alcohol consumption, and (5) chronic use of nonprescribed drugs or substance abuse. The risk of CL/P is found to be higher among pregnant women older than 35 years of age, as well as among teenaged pregnancies (Slavkin, 1992).

ASSESSMENT OF CLEFT LIP AND PALATE

Because clefting causes very obvious physical changes, diagnosis of the condition is straightforward. As ultrasound testing becomes increasingly common in

---

FYI

The cause of CL/P most often is attributed to a combination of genetic and environmental factors. However, a group of scientists at the University of Bonn in Germany recently found that a genetic variant on chromosome 8 occurs with significantly higher frequency in people with CL/P than those without a cleft. Although the exact gene on chromosome 8 has yet to be identified, these results point to genes playing a far more important role in the formation of CL/P than previously thought.

routine obstetric practice and its accuracy improves, prenatal diagnosis of CL/P is now a reality. Developments in ultrasound technology have enabled the identification of major facial anomalies as early as 12 weeks gestation. If the cleft has not been detected in an ultrasound prior to the baby's birth, a physical examination at birth of the mouth, nose and palate confirms the presence of CL/P. Aside from the obvious physical features which serve to confirm the assessment of CL/P, there are related areas that are also assessed in regard to the child's health status and these include: (1) feeding, (2) hearing, (3) dentition, and (4) communication.

Feeding

Normally, in order for an infant to feed (suck), he needs to squeeze the nipple with the lips between the tongue and alveolar ridge at the same time maintaining suction during the act of swallowing. The muscular motions of the jaw and soft palate at the back of the mouth allow suction to draw the milk. For an infant with CL/P, sucking is a much more difficult task. Depending on the location and severity of the cleft, it is a challenge for the infant to maintain suction of the breast or bottle. Swallowing air is likely, and babies with clefts need thorough burping. Most babies with CL/P are fed with a bottle, although breastfeeding is not precluded and may be attempted in some cases. It is possible the infant may need to wear a prosthetic palate called an **obturator** to help him or her eat properly. The infant needs to be positioned in a nearly upright position during feeding so as to prevent milk from coming through the nose (Figure 7.12). Positioning the baby upright also limits

FIGURE 7.12. Feeding a baby with a cleft lip and palate. The infant is positioned in an upright position to prevent milk from entering the nasal cavity.

choking and helps to decrease the risk of ear infections.

Hearing

Almost all babies with CL/P are likely to acquire **otitis media** (ear infections) at some point during the first year of life. The common occurrence of otitis media is due to the fact that the muscles that move the palate also open the **eustachian tube**, which runs from the back of the throat into the middle ear space (see Chapter 12). Its primary function is to ventilate the middle ear and also to drain any accumulated secretions or debris from the middle ear space. Among children with CL/P, these muscles are deficient or abnormal. Although short bouts of otitis media are common in most children, persistent otitis media may cause permanent hearing loss. Treatment for this problem typically involves careful observation by the family physician and audiologist. In most instances, **pressure equalization** (PE) tubes (sometimes called "grommets") are surgically inserted through the eardrum to improve ventilation in the middle ear. These temporary tubes enable the child to hear better and serve to decrease the number of ear infections (see also Chapter 13).

Dentition

Children with CL/P, particularly a cleft affecting the alveolar (gum) ridge are likely to develop dental problems such as missing or malformed teeth. These dental problems may occur unilaterally or bilaterally (depending on the cleft). Because the young infant is not born with teeth, and his first set of teeth will eventually fall out, special planning is needed to solve the functional and cosmetic dental problems that a cleft can create. In about 25% of children with a unilateral CL/P, the upper jaw (maxilla) growth does not keep up with the lower jaw (mandible) growth. If this occurs, the child may need **orthognathic** surgery. This type of surgery involves manipulation of various facial bones to restore the proper anatomic and functional relationship between the teeth and jaws. Fortunately, dental experts can successfully treat most problems resulting from CL/P.

Communication

It is common for children who are born with CL/P to have communication problems at some time in their young lives. Over half of them will require speech therapy at some point during early childhood. However, many children who are born with CL/P develop normal speech by 5 years of age. Children with CL/P are likely to experience problems in two domains of communication: (1) voice and (2) speech articulation.

Voice

The particular voice problem associated with CL/P concerns the ability to regulate air flowing through the nasal cavity during speech production. During normal speech production, the nasal cavity is typically closed off from the oral cavity by elevating the velum against the back of the throat (pharynx). This process is referred to as **velopharyngeal closure** (Figure 7.13). You can observe velopharyngeal closure by facing a mirror, opening your mouth, and saying "ahhh," as your doctor might have you say during a routine visit. At the precise moment of turning on your voice, you should observe the uvula elevate and press against the back of the throat.

In cases of CL/P, the palatal structures may be impaired resulting in a lack of closure between the two cavities. The inability to close off the nasal cavity from the mouth is called **velopharyngeal inadequacy (VPI)**. The end result is that excessive air flows through the nasal cavity, which is referred to as **hypernasal** speech. Children who have VPI may sound like they are "talking through their noses." Approximately 25% of children who undergo repair of a cleft palate may still show signs of VPI. Assessment of VPI can be accomplished in a number of ways. By placing a mirror directly below the nose, and having the child speak, one is able to determine whether excessive nasal airflow is occurring by simply noting whether the mirror fogs up. A second approach involves either directly listen-

A   B

FIGURE 7.13. Depiction of velopharyngeal opening (**A**) and velopharyngeal closure (**B**).

ing to nasal airflow or using an instrument to measure the amount of airflow exiting the nose during speech production (Figure 7.14).

Speech Articulation

Not only are the lips and palate essential for eating, but like the teeth, tongue, and other throat and mouth structures, they are also used to produce speech. When we speak, the stream of air from the lungs passes through the vocal tract and is shaped to produce the many different consonant and vowel sounds used to create strings of words. Nearly all of the sounds of English involve closure of the nasal cavity and the sounds are directed through the mouth. The only exceptions are the nasal consonants /m/ (e.g., me), /n/ (e.g., no), and /ŋ/ (e.g., sing), which all have a natural nasal quality to their production. In the case of VPI, the consonants and vowels that normally are produced through the mouth are now produced through the mouth *and* nose.

Due to advances in surgical techniques, speech articulation is seldom a problem. However if problems with speech articulation do exist, they are related to two particular classes of speech sounds. These are stop consonants (i.e., p, t, k, b, d, g) and fricative consonants (e.g., s, z, f, v, th, sh). These consonants require the buildup of a large amount of air pressure inside the oral cavity to be produced correctly. For stop consonants, air pressure is created behind a point of constriction (such as the closed lips for /p/) and then suddenly released. If the child is unable to maintain a sufficient amount of pressure at this point of constriction because of air escaping through the nose, the subsequent production of this consonant is likely to be weak. The child may acquire a **compensatory strategy** to this situation by producing a **glottal stop** (ʔ). A glottal stop is articulated deep in the vocal tract and thus bypasses any possible nasal emission that would occur in the forward flow of speech. Acoustically, it sounds like the break separating the syllables of the

A

FIGURE 7.14. Detecting velopharyngeal insufficiency (hypernasal airflow) through the use of a mirror (**A**), listening device (**B**), and an airflow detecting instrument (**C**).

B

C

interjection *uh-oh*. For the production of fricatives, high oral air pressure is required to maintain a forward flow of air "friction" (such as in the production of /v/). If the child is unable to maintain a sufficient amount of air pressure for fricatives, the sound will be substituted by some fricative sound made in the pharynx. This sound is called a **pharyngeal fricative** (ʕ) and is produced by vibrations set-up between the back of the tongue and the pharyngeal wall. Acoustically, the sound resembles the /h/ but it is made with increased friction in the back of the throat.

TREATMENT OF CLEFT LIP AND PALATE

A child with CL/P will need to see a variety of specialists who work together as a team to treat the condition and improve the quality of life. Treatment usually begins in the first few months of an infant's life, depending on the health of the infant and the extent of the cleft. Various forms of treatment can extend until the patient reaches early adulthood (Table 7.1). The need for assembling a team of heath professionals is related to the concept of the **whole child** and the many facets related to human growth and cognitive development that is found across various health disciplines. The use of a team also is an ideal way of managing complex medical problems and avoids rigid compartmentalization of various specialties in medical practice. The notion that many brains are better than one prevails in working with children who have complex needs. The concept of a **cleft palate team** was first developed by Herbert Cooper in 1939 and has continued to serve as the preferred model of health care for children with CL/P. The principal role of the multidisciplinary team is to provide integrated case management for the child and to ensure the quality and continuity of care and long-term follow-up. A typical cleft palate team consists of:

- Audiologist, who manages ongoing hearing status.
- Geneticist, who screens child for possible syndromes and counsels parents for future pregnancies.
- Orthodontist, who straightens the teeth and aligns the jaw.
- Otolaryngologist, who monitors middle ear problems.
- Pediatrician, who monitors the child's overall health and development.
- Pediatric dentist, who makes prosthetic devices for the mouth.
- Psychologist or social worker, to support the family and assess any adjustment problems.
- Speech-language pathologist, who treats communication and feeding problems.
- Surgeon, who manages the cleft repair.

FYI

Young children who have dental problems resulting from a CL/P are treated by a pedodontist. A pedodontist is a dentist specialized in handling children. Generally, treating a child may take two or three times longer than the same procedure for an adult.

Table 7.1. Typical Timeline of Treatment for a Child Born With Cleft Lip and Palate

Age	Treatment
1 month	Evaluation of feeding
	Hearing evaluation
	Dental evaluation
	Emotional support for families
	Planning for upcoming surgery
3 months	Repair of cleft lip
3–12 months	Continued dental evaluations
	Hearing evaluation
	Speech evaluation
1 year	Repair of cleft palate
	Insertion of pressure equalization tubes if required
1–5 years	Annual hearing and speech evaluation
	Dental evaluation
	Evaluation of child emotional development
	Occasional lip and palate revision surgery to minimize deformity
5–9 years	Orthodontic preparation before permanent teeth erupt
	Continued speech evaluations
9–20 years	Orthodontic treatment
	Minor lip and nose surgical revisions

All of the specialties contributing to the cleft palate team are important and provide a valuable contribution to the well-being of a child with CL/P. Specific forms of treatment offered by the surgeon, SLP, and psychologist are detailed below.

Surgery

Cleft palates have to be surgically repaired before the baby is ready to speak. There is no worldwide consensus on the surgical techniques for repair of CL/P. The decision as to when and how to repair a cleft lip or palate is based on a variety of factors such as facial growth, speech development, and psychological impact on the child and family. As a general rule, a child born with a cleft of the lip (with or without a cleft of the palate), usually has the lip repaired at approximately 3 months of age. Repair of the palate is usually performed between 9 to 15 months of age. The primary reason for repairing the lip earlier than the palate is to permit as near normal feeding as possible. Another reason is to improve the appearance of the child in regard to social acceptance. Repair of the palate is performed primarily for speech purposes. Without an intact hard and soft palate, it would be nearly impossible for the child to produce intelligible speech.

Other surgical treatments for cleft deformities occur during the teenage years, and may include nasal reconstruction and possible jaw alignment. However, this latter surgery is typically delayed until growth of the facial skeleton is complete. In addition to the surgical procedures that are designed to repair the palatal and facial structures, there are additional procedures performed to assist with speech production. Some children may continue to demonstrate VPI following initial palate repair. Sometimes the palate is still not able to close off the nose from the mouth. This may be because it is too short, does not stretch far enough backward and upward, or does not move quickly enough. A widely performed surgical procedure to eliminate VPI is the creation of a **pharyngeal flap**, and is usually performed between 6 to 12 years of age (Figure 7.15). Another surgical procedure is the sphincter **pharyngoplasty**. In this procedure, the surgeon moves tissue from the back of the throat closer to the back of the palate. This surgery is recommended when the surgeon decides that the palate is working as well as it can, but the back of the throat (pharynx) is not moving correctly (see Figure 7.15).

A frequently chosen surgical approach for improving velopharyngeal function is the option of a prosthetic device (i.e., **obturator**) for some patients. These speech aids are placed in the mouth, much like an orthodontic re-tainer. One common type of obturator is a speech bulb (Figure 7.16), which is designed to partially close off the space between the soft palate and the throat. An acrylic ball is attached to an acrylic (dental) retainer held by the teeth. The bulb is tailored to the vocal tract anatomy and physiology of the patient. Many professionals feel that prosthetic appliances work best in children who are at least 5 years of age.

Speech-Language Therapy

Since the early creation of the speech-language pathology profession, there has been high interest in the communication characteristics among individuals with CL/P. From 1940 to 1960, many SLPs believed that children with CL/P showed oral-motor problems that prevented them from producing clear speech. As a means of addressing this assumed problem, children with CL/P were asked to undergo a number of activities designed to strengthen the speech musculature. Some of these strengthening exercises involved swallowing, sucking, blowing, and whistling. Tasks such as these were later discredited during the 1960s and 1970s because research failed to substantiate an improvement in speech articulation. That is, the children may have shown improvements in their abilities to blow and whistle but these nonspeech activities did not transfer to speaking ability. We now know that a typical child with CL/P does not have oral motor problems.

Although current medical technology is not advanced enough to prevent the occurrence of CL/P, most of the speech problems associated with CL/P can be improved or even corrected. There is no doubt that a child with an

A

B

FIGURE 7.15. Illustration of pharyngeal flap (**A**) and pharyngoplasty (**B**).

unrepaired CL/P will experience severe speech difficulties. However, this is becoming the exception rather than the norm. Following surgery, only 10% of children are likely to experience a communication disorder. For those whom speech articulation difficulties may persist, the use of conventional articulation/phonology therapy approaches is preferred. A second area of concern is in regard to the child's voice, specifically the production of **hypernasal speech**. This condition may be corrected surgically (see previous section). However, in the event the child still demonstrates VPI, some form of therapy may be required. The use of devices that provide the child with visual or auditory

A
B

FIGURE 7.16. Example of a prosthetic device called a bulb obturator. The device is fit to the hard palate similar to a dental retainer. The bulb assists with maintaining velopharyngeal closure for speech production.

feedback regarding the amount of speech nasality has proven to be successful. The feedback guides the child in learning alternative strategies for maintaining appropriate closure between the oral and nasal cavities during speaking activities.

Psychology

Psychosocial issues are a critical part of the assessment and management of the child with CL/P and must be addressed from the onset of care. The birth of a child is always a time of great family adjustment, and it is especially stressful when the child is born with a birth defect such as CL/P. Parents often experience feelings of sadness, guilt, anger, and fear for their child's future social acceptance. Our society often focuses on people's appearance, which can make childhood, especially the teenage years,

an emotionally challenging time for someone with a physical difference. Depending on the severity of the cleft, quality of the surgery, and the effect on speech clarity, a child with CL/P may experience painful teasing or seclusion, which can damage self-esteem. Chan et al. (2006) summarized the research examining the psychosocial influences on CL/P and found that 70% of children with CL/P and their parents reported having to deal with teasing and ostracism because of their cleft. Teachers have been found to misjudge the intelligence of students with CL/P with more noticeable facial disfigurement, and this may lead to reduced teacher expectations and poor school performance. Teachers also have rated school-aged children with CL/P as more withdrawn and inhibited compared to children without CL/P, and this has been associated with academic underachievement of children with CL/P. Upon entering the workforce, people with CL/P have been viewed negatively by prospective employers. Although the majority of children and adults may not experience major psychosocial consequences as a result of CL/P, a recent large systematic review of the literature suggests that behavioral problems, depression, and anxiety are associated with the disorder for some individuals (Hunt et al., 2005). One role of the cleft palate team is to provide psychological and emotional support personnel who can help address emotional and social issues. A major goal for parents is to nurture their children so that they have a positive sense of self and ultimately make a contribution to their community.

CULTURAL CONSIDERATIONS AND CLEFT LIP AND PALATE

The management of children with CL/P may require special multicultural considerations. The cultural variations that are likely to exist in families should be recognized so as to encourage their participation in the team approach. Traditional religious, as well as philosophical, beliefs are known to affect the attitudes of various cultural groups toward birth defects such as CL/P. For example, there are reports that Chinese have misapprehensions and superstitions toward people with CL/P. Bebout and Arthur (1997) surveyed a group of Cantonese-speaking Americans and found that some individuals considered the speech produced by individuals with CL/P as indicative of an emotional disturbance and felt that persons with CL/P could "try harder" in order to speak in a less disordered manner. Meyerson (1990)

notes that Latinos from many geographic subgroups (Mexico, Central America) have attributed the cause of CL/P to a number of folk theories including: (1) an eclipse of the moon, (2) God's punishment of sins, (3) paternal alcoholism, (4) venereal disease, and (5) emotional stress during pregnancy. Even if folk explanations or folk treatments are rejected by members of the cleft palate team, it should not be viewed as negatively influencing the goals for the patient. Unless these alternative treatments are suspected of causing physical harm or mental harm to the patient, they should be viewed as an adjunct to the treatment plan.

In many countries there is limited medical and rehabilitation support for people with CL/P. Individuals may go through their entire lives with an unrepaired CL/P. In 1982, an American plastic surgeon, William Magee, and his wife Kathleen, a nurse and clinical social worker, traveled to the Philippines and volunteered their time to help repair facial clefts for those who did not have access to medical care. The country's demand for repair of clefts far exceeded what the couple was able to accomplish during their visit. In response to this initial visit to the Philippines, various volunteer agencies have since been established that are designed to provide assistance

FYI

The type of doctor who usual performs a CL/P operation is a craniofacial surgeon, which is a subspecialty of plastic surgery. Craniofacial surgery deals with congenital and acquired deformities of the skull, face, and jaws.

to some of the world's poorest countries in the management of CL/P. Two of the better known agencies are **Operation Smile** and **Smile Train**. Trained surgeons and other members of a cleft palate team donate their time and services to travel to various countries and quickly treat a high number of cases in a 1- to 2-week period. The stated mission of these organizations is to provide free CL/P surgery for millions of poor children in developing countries until there are no more children who need help and the problems contributing to CL/P have been completely eradicated.

CURRENT RESEARCH IN CLEFT LIP AND PALATE

Surgical Timing

Over 25 years ago, surgeons at the University of California (San Francisco) performed the first fetal surgery as a last-chance operation to save a dying baby. They partially removed the fetus from inside a pregnant woman's uterus, repaired a urinary obstruction, and then resealed the fetus into the mother's womb. Since then, fetal surgery has been performed on a number of occasions to repair a problem before a baby is born. Surgery before birth can be immediately

life saving for a fetus at risk, or it may alter the course of physical development, resulting in a more favorable condition after birth. Although it is not yet a reality, researchers are discussing the likelihood of fetal surgery in the management of CL/P (Berge et al., 2001). At the moment, surgeons are not clinically ready to repair fetal CL/P and the risks to the fetus and mother from the surgery are far too high. Fetal surgery for non-life-threatening conditions, such as CL/P, will become possible only when it is proven to be routinely safe for both mother and fetus. Ultimately, the likelihood of performing fetal surgery for CL/P will be based on the ability to accurately identify fetuses with clefts and exclude those that have severe associated anomalies.

Early Intervention

Over the years, much has been written about the communication problems associated with CL/P and the strategies that can be employed to remediate these problems. Traditionally, however, this research has focused on the voice and speech articulation problems demonstrated by preschool and school-age children. Past research assumed that CL/P did not affect the communication abilities of children until after they began

---

FYI

While most conditions of CL/P are of a congenital nature, it is possible for CL/P to be acquired. Oral cancer affecting either the hard or soft palate would necessitate removal of these structures, thereby creating a clefting condition. Cancer of either the hard or soft palate accounts for approximately 2% of all head and neck cancers.

producing meaningful speech. More recently, there has been a push to provide intervention to children at a much earlier age to lessen the impact of clefting on communication skills of children with CL/P (Hardin-Jones et al., 2006). Intervention techniques for infants and toddlers with CL/P include a variety of approaches depending on the age and linguistic level, and the profile of communicative strengths and weaknesses of the child. The techniques combine early language intervention methods with speech production strategies to facilitate accurate voice and speech articulation skills.

CLEFT LIP AND PALATE ON THE WORLD WIDE WEB

Listed below are Web sites that provide further information on the topic of cleft lip and palate. At the time of publication each Web site was freely accessible.

Cleft Palate Foundation
http://www.cleftline.org/

Smile Train Video
http://www.smiletrain.org

Operation Smile Video
http://www.operationsmile.org/

WebMD Video: Cleft Palate
http://www.webmd.com/video/new-cleft-palate-procedure

What to Do: Cleft Lip and Palate Video
http://www.5min.com/Video/What-to-do—Cleft-lip—Cleft-Palate-38562823

REFERENCES

Bebout, L., & Arthur, B. (1997). Attitudes toward speech disorders: Sampling the views of Cantonese-speaking Americans. *Journal of Communication Disorders, 30,* 205–229.

Bergé, S. J., Plath, H., Van de Vondel, P. T., Thorsten, A., Niederhagen, B., von Lindern, J. J., . . . Hansmann, M. (2001). Fetal cleft lip and palate: Sonographic diagnosis, chromosomal abnormalities, associated anomalies and postnatal outcome in 70 fetuses. *Ultrasound Obstetrics and Gynecology, 18,* 422–431.

Bzoch, K., & Williams, W. (1979). Introduction, rationale, principles, and related basic embryology, and anatomy. In K. Bzoch (Ed.), *Communicative disorders related to cleft lip and palate* (2nd ed.). Boston: Little, Brown & Co.

Chan, R., McPherson, B., & Whitehill, T. (2006). Chinese attitudes toward cleft lip and palate: Effects of personal contact. *Cleft Palate–Craniofacial Journal, 43,* 731–739.

Hardin-Jones, M., Chapman, K., & Scherer, N. J. (2006, June 13). Early intervention in children with cleft palate. *ASHA Leader, 11*(8–9), 32.

Hunt, O., Burden, D., Hepper, P., & Johnston, C. (2005). The psychosocial effects of cleft lip and palate: A systematic review. *European Journal of Orthodontics, 27,* 274–285.

Meyerson, M. (1990). Cultural considerations in the treatment of Latinos with craniofacial malformations. *Cleft Palate Journal, 27,* 279–288.

Rogers, B. (1971). History of cleft lip and palate treatment. In W. Grabb, S. Rosenstein, & K. Bzoch (Eds.), *Cleft lip and palate: Surgical, dental, and speech aspects,* (pp. 371–390). Boston: Little Brown.

Slavkin, H. C. (1992). Incidence of cleft lips, palates rising. *Journal of the American Dental Association, 123,* 61–65.

Acquired and Genetic Communication Disorders

VOICE DISORDERS

OBJECTIVES

After reading this chapter, the student should be able to:

- Demonstrate an understanding of anatomic, neurologic bases of vocal behavior, and physiologic processes of normal voice production.

- Demonstrate an understanding of the historical aspects of normal voice production and advances in the profession of otolaryngology.

- Demonstrate an understanding of current theories in voice production.

- Demonstrate an understanding of current research areas in the area of normal voice production and voice disorders.

- Demonstrate knowledge of the occurrence, classification, and symptoms of voice disorders.

- Describe appropriate counseling strategies and features of vocal hygiene.

- Demonstrate knowledge of laryngectomy including physiologic changes, and the various options for alaryngeal speech.

- Describe sociocultural influences in voice disorders.

INTRODUCTION

The use of **voice** is an integral part of communication. Dogs bark, growl, and howl. Cats purr and mew. Birds use different calls to warn other birds about threats or food. Each animal has a distinct voice and all animal species have some form of set vocal patterns that they use to communicate. The use of voice allows animals to recognize each other and convey messages like "get away," "danger," and "that feels good." Humans also use voice to communicate basic needs and wants. Because humans have also developed the capacity to use language, our use of voice has become more specialized. When we open our mouths to speak, the voice we use is uniquely special to us. Our voice is one of the defining features of our individuality, and it shares a lot of information about you. It tells others if you are happy or sad, healthy or unwell, young or old. Our voice can also reveal to others our background, such as the region of the world where we live, and even our social economic status. Although some people are expert at voice impersonations, our voice is what helps to define who we are. Indeed, many past and present celebrities are readily identifiable as a result of their voice. A list of some well-known voices is provided in Table 8.1. A "normal voice" is one that is pleasing to the ear, has a balance of sound through the mouth and nose, and matches a person's size, age, and sex. When a voice is produced that is perceived by others as unusual or strange and draws attention to the person who is speaking, it is quite likely the person is demonstrating a voice disorder.

Table 8.1. Unmistakable Voices of Well-Known and Some Not So Well-Known Celebrities

Humphrey Bogart	Actor
Bette Davis	Actor
Janeane Garofalo	Actor
Cary Grant	Actor
Arnold Schwarzenegger	Actor
Sylvester Stallone	Actor
Luciano Pavarotti	Singer
Elvis Presley	Singer
Justin Timberlake	Singer
Madonna	Singer
Kanye West	Singer
Bing Crosby	Singer
Barbra Streisand	Singer
Christopher Martin	Singer
Nat King Cole	Singer
Dan Castellaneta	Voice of Homer Simpson
James Earl Jones	Voice of Darth Vader
Andy Serkis	Voice of Gollum—Lord of the Rings
Frank Oz	Voice of Yoda—Star Wars
Mel Blanc	Voice of Looney Tunes cartoon characters
Don Pardo	Voice of Saturday Night Live introduction
Jim Henson	Voice of Kermit the Frog

Voice disorders occur in people of all ages. Voice disorders are also likely to be found among individuals whose occupation is dependent on having a healthy voice. These vocal performers work in a variety of settings such as the music industry, theatre, clergy, the courtroom, or the classroom. Voice disorders reflect a special form of communication disorder that involves a close working relationship between the patient, SLP, and medical personnel. Amazingly, most instances of voice disorders are preventable by simply taking the proper precautionary steps. The fact that many voice disorders could be prevented also makes this form of communication disorder unique.

TERMINOLOGY AND DEFINITIONS

The key anatomic structures required for the production of voice can be found within the framework of the larynx. The **larynx** consists of a number of muscles and cartilages that work cooperatively to produce voice. To appreciate the nature of various voice disorders it is necessary to reacquaint ourselves with the basic anatomy and physiology of the larynx that was covered in Chapter 3. The larynx is positioned between the base of the tongue and the top of the **trachea** (windpipe), the passageway to the lungs. The larynx is not designed for the daily wear and tear we place on it for the production of voice. The key function of the larynx is to protect the breathing airway from foreign matter (i.e., food, liquid) that may be heading toward the lungs. The primary muscle involved in the generation of voice is the **thyroarytenoid muscle**, which is the formal term for the **vocal folds**. The thyroarytenoid muscle is comprised of two bands of smooth muscle tissue that lie opposite each other and sit prominently over the trachea. One end of the muscle is inserted to the inside of the thyroid cartilage. The other end is attached to the arytenoid cartilages. When the vocal folds are **abducted** (open) a space forms between the two folds known as the **glottis**. During breathing, air flows in and out of the lungs and passes through the glottis. When the vocal folds are **adducted** (closed), the space (or glottis) disappears. During heavy duty activities such as lifting or pulling, as well as during moments of swallowing, the vocal folds are adducted. A depiction of the vocal folds in abducted and adducted positions is shown in Figure 8.1.

To produce voice, we "exploit" the structure of the larynx by deliberating adducting the vocal folds and cause them to vibrate. The technical term for the physiological process of generating voice is **phonation**. To produce voice, the brain precisely coordinates a series of events involving the three subsystems of voice: (1) respiration, (2) phonation, and (3) resonance. The respiratory

FYI

A bird's larynx, called a **syrinx**, is anatomically simpler than that found in humans. Instead of being located at the top of the windpipe (trachea), it is located at the bottom, much closer to the lungs. This close proximity to the lungs is what allows very small birds to sing so loudly.

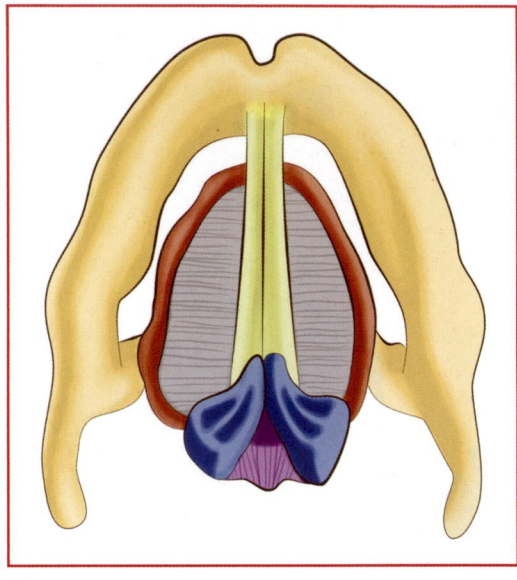

A **B**

FIGURE 8.1. A superior (*top-down*) view of the larynx depicting abducted (*open*) vocal folds (**A**) and adducted (*closed*) vocal folds (**B**).

system serves as the driving force of voice production. Without the forward (exhaled) flow of air from the lungs, we would not be able to produce voice smoothly. Upon exhalation of inspired air, the phonatory system is then responsible for closing the vocal folds in a deliberate but relaxed fashion. Once the vocal folds close, air from the lungs builds up underneath them until they are blown open, causing them to vibrate and produce sound. This sound then travels outward through the oral and nasal cavities, which serve to shape or resonate the sound quality as it leaves our mouth. The number of vocal fold vibrations per second determines the fundamental frequency (F_0) (or **pitch**) of our voice. A person's voice pitch can be high or low, variable (sing-song) or flat (monotonic). An individual might also demonstrate natural pitch breaks such as the case when young males undergo puberty. These hormonal changes can affect voice production as a young male's voice pitch begins to lower with age.

Voice **quality** refers to the subjective aspect of voice that is perceived by

FYI

A **castrato** is a male singer with an artificially created falsetto (high pitched) voice, the result of castration in childhood that stunts the growth of the larynx. The combination of the larynx of a boy and the chest and lungs of a man produced a powerful voice of great range and unique sound. Castrati were especially popular in churches and opera in Europe during the 17th and 18th centuries.

listeners. The size and shape of the vocal folds, as well as the size and shape of the oral and nasal cavities, help to determine the quality of voice. Terms such as a **breathy** voice (i.e., excessive and audible air leakage), **hoarse** voice (i.e., a grating voice with pitch breaks), or **hyper/hyponasal** voice (e.g., too much or too little voice through the nasal cavity) are examples of qualitative descriptions of voice. Another aspect of voice quality is the dynamic range or **register** of voice. A typical speaking voice has three registers that cover the low, middle, and high range of voice. The lowest register is called **pulse** register. The middle and high registers are called **modal**, and **falsetto**, respectively. Voice **loudness** is somewhat self-explanatory. A voice can be produced excessively soft or loud. The term **voiced sounds** encompasses all vowels, as well as approximately half of all consonants.

A voice disorder is a condition whereby which a person's voice pitch, quality, or loudness differs from that of people the same sex, age, geographic region, or cultural background. **Dysphonation** refers to any type of impaired voice and includes a condition called **aphonia**, which is the inability to produce any sort of voice. The term **phonatory disorder** is synonymous with a voice disorder. **Edema** refers to the buildup of fluid in tissue that is a natural, protective reaction to trauma or misuse. The vocal folds are a delicate muscle that is prone to edema, even under the slightest instances of misuse. Edema may also develop in tissue as a side effect to certain drugs. **Hyperfunctional** voice refers to speaking with excessive muscular effort and force resulting in a tense, high-pitched voice. **Hypofunctional** voice refers to inadequate muscle tone of the laryngeal

mechanism during the production of voice often resulting in a weak, low-pitched voice that may also sound breathy. An **otolaryngologist** is a surgeon who specializes in disorders of the ear, nose, and throat (i.e., ENT surgeon, or otolaryngology, head, and neck surgeon). These professionals provide the initial diagnosis of a voice disorder. Most recently, the physicist **Ingo Titze**, who is one of the world leaders in the scientific study of the human voice, coined the term **vocology** to reflect the practice of voice rehabilitation (Figure 8.2).

HISTORIC ASPECTS OF VOICE DISORDERS

Man has sung through the ages and so it is not surprising to find accounts of normal or unusual voice production

FIGURE 8.2. Ingo Titze. One of the world leaders in the scientific study of human voice. Permission granted by I. Titze.

dating back many centuries. **Hippocrates** described the importance of the lungs, trachea, lips, and tongue in phonation in the early 5th century BC. In 350 BC, **Aristotle** was the first to mention the larynx in his book, *Historia Animalium*, in which he describes the neck as the part between the face and the chest. He noted that the larynx was located at the front of the neck, and it was through this structure that speech and breathing occurred.

Claudius Galen (129–200 AD) of Pergamum (Figure 8.3) was a physiologist considered the most important contributor to medicine following Hippocrates, and the founder of laryngology and voice science. Because dissections of human corpses were against Roman law in the second century, Galen uncovered information about laryngeal physiology and anatomy based on dissections of apes and pigs. Galen was the first to recognize that the larynx was the primary organ of voice, as well as for the regulation of breathing, and called it "an instrument of pneuma." Galen theorized that the larynx functioned similarly to a flute, where the vocal folds were the beak (mouthpiece) and the trachea was the body of the flute. Even though Galen learned much about the larynx, he had no ability to observe how it worked in a living person; therefore, knowledge regarding the specific aspects of voice production would not come about for many centuries.

Julio Casserius (1552–1616) was an Italian anatomist who made a major contribution to the study of voice with his 1600 publication of *The Anatomy of Voice and Hearing*. The book contained plates of the anatomy of the larynx in humans and mammals that were remarkably accurate from an artistic standpoint.

In 1741, a French anatomist **Antoine Ferrein** (1693–1769) (Figure 8.4) concluded that the larynx functioned similarly to that of a stringed instrument, in which the loudness and variety of tones

FIGURE 8.3. Claudius Galen. The founder of laryngology and voice science.

FIGURE 8.4. Antoine Ferrein. The 18th century French anatomist who coined the term *vocal cords.*

produced by the voice were a result of different degrees of tension and length. The concept of a vibrating string led Ferrein to develop the term **vocal cords**.

Henri Dutrochet (1776–1847) (Figure 8.5) was a French botanist who was primarily interested in plant physiology. His research involved investigations of the mechanisms responsible for physical movement in plants that led to his discovery of cell biology. His interest in the natural biological movement of organisms also carried over to the examination of certain excitability responses in animals, namely the production of voice. In 1806, he published *A New Theory of Voice* and theorized about the manner in which the vocal folds vibrated. His view was different from that of Ferrein—he recommended dropping the term vocal cords in favor of the term vocal folds because of the observation that the vocal ligaments of the larynx

FIGURE 8.5. Henri Dutrochet. Theorized about the manner in which the vocal folds vibrated.

did not act as cords but like a reed of a clarinet.

In early days, the larynx was oftentimes singled out as the root cause of various diseases. The primary symptom of many diseases such as diphtheria, typhus, and tuberculosis was a marked change in voice or coughing. Because the voiced failed to function normally, considerable interest grew in examining the larynx from both a physiological and a clinical viewpoint. By the early part of the 19th century, there was an overwhelming curiosity to examine the interior of the larynx through the development of various types of viewing instruments. However, it was not until the Spaniard **Manuel García** (1805–1906), created the laryngeal mirror in 1855 that clear examinations of the larynx were possible. García was an opera singer who had a personal interest in the physiology of voice production. Using a dentist's mirror, he placed the mirror in the back of the throat, and by positioning it at a proper angle, he was able to see the reflection of his vocal folds in an opposing mirror (Figure 8.6). The procedure was originally referred to as autolaryngoscopy but today is referred to as **indirect laryngoscopy**. García was hardly the first to look into the physiology of voice but what made his work different was that he experimented on himself, seeking the cause of his own voice disorder.

Elizabeth Blackwell (1821–1910) was the first woman to obtain a medical degree in the United States by graduating at the top of her class from the Geneva Medical College of New York. Blackwell enabled many more women to follow in her footsteps, including one of the first female otolaryngologists, **Margaret F. Butler** (1861–1931) (Figure 8.7). Dr. Butler initially decided to specialize in

FIGURE 8.6. Manuel García performing an indirect laryngoscopy. Note that the light source is an oil lamp.

FIGURE 8.7. Margaret Butler. One of the first female otolaryngologists. Photo courtesy of Archives and Special Collections on Women in Medicine and Homeopathy, Drexel University College of Medicine.

gynecology, but recognized the need for her skills in otolaryngology. She was a clinical professor of laryngology and chief of the Nose and Throat Department at the Woman's Medical College of Pennsylvania in 1906. She was the sole representative from the United States at the First International Congress of Rhinolaryngology held in Vienna in 1908. She invented a number of ENT surgical in-

---

FYI

As late as 1947, there were 77 approved medical colleges in America with four still closed to women, including the world-renowned Harvard Medical College. Of the colleges that accepted both women and men during that time, most limited their enrollment of women to 5%.

struments, including a device to remove tonsils, called the Butler tonsil snare.

The assessment and management of voice disorders remained exclusively within the domain of otolaryngologists or singing teachers throughout the 19th century and the early 20th century. **Friedrich Brodnitz** (1899–1995) was a German physician who introduced the concept of **phoniatrics** (i.e., voice science) in the late 1930s (Figure 8.8). When he arrived in the United States in 1937, he was something of a novelty among ENT surgeons, having been trained in both otolaryngology and speech therapy. Prior to this time, there was little interest in the field of voice disorders among otolaryngologists. He established one of the first clinics in the United States for voice disorders, and devoted his life to problems of the voice, especially if they interfered with the livelihood of opera singers, actors, or other professional voice users. Dr. Brodnitz was a pioneer in the so-called chewing method, which were exercises designed to strengthen and realign the throat muscles to produce less strain and better control of the vocal folds.

The development of the speech-language pathology profession served to greatly advance assessment and treatment approaches to voice disorders. Two textbooks were published in the 1930s that contained material concerning voice disorders that were specifically designed for use by SLPs in their clinical practice. The first of these books was *The Rehabilitation of Speech* (West et al., 1937), followed by *Speech Correction: Principles and Methods* (Van Riper, 1939).

FIGURE 8.8. Friedrich Brodnitz. German physician who introduced the concept of *phoniatrics*.

TYPES OF VOICE DISORDERS

It is rare for a voice problem to occur instantaneously; they do not occur overnight. Rather, it is likely for a voice disorder to result from daily lifestyle behaviors, including occupational or social demands on the voice, as well as issues related to overall health. Voice disorders are classified according to the causal basis of the disorder. Colton et al. (2006) have organized voice disorders into three categories, those resulting from: (1) vocal misuse, (2) nervous system involvement, or (3) organic disease and trauma. Some of the more frequently encountered voice disorders found in each of these categories are highlighted below. A comprehensive list of the wide range of voice disorders can be found in Table 8.2.

Table 8.2. Types of Voice Disorders and the Vocal Quality Associated With Each Disorder (from Colton et al., 2006)

Classification	Type and Vocal Quality
Vocal Misuse/Phonotrauma	*Nodules*—breathiness and lowered pitch
	Polyps—breathiness and lowered pitch
	Edema—lowered pitch
	Laryngitis—breathiness and lowered pitch
	Aphonia—total loss of voice in spite of apparent normal vocal anatomy
	Puberphonia—unusually high pitch in spite of normal vocal anatomy
Nervous System Involvement	*Parkinson Disease*—monopitch and reduced loudness
	Myasthenia Gravis—breathiness
	Spasmodic Dysphonia—vocal strain/struggle
	Lesions of Peripheral Nerves—breathiness
	Huntington's Chorea—hoarseness
	Motor Neuron Disease—hoarseness or strain/struggle
	Multiple Sclerosis—impaired loudness control and hoarseness
Organic Disease and Trauma	*Laryngeal Granuloma*—hoarseness
	Contact Ulcer—hoarseness
	Papilloma—hoarseness
	Vocal Fold Hemorrhage—hoarseness and intermittent aphonia
	Laryngeal Web—hoarseness
	Inhalation Trauma—hoarseness
	Carcinoma—hoarseness

Vocal Misuse

The first type of voice disorders are those related to vocal misuse. In these particular disorders, the basic anatomy of the larynx is normal but the manner in which the larynx is being used contributes to a voice disorder. Vocal misuse (also called **phonotrauma**) is any improper or inefficient speaking behavior that can damage the vocal folds and cause temporary or permanent changes in vocal function, voice quality, and possible loss of voice. Examples of vocal misuse include excessive talking, throat clearing, coughing, inhaling irritants, smoking, screaming, or yelling. The term **vocal misuse** is preferred over vocal abuse because "abuse" places blame for the disorder on the patient due to purposeful damaging actions. In reality, there are instances when the patient is simply using their voice incorrectly with little knowledge as to any vocal wrongdoing. Disorders of vocal misuse are the most prevalent and preventable types of voice disorders as people of all ages who use their voice excessively may experience phonotrauma. Young children, teachers, lawyers, cheerleaders, and professional voice users such as singers and actors are prone to voice disorders of this nature. Some disorders resulting from vocal misuse are laryngitis, vocal nodules, and vocal polyps. Each of these various disorders of vocal misuse represents a form of hyperfunctional voice disorder.

Laryngitis

Inflammation or swelling of the vocal folds results in **laryngitis** (Figure 8.9). Some symptoms associated with laryngitis are a sore throat and swallowing difficulty. The condition may be caused by excessive use of the voice, bacterial or viral infections, or irritants, such as inhaled chemicals or the backup of stomach acid into the throat (i.e., reflux). The voice of someone with laryngitis will often sound breathy and hoarse. Laryngitis occurs in two forms: (1) **acute**, which lasts only a few days, and (2) **chronic**,

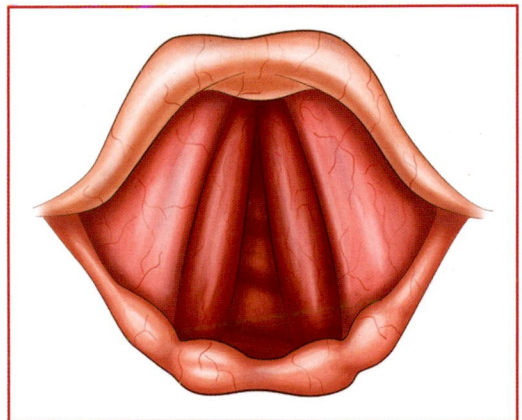

FIGURE 8.9. Example of laryngitis.

which persists over a period of weeks or months. Chronic laryngitis can result in the development of a more severe and long-lasting voice disorder. In addition, children who experience severe forms of laryngitis can run the risk of breathing difficulty because inflamed vocal folds can serve to narrow the air passage leading to the lungs.

Vocal Nodules

Small, benign (noncancerous) callus-like bumps that form on the vocal folds are called **vocal nodules** (Figure 8.10). They can form on one or both of the folds, are located on the front one-third of the vocal folds, and range in size from a pinhead to a split pea. Nodules develop from irritation caused by repeated pressure on the same area of the vocal

---

FYI

Whistle register is the highest register of the human voice. The sound in this register resembles a flute. The ability to produce a voice in this register is believed to be rare. A famous pop artist who uses this register in her music is Mariah Carey.

FIGURE 8.10. Example of vocal nodules.

FIGURE 8.11. Example of vocal polyp.

folds much like a callus forms on areas of a person's hands or feet following repeated physical activity. During normal voice production, the vocal folds should naturally meet together at a midline position. However, when a vocal nodule is present, the vocal folds are unable to close completely, resulting in excessive air escaping during the production of voice. The voice of a person who has vocal nodules usually sounds hoarse, low-pitched, and slightly breathy. Vocal nodules are a prevalent type of voice disorder resulting from vocal misuse. This condition is also referred to as "singer's nodes" because it is a frequent problem among professional singers. The inability to sing high notes is a hallmark feature of nodules. When the individual tries to sing in a high voice, there is a delay in the onset of the sound with an audible escape of air.

Vocal Polyp

A small, noncancerous growth on one or both of the vocal folds results in a **vocal polyp** (also termed polypoid degeneration). Just as a vocal nodule is much like a hard callus, a vocal polyp is much like a soft blister (Figure 8.11). Symptoms of vocal polyps include abnormal voice quality, vocal fatigue, and the sensation of a lump in the throat that involves constant throat clearing. A polyp typically forms on only one vocal fold. Although polyps occur most often as a result of sudden vocal trauma, a specific type of polyp (known as Reinke's edema) results from long-term cigarette smoking, creating the well-known **smoker's voice**. People who develop a vocal polyp usually have a low-pitched, hoarse, breathy voice, similar to the voices of people who have vocal nodules.

Puberphonia

A fourth type of vocal misuse is **puberphonia**, also called mutational falsetto. Puberphonia refers to a condition in which an adult (usually an adolescent male) continues to speak with a high-pitched voice well after the age when a natural lowering in voice pitch should have occurred. The condition is rare and is believed to reflect a form of **psychogenic** disorder. A psychogenic voice disorder is thought to result from an underlying psychological disturbance. In the case of puberphonia, there is no structural reason for the voice disorder. However, since the voice is not being used normally, a condition such as puberphonia is classified as a disorder of vocal misuse.

Nervous System Involvement

The nervous system consists of the brain, spinal cord, and an enormous network of sensory and motor nerves that course throughout the body. Malfunctions of the nervous system may result from disease, abnormal growths, or trauma. Nervous system damage can also impair normal voice production. Two particular conditions that reflect voice disorders having a nervous system origin are: (1) neurogenic disorders and (2) spasmodic dysphonia. These disorders are not related to trauma, as this forms the basis of organic voice disorders (see later section).

Neurogenic Voice Disorders

Two examples of voice disorders having a neurogenic origin are **Parkinson disease** (PD) and **Amyotrophic Lateral Sclerosis** (ALS), also known as motor neuron disease. The condition of PD is a progressive neurologic disorder affecting movements such as walking, talking, and writing. The disease generally affects people beyond the age of 40 years. The three main symptoms of PD are tremor, stiffness, and bradykinesia (i.e., slowness of movement). These conditions can carry over into the production of voice, with approximately 50 to 80% of all patients with PD demonstrating a

voice disorder. The voice features found in PD are **monotonic voice** and a low-pitched voice, as well as considerable variation in the loudness of voice. The condition of ALS is a progressive chronic disease of the nerves that are responsible for supplying electrical stimulation to the muscles used for any and all movement. The disease causes gradual muscle weakness and wasting. The disease generally affects people over the age of 40 years with a typical lifespan of less than 3 years from the date of diagnosis. The muscles responsible for the production of voice are not spared among individuals with ALS. Early symptoms include a hoarse voice accompanied by vocal spasm. As the disease progresses, the voice becomes weaker and is characterized by **breathiness** and **hypernasality**. The increase in nasality results from weakness in the muscles responsible for closing off the nasal cavity from the oral cavity during normal voice production.

Spasmodic Dysphonia

A spasm is an involuntary and abnormal contraction of a muscle. In the case of **spasmodic dysphonia**, the particular voice disorder appears to be one of involuntary and abnormal functioning of the muscles responsible for voice production. Spasmodic dysphonia is perhaps the most mysterious of all voice disorders because we still do not know what causes it and how best to treat it. The disorder was originally thought to be a type of psychogenic condition, and because there was no identifiable physical cause to the problem, researchers believed it must result from some level of mental distress. This way of thinking is evident in use of the term hysterical dysphonia, which has since been dropped in favor of the term spasmodic dysphonia. Research over the past 30 years now indicates that the disorder probably reflects a motor disturbance deep in the brain.

There are two types of spasmodic dysphonia, based on whether the spasm affects the closing or opening phases of vocal fold vibration. **Adductor type** spasmodic dysphonia results in a severe hyperfunctional voice. The patient demonstrates obvious struggle in attempting to produce a clear voice. The vocal folds show intermittent spasms causing them to close and stiffen. Patients find it difficult, if not impossible, to shout, but surprisingly the spasms are usually absent while laughing, singing, or speaking on inhalation. **Abductor type** spasmodic dysphonia is more rare and essentially the opposite to that of the adductory type. In abductor spasmodic dysphonia, sudden involuntary muscle movements or spasms cause the vocal folds to open. The vocal folds are unable to vibrate when fully abducted causing periods of aphonia. The open position of the vocal folds also allows air to escape from the lungs during speech. As a result, the voices of these individuals sound weak and breathy. As with adductor spasmodic dysphonia, the spasms are often absent during activities such as laughing or singing. The prevalence of either type of spasmodic dysphonia in the general population is unknown. There is no difference in regard to its occurrence in men and women. The disorder is rarely found in children and young adults, with most cases occurring in middle-aged adults.

Organic Disease and Trauma

The third type of voice disorders are those that affect the structure of the vocal mechanism as a result of an organic disease state or some form of physical trauma. Two voice disorders resulting from these conditions are: (1) papilloma and (2) cancer of the larynx.

Papilloma

Papillomas are benign epithelial (surface-level) tumors caused by infection with the human papilloma virus (HPV). The tumors can develop in various parts of the body, including the larynx. Laryngeal papillomas appear as numerous warty growths on the surface of the vocal folds (Figure 8.12). Laryngeal papillomas are most often found among children, and between 60 to 80% of cases occur in children, usually before the age of three. Although papillomas are benign, their rapid growth on the vocal folds can cause obstruction of the airway that could potentially lead to asphyxiation if not promptly treated. Like warts, papillomas are very stubborn lesions that tend to grow back no matter how completely they are removed. This is particularly the case among children. In adults, laryngeal papillomas tend to be less aggressive. Papillomas generally

FIGURE 8.12. Example of vocal papilloma.

cause no physical pain with the most obvious symptom of the disorder being a hoarse-sounding voice.

Carcinoma

Cancer can develop in any part of the body and the larynx is no exception (Figure 8.13). **Laryngeal cancer** comprises approximately 5% of all forms of cancer. If allowed to develop without treatment, the condition can be life threatening. The primary cause of laryngeal cancer is smoking. In addition to laryngeal cancer, smoking is the major cause of cancers of the lungs, oral cavity, and esophagus. The ratio of men to women who develop laryngeal cancer is 5 to 1, although this ratio is rapidly decreasing with the rise in smoking among women. Smoking serves as an irritant to the vocal folds causing edema. It also decreases lung function, and without good lung power, more stress is placed upon the larynx when speaking or singing. This is why heavy, long-term smokers' voices are often hoarse and low in pitch. These voice features are also the prime symptoms or warning signs of laryngeal cancer.

FIGURE 8.13. Example of vocal carcinoma.

CURRENT THEORIES OF VOICE DISORDERS

One of the earliest modern theories of normal voice production was proposed by the French scientist **Raoul Husson** in 1950, who sparked considerable debate as far as the physiology of the vibration of the vocal folds is concerned. In his **neurochronaxic theory**, he suggested that the frequency of vocal fold vibration was dependent on excitation of nerve cells from the laryngeal nerve (part of cranial nerve X). For example, if the vocal folds were to vibrate at a rate of 200 Hz, this theory suggests that 200 nerve impulses per second are sent to the thyroarytenoid (vocal fold) muscle. Husson's theory was eventually found to be invalid because we now know that nerves are unable to discharge at such high rates. This theory was eventually replaced by the **myoelastic aerodynamic theory of phonation** in 1959 by the Dutch scientist, **Janwillem van den Berg** (1926–1985) (Figure 8.14). The title of the theory is self-explanatory in regard to the process of producing voice—the theory is that normal vocal fold vibration involves coordination of muscle tension and breath pressure. In order to produce voice, there needs to be air pressure and flow. Elastic muscular movement of the structures comprising the vocal mechanism is also necessary, and the entire process is dynamic, involving movement and change. Over the past 50 years, the various intricate steps in vocal fold vibration have been more critically examined; however, the general concept of producing voice is still captured within the myoelastic aerodynamic theory of phonation.

Recently, Roy and Bless (2000) proposed a **personality and emotional**

FIGURE 8.14. Janwillem van den Berg. Proposed the myoelastic aerodynamic theory of phonation.

ASSESSMENT OF VOICE DISORDERS

At any given time, approximately 6% of the general population experience a voice disorder and a majority of these individuals tend to be female (Roy et al., 2005). Approximately 30% of the entire population will experience a form of voice disorder, either fleeting or long term, at some point in their lives. Most instances of voice disorders occur in people between the ages of 40 to 60 years, although voice disorders are also found in children. Among children, there is a greater likelihood of voice disorders in boys compared to girls, with boys more often implicated in vocally abusive behaviors, such as shouting and screaming. Anyone who experiences vocal discomfort for more than two weeks should consider seeking an assessment of their voice. In some cases, the SLP may be the first individual to encounter a patient complaining of a voice problem. The SLP may perform an initial evaluation of the patient's voice; however, appropriate ethical practice requires the SLP to immediately refer the patient to an otolaryngologist. The otolaryngologist will examine the individual's vocal folds and determine if a medical condition is causing the voice problem.

The assessment of voice disorders involves subjective and objective procedures. Both approaches are essential to obtaining the detail necessary to accurately diagnose the cause, type, and severity of voice disorder. A **subjective assessment** of voice entails listening and observing the patient while they are speaking, and the collection of a case history. When listening to the patient's voice, the SLP will complete a **rating** of the patient's voice quality, which is

adjustment theory of voice disorders. The premise of the theory is that an individual's personality and behavioral patterns may contribute to the eventual development of a voice disorder such as nodules. In turn, the subsequent voice disorder that develops creates further emotional problems and personality effects for the individual with the disorder. For example, a person with an impulsive, preservative personality who is misusing their voice may be unable to normally cease in misusing their voice, thereby contributing to a more long-lasting voice disorder. The role of personality and issues such as impulsivity have not been considered in previous theories concerning voice disorders. If personality issues are found to show a direct link to some voice disorders, advancements in the diagnosis and treatment of these disorders will likely occur.

based on having the patient prolong isolated vowels, read aloud, and speak in a conversational setting. This is where the SLP may use terms such as "breathy" or "hoarse" to describe the patient's voice. The SLP will also observe the patient's general **body movements** during speaking, in particular, examining for excessive neck tension and irregular breathing patterns. Obtaining a patient's **case history** provides the SLP with background information that may hold relevance to diagnosing the voice disorder. The SLP collects information about the patient's occupation, daily use of voice, onset and duration of the voice problem, and expectations for improving their voice. An example of a voice case history form is provided in Table 8.3.

Objective assessments involve use of instruments to examine the dynamic process of voice production. Two frequently employed instrumental approaches in voice diagnosis are indirect and direct laryngoscopy (Paparella & Shumrick, 1991). Both approaches are illustrated in Figure 8.15. The steps to performing an indirect laryngoscopy have changed little since the original method established by Manuel García in 1855. The patient is seated upright and the otolaryngologist inserts a small hand mirror to the back of the throat. Prior to inserting the mirror, an anesthetic is sprayed in the back of the throat to prevent gagging. A light is projected into the throat and deflected off the mirror toward the vocal folds. The same mirror is also used to visualize the vocal folds. The patient is asked to sustain vowels ("say eee") during the examination. A **direct laryngoscopy** is

---

Table 8.3. Example of a Case History Form Used in the Assessment of Voice Disorders

Voice History Form

Name: _____ Age: _____   Sex: ☐ Female ☐ Male

Did concern over your voice begin with: ☐ Illness ☐ Trauma (injury) ☐ Surgery?

Voice History

Please list previous voice problems: _____

Please list previous voice treatments: _____

Current Status of Voice

Is your voice today typical of how it sounds since the voice problem began? ☐ Yes ☐ No

Does your voice vary with: ☐ Seasons/Weather? ☐ Time of day?

Do you ever experience voice loss where you are only able to whisper? ☐ Yes ☐ No

continues

Table 8.3. *continued*

Medical History

Do you currently have or have you ever had any of the following conditions?

☐ Pain, tightness in throat ☐ Sinus ☐ Allergies ☐ Breathing difficulties

Please list current medications: _____

How much caffeine (coffee, tea, soft drinks, etc.) do you drink per day? Cups: _____

How much alcohol do you drink? _____

Do you smoke? ☐ Yes ☐ No How much? _____

Are you frequently in a situation where you are breathing noxious fumes? ☐ Yes ☐ No

Voice Use

How many hours do you spend?

- In conversation (friends, family, work, etc.): _____

- Talking in noise (work, machines, restaurants, taverns, crowds, etc.): _____

- Yelling (sporting events, coaching, etc.): _____

- Teaching, instructions or training: _____

- Singing: _____

Are you using your voice less than usual because of the problem? ☐ Yes ☐ No

Self-Perception of Voice Concern

Please rate the importance of the following:

Use of voice for work: ☐ Unimportant ☐ Somewhat Important ☐ Very Important

Use of voice for socializing: ☐ Unimportant ☐ Somewhat Important ☐ Very Important

Please rate each of the following potential problems which most closely apply to you.
(1 = No problem, 2 = Slight problem, 3 = Moderate problem, 4 = Severe problem)

- My voice is not loud enough for people to hear me in some situations. _____

- My voice is too loud for some situations. _____

- My pitch is too high. _____

- My pitch is too low. _____

- My voice quality is not good. I sound harsh or hoarse. _____

- I'm bothered by the way people react to my voice. _____

- My voice gets tired and fatigued with talking. _____

A **B**

FIGURE 8.15. Examples of indirect and direct approaches to examining the larynx (**A**). An indirect examination of the larynx using a lamp and head mirror. (**B**) Direct examination of the larynx using a flexible fiberoptic endoscope.

most often performed after the indirect method to allow for viewing of a greater area of the larynx. Direct laryngoscopy is easily accomplished using a **flexible endoscope**, which consists of hundreds of fiberoptic strands that serve as both a light source for illumination, as well as a camera for examination. The scope is inserted through one of the nostrils and is guided toward the back of the throat and rests slightly above the vocal folds. This particular view is valuable for direct examination of the vocal folds and any existing vocal pathology.

TREATMENT OF VOICE DISORDERS

The wide range of possible voice disorders and their occurrence in children and adults results in treatment programs varying from one patient to the next. The general goal of voice therapy is to restore the best voice possible. An acceptable voice is one that is functional

for purposes of general communication. Ideally, the best form of treatment is one aimed at eliminating the vocal behavior that created the voice disorder in the first place. Voice therapy with singers involves working on both the speaking and singing voice and generally a program of therapy helps to achieve an easy natural voice without strain. When the healthiest possible voice is achieved, the SLP may refer the patient to a singing teacher, whose role is to provide advice on singing style and technique. Four approaches to the management of voice disorders are: (1) indirect therapy, (2) direct therapy, (3) phonosurgery, and (4) prevention. These approaches seek to eliminate potentially harmful vocal behaviors, enhance vocal fold tissue healing following injury, and/or alter the manner of voice production.

Indirect Therapy

Techniques associated with indirect therapy include voice rest and patient education. **Voice rest** is the process of resting the vocal folds by not allowing any form of speaking, singing, or whispering for several days. Voice rest in itself is not a cure for most disorders. The purpose of voice rest is to hasten recovery time in conditions where the vocal folds have been traumatized. It is generally believed that if a person must absolutely speak during a prescribed period of vocal rest, regular phonation is preferred over whispering. The use of whispering does not allow the voice to rest and actually may have an irritating effect on the vocal folds. **Patient education** consists of informing the patient about the manner in which voice is produced, including a simplified interpretation of the myoelastic aerodynamic theory of phonation. As well, the patient is educated about the subsequent long-term vocal damage that may result from not producing voice normally.

Direct Therapy

The use of direct therapy involves alteration of a patient's existing speaking behavior in an attempt to increase vocal efficiency and improve voice quality.

Four examples of direct therapy are: (1) vocal function exercises, (2) respiratory training, (3) use of confidential voice, and (4) the **Lee Silverman Voice Treatment** (LSVT). **Vocal function** exercises are a form of calisthenics designed to strengthen and improve coordination of laryngeal musculature. Examples of vocal function exercises include maximum vowel prolongations and smoothly raising and lowering pitch along a musical scale. **Respiratory training** is one of the major methods for enhancing vocal function. Respiratory retraining focuses on coordinating muscles used for breathing and vocalizing. Professional singers are well aware of the importance of respiration in maintaining a normal healthy voice. **Confidential voice** therapy involves using a soft, breathy voice. The term is based on the concept of speaking softly with another individual so as to not be too obvious. From a physiological standpoint, speaking with soft voice reduces laryngeal muscle tension. Somewhat opposite to confidential voice therapy is LSVT. The LSVT is a structured, programmatic approach to voice therapy. The premise of the approach is to encourage a full, loud speaking voice to improve overall voice quality as well

FYI

The term **ventriloquism** comes from Latin *venter* and *loqui*, which translates to "belly-speaking." It actually is not possible to throw your voice across the room. Rather, the effect used by ventriloquists is to disguise their voice to make it appear that it is coming from another voice (i.e., a dummy). This unusual manner of speaking can place strain on the voice.

as to improve aspects of speech clarity. The treatment has gained widespread acceptance for working with individuals with Parkinson disease (see also Chapter 9).

Phonosurgery

In some instances, indirect or direct therapy is not sufficient to improve one's voice. In these cases, an operation may be necessary to repair the vocal folds or remove growths from the vocal folds. The term **phonosurgery** denotes restoration of voice by using various surgical techniques. The term was original used by the otolaryngologist **Hans von Leden** (b. 1918) in the 1950s to describe any surgery performed specifically to improve voice. In most cases, some form of postoperative voice therapy is required following surgery. Two routine types of phonosurgeries performed by an otolaryngologist are: (1) phonomicrosurgery and (2) injection laryngoplasty. Both surgeries take place in an operating room with the patient asleep. Phonomicrosurgery involves use of a microscope to view the area of surgery and the operation is carried out using special microinstruments and lasers (Figure 8.16). **Phonomicrosurgery** is performed to remove vocal nodules and polyps. A guiding principle of this surgery is to maintain normal vocal function by only removing the growth found on the superficial tissue of the vocal folds. It is seldom performed on children's voices because nodules and polyps often reappear in developing children so repeated phonosurgery would likely cause long-lasting damage to the vocal folds. Injection laryngoplasty entails use of a syringe to insert material (such as **collagen**) into one or both of the vocal folds to "plump

A

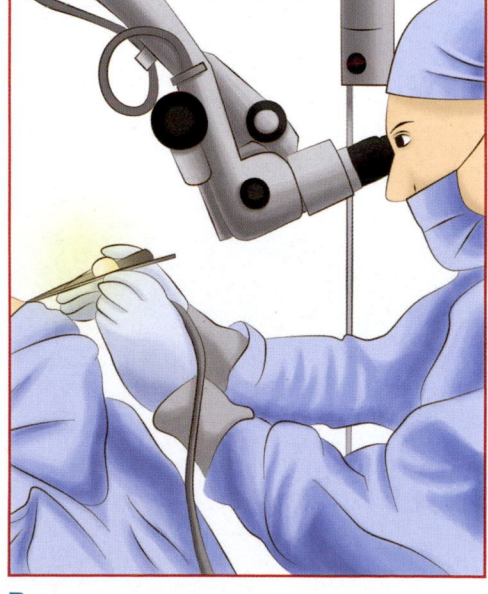

B

FIGURE 8.16. The process of phonosurgery. The surgeon uses delicate instruments to remove a growth from the vocal folds.

up" the overall size and shape of the muscle. Injection laryngoplasty has been successfully used to treat vocal fold paralysis. An effective treatment for reducing the symptoms of spasmodic dysphonia is injections of very small amounts of botulinum toxin (**Botox**) directly into the affected muscles of the larynx. The toxin weakens muscles by blocking the nerve impulses to the muscle, thereby freeing up the muscle to vibrate in a more normal fashion. Botox injections improve the voice for a period of four months after which voice symptoms gradually return. This treatment requires continual injections to maintain a good speaking voice.

A **laryngectomy** is the complete surgical removal of the larynx, most likely resulting from cancer of the larynx. In nearly all cases of laryngectomy, the individual was a cigarette (or cigar) smoker. A person who has undergone a laryngectomy no longer breathes through the nose or mouth, but through an opening in the neck called a **stoma**. The individual is incapable of producing a normal voice because the primary laryngeal structures need to generate voice have been removed (Figure 8.17). Several alternative methods exist for producing **alaryngeal** speech. One of these methods involves use a small handheld device known as an **electrolarynx** (see Figure 8.17). The device produces a buzzing sound that is transferred into the vocal tract by holding it firmly against the neck. The patient learns to modulate this sound by shaping the lips, tongue, and jaw as they normally would if they still had a larynx. The quality of the sound is unnatural but many patients use the device for basic communication needs. Another method for producing speech is referred to as esophageal speech. **Esophageal speech** is a type of speaking in which air is purposely injected into the back of the esophagus in a man-

A

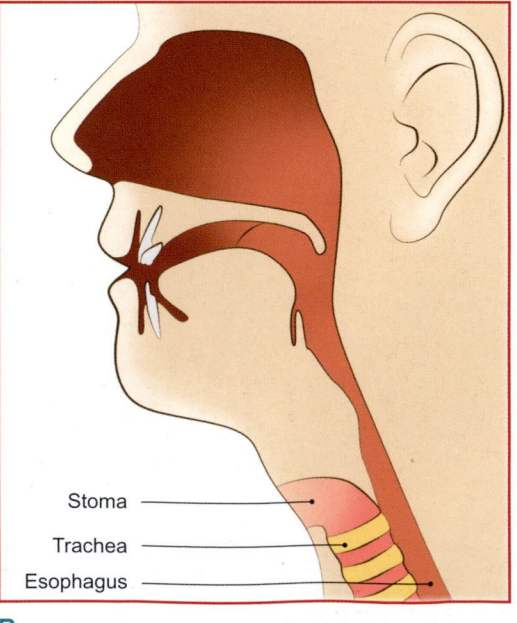

B

FIGURE 8.17. Depiction of vocal anatomy before (**A**) and after (**B**) a laryngectomy.

ner similar to burping to create speech. This form of speaking is difficult to master. Although most of us are probably able to utter one or two words on a single burp, a skilled esophageal speaker is able to produce short phrases. A very popular method of speech used following laryngectomy is **tracheoesophageal speech**, which is similar to esophageal speech, but uses a device to redirect air from the trachea into the esophagus. This is done through a small shunt placed through an opening made between the

trachea and esophagus called a tracheoesophageal puncture (TEP). A small one-way valve placed into this opening allows the patient to force air from their lungs into the mouth to create speech (Figure 8.18).

Prevention

Most voice disorders are preventable. Strategies that raise a person's awareness of voice disorders and vocal health

---

FYI

Each of us has a **habitual pitch**, or level at which we speak most frequently, and an **optimum pitch**, or the level at which we can produce our strongest voice with minimal effort. One way to determine your optimum pitch is through the yawn-sigh technique. Do just what the technique describes: yawn (or take a deep breath), and then sigh (usually we sigh, "ahh"). The pitch of the sigh is your optimum pitch.

A

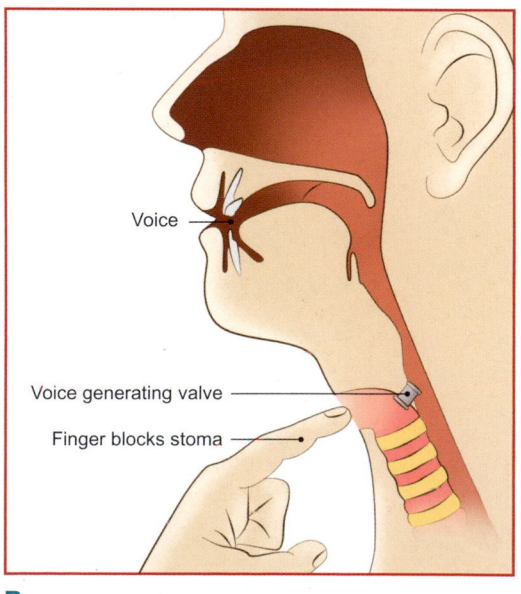

B

FIGURE 8.18. Use of an electrolarynx following a laryngectomy (**A**), and use of tracheoesophageal speech (**B**).

are essential to the prevention of voice disorders. **Vocal hygiene** refers to the healthy habits that patients should follow to take care of their voices. Examples of good vocal hygiene are listed in Table 8.4. The various examples can be summarized using the acronym developed by voiceproblem.org, VOICE:

V = Value your voice through healthy diet and lifestyle.

O = Optimize your voice with vocal warm-ups before use.

I = Invest in your voice with training in proper voice technique.

C = Cherish your voice by avoiding voice misuse, overuse, and abuse.

E = Exercise your voice to increase endurance and power.

CULTURAL CONSIDERATIONS AND VOICE DISORDERS

The occurrence of various types of voice disorders does not appear to differ significantly across racial and ethnic groups. However, a combination of social and cultural factors seems to influence voice and the subsequent development of voice disorders. For example, Japanese women tend to speak with a higher pitch (F_0) level than western female counterparts. The high-pitch voice is assumed to project a vocal image associated with femininity. In contrast, Japanese men tend to use a lower pitch level compared to western males that is used to emphasize masculinity. In both of these situations, the differences in F_0 are not due to anatomical differences in size of the larynx. Rather, the use of F_0 is altered

Table 8.4. Examples of Good Vocal Hygiene

- Control the amount of shouting or yelling.
- Minimize or avoid using a whispered voice.
- Control the amount of caffeine and alcohol consumption.
- Reduce and avoid excessive coughing and throat clearing.
- Minimize grunting or vocalization during exercise.
- Limit the amount of talking in loud and noisy environments.
- Do not smoke and limit your exposure to second-hand smoke.
- Conserve your voice during periods of excessive fatigue and stress.
- Keep hydrated by drinking water every day.
- Maintain a healthy diet and minimize laryngopharyngeal reflux.
- Be aware of potentially traumatic vocal behaviors.

due to sociocultural reasons. Presumably, this somewhat unnatural use of F_0 may place Japanese speakers at a higher risk for voice disorders due to possible misuse of the voice.

Society and culture also impact individuals who have undergone a sex change and require a subsequent change in speaking voice. Gender typically is demonstrated in a number of physical and behavioral ways, one of which is speaking voice. Transsexual individuals frequently undertake voice therapy as part of a female/male gender transition in order to make their voices sound appropriate and therefore facilitate their entrance (and acceptance) as females/males in society. **Voice feminization** is the desired goal of changing a perceived male sounding voice to a perceived female sounding voice. **Voice masculinization** is the opposite of voice feminization—the change of a voice from feminine to masculine. There is a greater likelihood of vocal misuse occurring in the process of voice feminization compared to masculinization due to the need to consistently maintain hyperadducted vocal fold behavior when speaking.

Other examples of society and culture influencing voice production can be found from the **music industry** and **sporting events**. A common anthem shared by today's youth is, *"If it's too loud—you're too old."* Examples of this perspective can be found in musical groups whose song lyrics tend to verge on shouting and yelling. While this form of music may be accepted culturally and socially, there are clear risks of entertainers developing phonotrauma. Most sporting events consist of teams of athletes competing against each other, with the added sideline attraction of cheerleaders (both male and female). There is a cultural and social expectation that cheerleaders shout and yell as a means of supporting their team. Not surprisingly, cheerleaders are at high risk of developing voice disorders due to vocal misuse.

CURRENT RESEARCH IN VOICE DISORDERS

Teachers

Research is currently underway evaluating strategies for reducing the high occurrence of voice disorders among teachers. The use of one's voice is vital to the profession of teaching. Teachers are required to speak for several hours each day, often in noisy and poorly soundproofed environments. A teacher's voice is put under a great deal of strain on a regular basis. Several studies completed in Australia, Europe, and the United States have shown that voice

---

FYI

Adult men have a lower speaking voice (F_0) than adult women; however, among some elderly individuals the reverse can be found. The increase in pitch among elderly men is attributed to a stiffening (calcification) of the vocal folds. The decrease in pitch among elderly women is attributed to a thinning and loss of elasticity (tension) of the vocal folds.

problems occur more frequently with teachers than with any other occupation. In the United States, for example, the prevalence of voice disorders among teachers is 12% compared to the 6% occurrence found in the general population (Roy et al., 2005). The occurrence of a voice disorder can trigger a whole series of problems including: (1) loss of the ability to communicate normally, (2) loss of employment, (3) loss of income, and subsequently (4) loss of professional identity.

Spasmodic Dysphonia

The mystery surrounding the causes of spasmodic dysphonia (SD) is also a current area of research. As of 2006, the U.S. National Institute of Neurological Disorders and Stroke has been sponsoring a large-scale research project examining the neuropathologic basis of SD. The precise cause of this fascinating voice disorder remains unknown. This particular project is designed to look for abnormalities in the brain of persons affected with SD by comparing results of magnetic resonance imaging (MRI) to those of nondisordered individuals (Simonyan et al., 2008).

Phonotrauma

Scientists are also examining a wide range of issues related to phonotrauma. A majority of this research is based on in-depth examination of the tissues of the vocal folds to determine how various types of stress affect these delicate tissues. Researchers are particularly interested in discovering why similar amounts of vocal misuse may cause some individuals to develop vocal nodules, whereas others may only develop

a mild case of laryngitis, or perhaps no voice disorder (Welham et al., 2008).

VOICE DISORDERS ON THE WORLD WIDE WEB

Listed below are Web sites that provide further information on the topic of voice disorders. At the time of publication each Web site was freely accessible.

Index of Voice Disorders Videos
http://homepage.mac.com/changcy/voice3.htm#index

The Voice Foundation
http://www.voicefoundation.org/

The Voice and Swallowing Center Videos
http://www.voiceandswallowing.com/

The Voice Problem Web site
http://www.voiceproblem.org/

Voice Disorders Resources
http://www.voicedoctor.net/

REFERENCES

Colton, R. H., Casper, J., & Leonard, R. (2006). *Understanding voice problems: A physiological perspective for diagnosis and treatment* (3rd ed.). Philadelphia: Lippincott Williams & Wilkins.

García, M. (1894). *New and revised treatise on the art of singing.* London: Lowe & Brydone.

Paparella, M. M., & Shumrick, D. A. (1991). *Otolaryngology* (3rd ed.). Philadelphia: Saunders.

Roy, N., & Bless, D. M. (2000). Personality traits and psychological factors in voice pathology: A foundation for future research. *Journal of Speech, Language, and Hearing Research, 43,* 737–748.

Roy, N., Merrill, R. M., Gray, S. D., & Smith, E. M. (2005). Voice disorders in the general population: Prevalence, risk factors, and occupational impact. *Laryngoscope, 115,* 1988–1995.

Simonyan, K., Tovar-Moll, F., Ostuni, J., Hallett, M., Kalasinsky, V. F., Lewin-Smith, M. R., . . . Ludlow, C. L. (2008). Focal white matter changes in spasmodic dysphonia: A combined diffusion tensor imaging and neuropathological study. *Brain, 131*(Pt. 2), 447–459.

Van Riper, C. (1939). *Speech correction: Principles and methods.* New York: Prentice-Hall.

Welham, N. V., Marriott, G., Tateya, I., & Bless, D. M. (2008). Proteomic changes in rat thyroarytenoid muscle induced by botulinum neurotoxin injection. *Proteomics, 29,* 1933–1944.

West, R., Kennedy, L., & Carr, A. (1937). *The rehabilitation of speech: A textbook of diagnostic and corrective procedures.* New York: Harper and Bros.

NEUROGENIC COMMUNICATION DISORDERS

OBJECTIVES

After reading this chapter, the student should be able to:

- Demonstrate knowledge concerning neuroanatomy, neurophysiology, and their relationship to speech and language.

- Identify individuals who have made historic contributions to the fields of neurology and neurogenic communication disorders.

- Demonstrate theoretical and clinical knowledge of neurogenic communication disorders in the adult population.

- Describe etiologies and characteristics of neurogenic communication disorders, including site of lesion.

- Describe current approaches to the assessment of adults with neurogenic communication disorders.

- Identify current professional issues relevant to treatment and intervention of adult neurogenic disorders.

- Demonstrate knowledge concerning the multicultural aspects of neurogenic communication disorders.

- Describe current theories in neurogenic communication disorders.

INTRODUCTION

Individuals who have a neurogenic communication disorder are often clients of SLPs who work in a health care setting, ranging from acute care hospitals to long-term (nursing home) settings. The term **neurogenic** refers to having its origin or starting with the nervous system. Therefore, a neurogenic communication disorder is usually a brain-based disorder. Although the brain is likely to be involved in nearly all types of communication disorders, neurogenic disorders represent a special set of communication difficulties that are attributed to disease or damage of the nervous system, of which the brain is a major component. These particular disorders can affect speech sound articulation and/or language formulation and production. Neurogenic communication disorders typically are acquired disorders. That is, they reflect a disorder that occurred later in life and following a period of normal communication behavior. Although neurogenic communication disorders can be found in children, the majority of cases tend to be adults.

TERMINOLOGY AND DEFINITIONS

When the nervous system is compromised due to developmental abnormalities, acquired damage, or illness, communication is often compromised as well. To fully appreciate the nature of neurogenic communication disorders, understanding the anatomy and physiology of the nervous system is essential. The detail of the human nervous system is immense and cannot be adequately covered in an introductory textbook on communication disorders; therefore, the terminology covered in this section is somewhat abbreviated and simplified.

The human nervous system can be grossly divided into two parts: the central nervous system (**CNS**) and the peripheral nervous system (**PNS**). An illustration of the basic division of the nervous system is shown in Figure 9.1. The CNS is made up of the cerebrum, brainstem, cerebellum, and spinal cord. The **cerebrum**, which is most commonly referred to as the brain, is a major landmark of the CNS. The brain allows humans to engage in high level functions such as thinking and learning. The brain has specialized areas that are designed for purposes of receiving, organizing, and producing language. The surface of the cerebrum is called the **cortex**, which has a variety of ridges and grooves. The ridges are called **gyri**, and the grooves are referred to as either a **sulcus** (i.e., a shallow groove) or a **fissure** (i.e., a deep groove), depending on the depth of the groove. On the basis of the grooves along the surface of the cortex, the cerebrum can be divided into two halves, known as the left and right **hemispheres**. The grooves in each hemisphere serve to further subdivide the cerebrum into four parts, or lobes. Each of these lobes is found in both the left and right hemispheres of the cerebrum.

The **frontal lobes**, as aptly named, are found in the front of the cerebrum and play a major role in the planning of physical (i.e., motor) movement for all parts of the body. An important language feature of the frontal lobe is **Broca's area** which is found in the left hemisphere only. As detailed below, Broca's area plays a pivotal role in the production of speech. The left and right

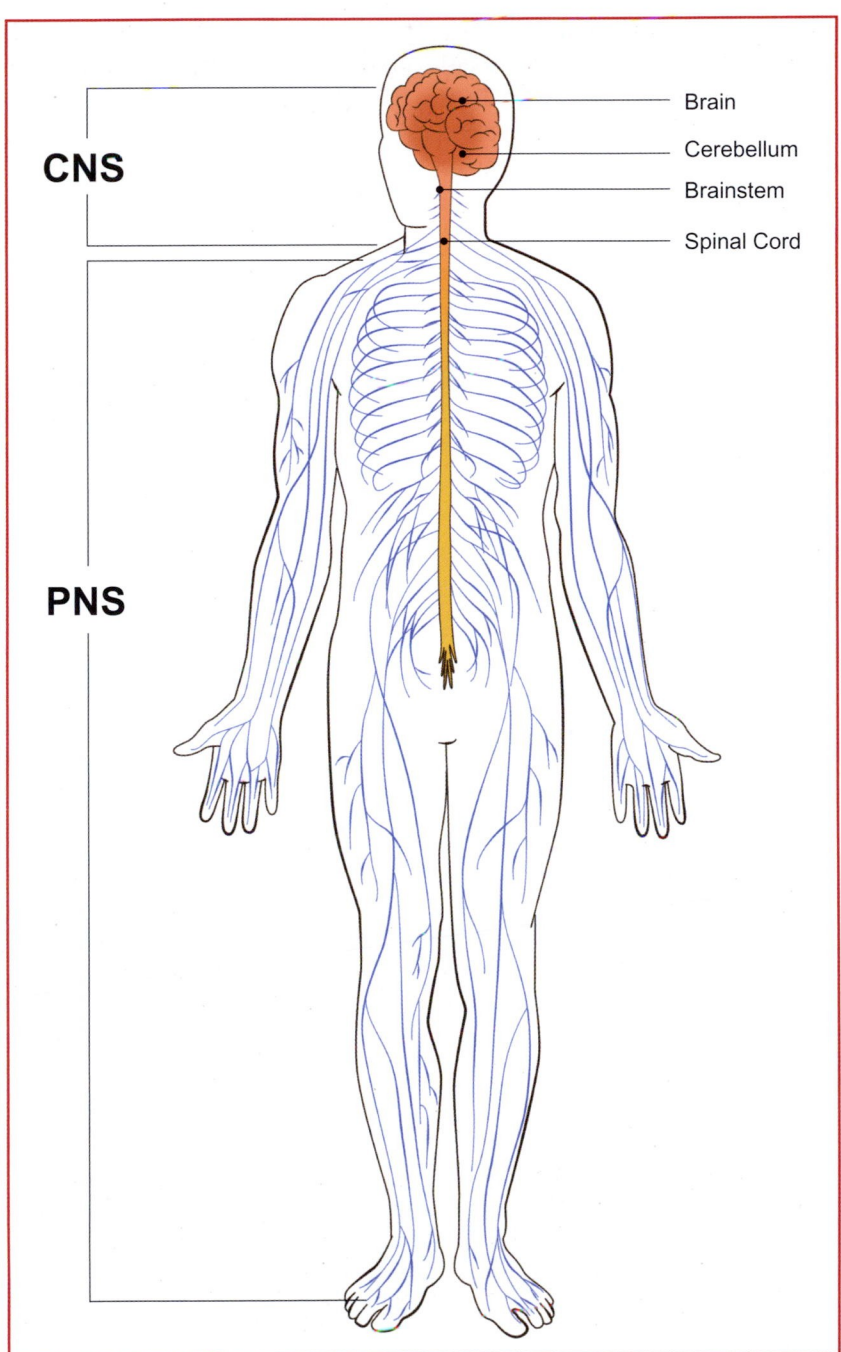

CNS

PNS

Brain
Cerebellum
Brainstem
Spinal Cord

FIGURE 9.1. Illustration of the nervous system consisting of the central nervous system (CNS) and the peripheral nervous system (PNS).

parietal lobes are located at the top of the cerebrum, behind the frontal lobes. The role of the parietal lobes is to process incoming sensory information (e.g., the mental sensation of touching something hot or cold). The **temporal**

lobes are located along the side of the cerebrum. There are two important landmarks in the temporal lobes that are relevant to communication. The first of these is the **primary auditory center** (also called Heschl's gyrus) found in both left and right temporal lobes. This is the endpoint location in the brain responsible for hearing. Sound initially entering the ears travels along a specific nervous system pathway and terminates in the primary auditory center. Further information regarding the anatomy and physiology of hearing can be found in Chapter 3. The second landmark of the temporal lobe is **Wernicke's area**. As noted below, Wernicke's area is only found in the left temporal lobe and is responsible for the understanding (or comprehension) of language. The fourth lobes are the **occipital lobes** and are found at the back of the cerebrum. A major function of the occipital lobes is the processing of incoming visual information. Deep within the cerebrum is an area known as the **limbic system** (or lobe) that includes part of most of the other lobes (i.e. frontal, parietal and temporal). The limbic system is involved in affective behaviors such as emotion and motivation. An illustration of the lobes of the cerebrum is provided in Figure 9.2.

The remaining parts of the CNS include the brainstem, spinal cord, and cerebellum. These structures contain bundles of nerve fibers (or pathways) that transmit sensory and motor information. Sensory pathways are those that carry information from the periphery toward the cerebrum. Motor pathways carry information away from the cerebrum towards the peripheral regions of the body. Damage to these structures can have an adverse impact on speech and language because these pathways either originate or terminate in the brain.

The peripheral nervous system (PNS) consists of all of the remaining nerves that lie outside the cerebrum, brainstem, and spinal cord. The PNS connects the brain to the outside world. Foremost among these nerves are a collection of **spinal nerves** and **cranial nerves**. There are 31 pairs of spinal nerves that are connected to the spinal cord and pass into the CNS where neural signals are processed. There are 12 pairs of cranial nerves that emerge from

FIGURE 9.2. Depiction of the four lobes of the left hemisphere of the cortex. The location of the cerebellum is also shown.

the base of the brain and are commonly identified by the Roman numerals I through XII. Several cranial nerves (CN) are involved in various aspects of speech, hearing, and swallowing, particularly CNV, CNVII, CNVIII, CNIX, CNX, CNXI, and CNXII (Table 9.1). So, damage to any of these cranial nerves could have a negative effect on communication and swallowing.

There are a wide range of conditions that can contribute to neurogenic communication disorders. These conditions result from damage to either the CNS or PNS, and sometimes both. Foremost among these damaging conditions is a **cerebrovascular accident** (CVA), or what physicians commonly refer to as a **stroke**.

A stroke is an injury to blood vessels in the brain (not the heart), usually in the form of a clot or hemorrhage (i.e., bleeding). Because blood is the means by which oxygen is transferred to the brain, injury to a blood vessels results in a lack of oxygen to brain cells that can lead to brain cell death within only a few minutes. There are two types of blood clots: (1) **thrombosis**, which is a stationary blood clot and (2) **embolism**, which is a blood clot that is carried to a brain artery where it lodges permanently. Approximately 80% of strokes result from a blood clot. A **hemorrhage** is a condition where a blood vessel bursts, resulting in internal bleeding in the brain. This condition comprises 20% of all

Table 9.1. The 12 Cranial Nerves Comprising the Peripheral Nervous System (The primary function associated with each nerve is shown.)

Cranial Nerve	Function
Olfactory (I)	Smell
Optic (II)	Vision
Oculomotor (III)	Eye movement (opening)
Trochlear (IV)	Eye movement (closing)
Trigeminal (V)	Facial sensation and chewing
Abducent (VI)	Eye movement
Facial (VII)	Facial expression and taste
Auditory (VIII)	Balance and hearing
Glossopharyngeal (IX)	Taste and salivation
Vagus (X)	Swallowing and talking Taste and respiration
Accessory (XI)	Pharynx/larynx muscles Neck and shoulder movement
Hypoglossal (XII)	Tongue movement

strokes. The occurrence rates for stroke show that men are at a slightly higher risk than women. The occurrence of stroke increases with age—approximately 75% of all strokes occur in people over the age of 65 years. Stroke is the second single most common cause of mortality worldwide. Strokes are typically unilateral, affecting only one side of the brain. There is no difference in the frequency of occurrence of left-hemisphere and right-hemisphere strokes. When a stroke is not fatal, it leaves people physically impaired (Figure 9.3).

Aside from strokes, there are various diseases affecting the nervous system that contribute to communication disorders. **Parkinson** disease causes a progressive loss of nerve cell function in the part of the brain that controls muscle move-

---

FYI

Many famous people have died from stroke including Carol Barnes (newsreader), Winston Churchill (politician), Charles Dickens (writer), Catherine the Great (Empress of Russia), Rob Guest (entertainer), Isaac Hayes (singer), Curly Howard (one of the Three Stooges), Judy Mazel (author), Kirby Puckett (baseball star), Franklin Roosevelt (politician), Joseph Stalin (politician), and Luther Vandross (singer).

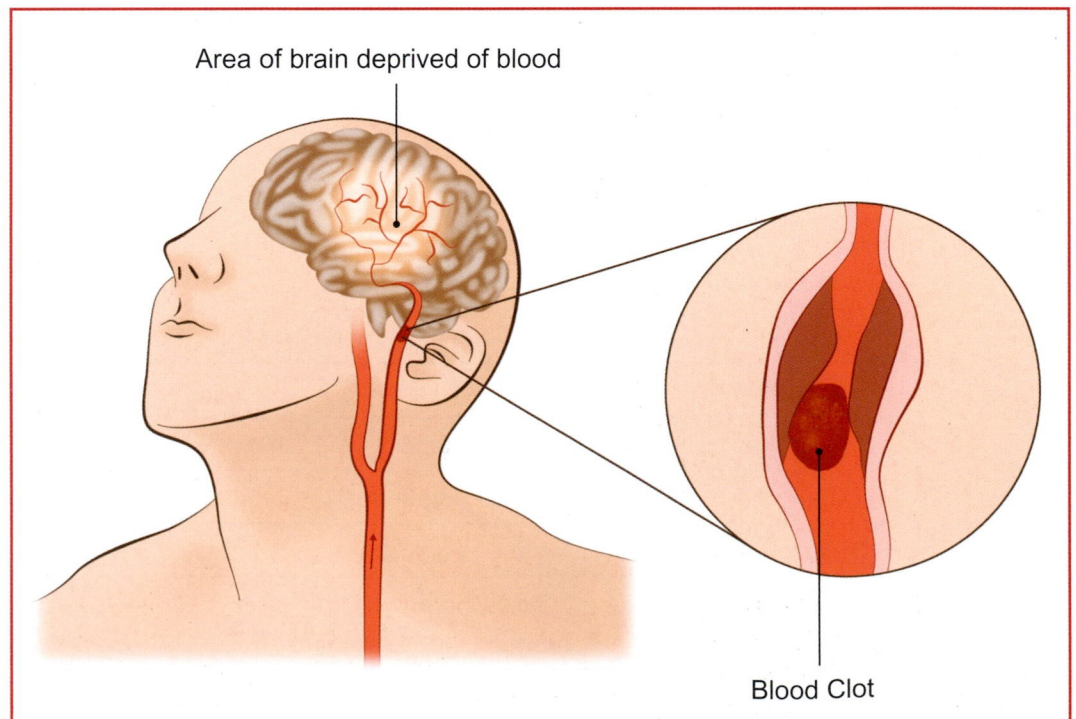

Area of brain deprived of blood

Blood Clot

FIGURE 9.3. Illustration of a cerebrovascular accident (i.e., stroke). A blood clot prevents the flow of blood and oxygen to the brain.

ment, and usually affects people over the age of 50 years. Progressive means that the effects of this disease worsen over time. The four primary symptoms of Parkinson disease are: (1) limb and facial tremor, (2) stiffness of the limbs and trunk (3) **bradykinesia** (i.e., slowness of movement), and (4) postural instability, or impaired balance and coordination. As these symptoms become more pronounced, patients may have difficulty walking and talking.

Alzheimer disease is a frequent form of dementia among older people. **Dementia** is a brain disorder that seriously affects a person's ability to carry out daily activities. The disease begins slowly and initially involves the parts of the brain that control thought, memory, attention, and language. Over time, symptoms get worse and people may not recognize family members or have trouble speaking, reading, or writing.

Multiple sclerosis (MS) is a nervous system disease of the brain and spinal cord that is a result of damage to the **myelin sheath**, the material that surrounds and protects nerve cells. This damage slows down or blocks electrical impulses between the brain and body. The condition is characterized by sporadic episodes of symptoms that may last for weeks or months and then periods where symptoms diminish or disappear (i.e., remissions). The disease occurs most often among women between the ages of 20 to 40 years. There are a variety of symptoms of MS due to the different ways it can affect the central nervous system, including lack of energy, fatigue, clumsiness, vision problems, and speech difficulties such as slurred speech.

Amyotrophic lateral sclerosis (ALS) also referred to as **motor neuron disease** or Lou Gehrig's disease (because it affected this well known American baseball player), is a nervous system disease that attacks nerve cells which transmit messages from the brain and spinal cord to voluntary muscles such as the arms and legs. The disease generally appears between the ages of 40 to 60 years and affects males more often than females. The disease leads to severe impairments in all motor activities including walking, writing, and speaking. The disease is fatal and on average runs its full course between 3 to 5 years following diagnosis. The disease eventually affects breathing ability, leading to respiratory failure.

Traumatic brain injury (TBI), also called a head injury, occurs when a sudden blow to the head causes damage to the brain. TBI can result when the head suddenly and violently hits an object, or when an object pierces the skull and enters brain tissue. Most TBIs are caused by motor vehicle accidents, falls and assaults account for the remaining cases.

FYI

Cerebral palsy is a form of brain damage that occurs at birth. The damage affects the ability to perform voluntary motor movements. This condition is often accompanied by involuntary spasms. Dysarthria is a common feature of cerebral palsy. The severity of the speech disorder is dependent on the degree of motor damage. Cerebral palsy occurs in roughly 2.5 out of every 1,000 births.

FYI

Long-term alcohol consumption could possibly lead to the development of a cognitive-communication disorder. Brain damage is a common and potentially severe consequence of regular alcohol consumption. Even mild-to-moderate drinking can adversely affect cognitive functioning, including memory loss and various language processes.

Symptoms of a TBI can be mild, moderate, or severe, depending on the extent of the damage to the brain. If various centers of the brain that affect speech, language, or hearing are affected by trauma, it is likely that a communication disorder will occur. TBI has been referred to as a silent epidemic because the condition does not receive much public attention and the results are not visible to the naked eye. Yet, TBI is a major public health problem and is a leading cause of disability among children and young adults, particularly males because they tend to be higher risk takers than females, leading to sometimes devastating consequences. Many face lasting impairments that affect their independence and daily lives.

HISTORIC ASPECTS OF NEUROGENIC COMMUNICATION DISORDERS

The history of neurogenic communication disorders has its origins in the discipline of neuroscience. A key issue in the historical developments of neuroscience was the debate over the functioning of the brain, particularly, whether areas of the brain had specific functions (**localism theory**) or whether the brain functioned as a single organ (**holism**

theory). **Franz Joseph Gall** (1758–1828), was a German anatomist and an early advocate of localism (Figure 9.4). He developed a theory in 1800 known as **phrenology**, in which he claimed that character and personality traits, as well as criminal intentions, could be determined based on the shape of the head. That is, a person's mental characteristics were physically engraved in the brain, and were signified by bumps on the surface of the head. Reportedly, Gall was jealous of a friend who showed outstanding memory skills and language proficiency. Because this friend had big bulging eyes, Gall thought the brain was particularly large at this location in the head, thus the brain functions for language and memory must be located behind the eyes. Gall's theory was very popular in the 19th century. A phrenology example is provided in Figure 9.4.

Paul Broca (1824–1880) was a French neurologist and surgeon who also believed that the brain functioned in a localized matter; however, he rejected phrenology (Figure 9.5), and instead was part of a group of scholars who thought there were specific centers within the brain responsible for specific motoric functions. This perspective was referred to as cortical localization. Broca became convinced of localization based on observations of two of his patients. The first was a 30-year-old who had progressive neurologic problems. Near the time of

A   **B**

FIGURE 9.4. Franz Joseph Gall (**A**) and his model of phrenology (**B**).

FIGURE 9.5. Paul Broca. Identified a region in the frontal lobe of the left hemisphere responsible for language formulation and production.

his death, at the age of 51, the man was only able to utter the word, "tan." The second patient was an 84-year-old who lost his speech after falling down a flight of stairs (most likely due to the sudden occurrence of a stroke). After the accident, the individual could only utter four words, "yes," "no," "always," and "three." Upon each person's death, Broca performed an autopsy of the brain and found specific damage to a region of the frontal lobe on the left hemisphere. Broca deduced that this particular region of the brain, which was later termed Broca's area, must be responsible for the production of speech.

Karl Wernicke (1848–1905) was a German neurologist (Figure 9.6). In 1873, Wernicke examined a patient who had suffered a stroke. Although the man was able to speak, he showed considerable difficulty understanding what was said to him. He also showed difficulty understanding written language. When the man died, Wernicke performed an autopsy of his brain and found a lesion in the temporal lobe of the left hemisphere. Wernicke deduced that this particular region in the brain must be localized for understanding language. This unique and highly specialized area of the brain was later termed Wernicke's area.

Korbinian Brodmann (1868–1918) was a German neurologist who supported the theory of localism. By staining tissues in various parts of the brain, he was able to show that different cell types (i.e., the histology) of various brain regions differed. In total, he was able to categorize the brain into 52 distinct areas (now referred to as **Brodmann's areas**) based on the cellular organization of the cortex. A map of Brodmann's areas is shown in Figure 9.7. Brodmann's research career was influenced by his close working relationship with another German neurologist, **Alois Alzheimer** (1864–1915) who is credited with publishing the first case of senile dementia (later known as Alzheimer disease).

FIGURE 9.6. Karl Wernicke. Identified a region in the temporal lobe of the left hemisphere responsible for language comprehension.

A

B

FIGURE 9.7. Korbinian Brodmann (**A**) and an illustration of the Brodmann numbering system for various brain functions (**B**).

Augusta Déjerine-Klumpke (1859–1927) was a renowned American neurologist, neuroanatomist, and an eminent physician of her time (Figure 9.8). She was a pioneer of rehabilitation therapy after spinal cord injuries and contributed much to our current knowledge of spinal cord diseases. She distinguished herself as being the first woman allowed to practice in the hospitals of Paris.

Karl Lashley (1890–1958) was an American psychologist who believed that certain parts of the brain were indeed holistic based on his search for the location in the brain responsible for memory (Figure 9.9). From work with rats, he reasoned that memory is not found in a specific location within the brain but rather the sum of many locations throughout the brain.

FYI

A **coma** is a deep state of unconsciousness, during which an individual is not able to react to his or her environment, and often can occur following a brain injury. The **Glasgow Coma Scale** is the most widely used scoring system used in quantifying the level of consciousness following traumatic brain injury. The scale is based on evaluating the complexity of the patient's eye movements, verbal behaviors, and motor responses.

FIGURE 9.8. Augusta Déjerine-Klumpke. Eminent neurologist who was a pioneer of rehabilitation therapy resulting from spinal cord injury.

FIGURE 9.9. Karl Lashley. American psychologist who believed that certain types of brain functioning involved holistic brain activity.

Hildred Schuell (1906–1970) received her PhD from the University of Iowa in 1946. Shortly after she graduated, she joined the Minneapolis veteran's hospital where she worked for most of her professional life. She was interested in both the evaluation and treatment of aphasia, and over her career she became known world wide for her research in the area of aphasia. She published *Differential Diagnosis of Aphasia with the Minnesota Test*, portions of which are still used today. Schuell was also known as a skilled clinician, working with many war veterans who had experienced aphasia. Her philosophy was that most individuals with aphasia could make progress in their communication abilities under the right conditions.

Finally, **Wilder Penfield** (1891–1976) was an American neurosurgeon who was an expert in the area of epilepsy (i.e., a brain disorder involving recurrent seizures). While performing brain surgery in a number of patients, Penfield would stimulate different sections of their cerebrum. He found that by stimulating very specific regions of the brain, the patients would provide a very specific response. Based on this very direct brain stimulation, he provided compelling support for the view of brain localism (Figure 9.10).

The debate over brain localism and holism has long since subsided. With advances in technology we are now able to identify and visualize many aspects of brain functioning. The results have shown that it is incorrect to assume a one-to-one mapping between brain structure and function. The preferred term regarding the functions of the brain is now **connectionism**. This view essentially supports a mix of both localized and holistic functions in the brain. Lower level or primary sensory and motoric

FIGURE 9.10. Wilder Penfield. Neurosurgeon who provided compelling support for the view of brain localism.

functions seem to be strongly localized but higher-level functions, such as memory and language are the result of interconnections between brain areas.

TYPES OF NEUROGENIC COMMUNICATION DISORDERS

Neurogenic communication disorders can affect speech and/or language components of communication. Two disorders that reflect impairments in speech sound production are **dysarthria** and **apraxia**. These particular conditions are sometimes referred to as **motor speech disorders**. Two disorders that reflect impairments in language are **aphasia** and **cognitive-communication disorder**. There are also a collection of disorders that have a neurogenic basis but are less well defined. The general distribution of the various neurogenic communication disorders is displayed in Figure 9.11 (Duffy, 2005).

Dysarthria

The disorder of dysarthria is an impairment of the motor control for speech caused by weakness, paralysis, slowness, or incoordination of the muscles responsible for producing speech sounds.

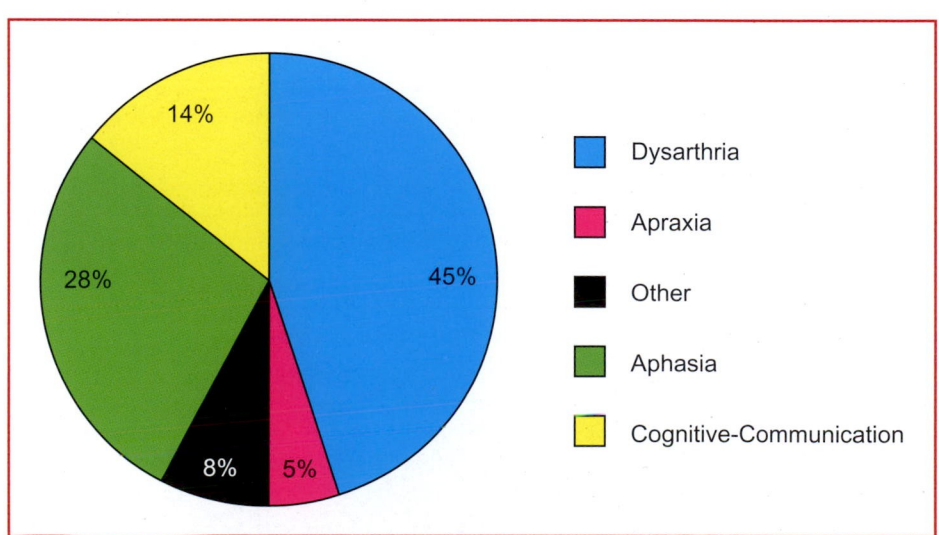

FIGURE 9.11. Distribution of neurogenic communication disorders.

Dysarthria is not a language disorder; however, a language disorder often may coexist with this condition. Individuals with dysarthria understand language and know what they want to say, but may have trouble moving the muscles necessary to clearly produce vowels and consonants. At least six different types of dysarthria have been reported in the research literature. Each type of dysarthria reflects an impairment of a specific location in the nervous system. A detailed description of the various types of dysarthria is shown in Table 9.2. The most frequently seen form of dysarthria is **mixed dysarthria**, reflecting more diffuse damage of the nervous system compared to other forms of dysarthria. Collectively, the six types of dysarthria account for approximately 45% of all neurogenic communication disorders. Common speech problems found in dysarthria are slow and sluggish speech that is often slurred and may be accompanied by drooling. There is reduced vocal loudness and a lack of intonation (i.e., monotone). Three nervous system diseases that show dysarthria are Parkinson disease, MS, and ALS.

Apraxia

The term apraxia is derived from the Greek word *praxis*, which means to work or perform. The condition of apraxia, therefore, refers to an inability to voluntarily perform skilled motor movements

Table 9.2. The Six Types of Dysarthria

Type of Dysarthria	Cause and Features
Hyperkinetic	• Results from damage to the basal ganglia (deep in the brain). • Problems with involuntary movement.
Hypokinetic	• Results from damage to the substantia nigra (a small region in the brainstem). • Condition most often associated with Parkinson disease.
Spastic	• Results from damage to the pyramidal (motor) tract of the nervous system. • Problems with executing fine motor movements.
Flaccid	• Results from damage to the cranial nerves involved in speech. • Problems with vocal fold movement (paralysis).
Ataxic	• Results from damage to the cerebellum. • Problems regulating the force, timing, rhythm, speed, and overall coordination of movement.
Mixed	• Results from simultaneous damage to two or more motor components of the nervous system. • Condition most often associated with motor degenerative diseases such as Lou Gehrig disease.

that are not a result of muscle weakness. The term dyspraxia is probably a more accurate description of the condition because there is not a complete loss of volitional movement, as might be expected in true apraxia. Conditions of apraxia are found for a variety of movement behaviors such as hand and leg movements. Apraxia of speech is a motor speech disorder resulting from impairment in the ability to mentally organize the speech muscles and articulators for volitional production of speech sounds. There are two types of speech apraxia: **developmental** and **acquired**. Developmental apraxia of speech occurs in children and is present from birth for most affected individuals. Further details concerning developmental (childhood) apraxia of speech can be found in Chapter 5.

Acquired apraxia typically occurs in adults and results from an identifiable neurological impairment. Acquired apraxia of speech accounts for approximately 5% of all neurogenic communication disorders. The condition often co-occurs with language problems among individuals who have a form of nonfluent aphasia (to be discussed in a following section). The condition is also apparent in degenerative diseases of the CNS, such as ALS or Creutzfeld-Jacob ("mad cow") disease. Individuals with speech apraxia will report that they know the words they want to say but they will not come out the right way. A primary feature of speech apraxia is inconsistent and variable speech misarticulations. In some instances, a person may clearly articulate words, whereas in other instances there is a breakdown in speech articulation (either substituting one consonant for another or completely deleting consonants). Correct ar-
" troublesome than monosyllabic

words. Apraxic speakers grope for the correct word. They may make several attempts at a word before they are able to accurately articulate the word. Individuals might also show oral (i.e., nonverbal) apraxia, which is characterized by an inability to imitate or follow commands to perform volitional movements of the speech structures. For example, a patient may have difficulty whistling, coughing, or blowing out a match on request, but minutes later, when not consciously thinking of the task, can naturally cough to clear his or her throat.

Aphasia

Aphasia is a language disorder associated with brain injury, usually a stroke. Aphasia refers to a collection of clinically diverse disorders that affect the production and comprehension of language and the ability to read, write, or calculate. This disorder accounts for approximately a quarter of all neurogenic communication impairments. There are four primary types of aphasia, each of which involves damage to the left hemisphere of the cerebrum, and are categorized according to the fluency of language expression (Table 9.3). People with **fluent aphasia** have major problems understanding spoken and written language, although their language expression seemingly appears to be within normal limits. **Wernicke's aphasia** and **anomic aphasia** are examples of fluent aphasia. People with **nonfluent aphasia** have difficulty expressing themselves when speaking or writing, although their ability to understand language seems to remain relatively intact. **Broca's Aphasia** and **mixed (or global) aphasia** are examples of nonfluent aphasia.

Table 9.3. Various Types of Aphasia	
Type of Aphasia	**Language Examples**
Fluent Aphasia: Wernicke	• May say words that make little sense. • May use made-up words such as "frangle" and are not aware of doing so. • May produce a full-length sentence that has no meaning. It sounds like a sentence but there is no content to what is being spoken.
Fluent Aphasia: Anomia	• May have difficulties naming certain words. • Patients tend to produce grammatically correct, yet semantically empty, speech. • Language comprehension tends to be preserved.
Nonfluent Aphasia: Broca	• May struggle to say words and form a sentence. • Affected people often omit small words such as "is," "and," and "the." • Often aware of their difficulties and can become easily frustrated by their speaking.
Nonfluent Aphasia: Mixed (or Global)	• May be completely nonverbal, and/or only use facial expressions and gestures to communicate. • May only understand some words.

Wernicke's aphasia is so named because of the location in the brain where damage has occurred. Wernicke's area is found in the temporal lobe of the left hemisphere at Brodmann area 22 (Figures 9.7 and 9.12). The lesion does not damage the frontal region of the brain, which is responsible for all motor behavior. Therefore, one obvious feature of Wernicke's aphasia is that there are no signs of body paralysis. The condition is characterized by fluent language expression but impaired language comprehension. To a naïve listener, the individual with Wernicke's aphasia may seem to have no expressive language difficulty because the speech is effortless. However, when listening closely, it be-

comes evident that the content of what is being spoken about may be impaired. Anomic aphasia generally results from damage to a very isolated region in Wernicke's area of the brain. Similar to Wernicke's aphasia, there are no obvious signs of body paralysis. This particular communication disorder is characterized by difficulty in word retrieval. The patient's speech is essentially fluent; however, there are high instances of **circumlocutions** (i.e., roundabout talking) due to word-finding problems.

Broca's aphasia results from a lesion to Broca's area which is in the left frontal lobe at Brodmann area 44 (see Figures 9.7 and 9.12). This lesion is accompanied by some sort of one-sided body weak-

FIGURE 9.12. Location of Broca's Area, Heschl's gyrus, and Wernicke's area. Broca's area and Wernicke's area are found only in the left hemisphere of the brain.

ness or paralysis (i.e., **hemiparesis**). This particular type of aphasia is characterized primarily by fairly intact language comprehension skills but nonfluent expressive language. The nature of the expressive language is confined to short utterances of approximately four words or less, and speech articulation is likely to be slow and labored as a result of dysarthria co-occurring. Mixed aphasia and global aphasia are nonfluent forms of aphasia that relate more to the sever-

ity of the brain lesion rather than the distinctive communication disorder. The lesion is usually deep and covers portions of both Wernicke's and Broca's areas. In mixed aphasia, the problems with expressive and receptive language are generally no more than moderate in severity. Global aphasia reflects a severe to profound communication disorder due to a massive brain lesion. In mixed and global aphasias, speech dysarthria is likely to be present as well.

Cognitive-Communication Disorders

The term, cognitive-communication disorder, is used to describe a broad range of communication problems that can result from damage to the frontal lobe regions of the brain. Along with controlling motor movement, this region of the brain also controls our ability to think (i.e., cognition). Damage to this part of the brain results in impairment in the ability to transform thoughts into meaningful expressive language. The impairment is also found in the use of gestures and written language. This language disorder should not be confused with aphasia. ASHA (2004) defines cognitive-communication disorders as problems with attention/concentration, memory, organization, reasoning, and social skills that impact communication. A cognitive-communication disorder can result from damage to the **right hemisphere**, as well as the left hemisphere; they comprise approximately 14% of all neurogenic communication disorders.

Symptoms of cognitive-communication disorders vary widely depending on the type and cause of brain damage, and the communication problems can range from minor to severe. Individuals who have experienced a traumatic brain injury (TBI) are at a high risk for developing a cognitive-communication disorder. Injury to the frontal lobes can occur in a number of ways, including: (1) laceration, (2) concussion, and (3) contrecoup. A **laceration** is a wound or cut to the brain that involves direct tearing of brain tissue. A **concussion** is a direct blow to the head that may result from violent shaking of the head, or a whiplash type of injury. A **contrecoup** injury involves a secondary injury that is opposite to the primary injury, whereby

the brain essentially rocks back and forth. Examples of the types of TBI are illustrated in Figure 9.13. Individuals with Alzheimer disease or those with a history of drug and/or alcohol abuse can also develop a cognitive-communication disorder.

CURRENT THEORIES REGARDING NEUROGENIC COMMUNICATION DISORDERS

One unique aspect of brain injury relates to a concept known as **spontaneous recovery**. This concept concerns a patient's natural re-establishment of skills that initially were lost immediately following the brain injury. Spontaneous recovery is not specific to communication but for motor and sensory abilities as well. All patients are expected to show some level of spontaneous recovery as a result of brain healing (e.g., reduction in swelling). Yet, no two patients are alike as to the amount of their spontaneous recovery. Patients may fully recover their communication abilities, a portion of their abilities, or show very minimal recovery. In addition, the time span of spontaneous recovery varies, ranging from a few days to several years post-injury. The investigation of spontaneous recovery is linked to one of the most fascinating areas of current neurobiological research known as neuroplasticity (Cappa, 2000). **Neuroplasticity** refers to the changes that occur in the organization of the brain as a result of trauma. A dedicated area in the brain associated with a given function can transfer to a different location in the brain as a consequence of brain damage/recovery. In regard to aphasia, researchers are in-

FIGURE 9.13. Types of traumatic brain injury including (**A** through **C**): laceration, concussion, and contrecoup.

trigued as to why and how recovery from aphasia takes place. One of the earliest hypotheses about neuroplasticity was that, as a result of damage (e.g., stroke) to left hemisphere, the right hemisphere simply takes over all linguistic functions that normally would have occurred in the left hemisphere.

FYI

An individual who experiences a stroke in the right hemisphere can acquire a condition known as **left neglect**. This is a type of attention disorder where the individual no longer acknowledges the left side of the body, or any environmental space that is in the person's left visual field. The person may not shave the left side of their face, or avoid eating food on the left side of the plate. The neglect is also found in their reading behavior.

The **right hemisphere theory of recovery** is still a popular theory, and with advances in functional imaging of the brain, the specific role of the right hemisphere as part of spontaneous recovery can be examined more directly.

There are numerous theories as to the cause of acquired apraxia of speech. Because of the inconsistency in speech sound misarticulations, and the tendency for these misarticulations to occur on words containing multiple syllables, the disorder is assumed to be related to difficulty sequencing the speech articulators (e.g., lips, tongue, jaw). The prevailing theory is that acquired apraxia is a **phonetic-motoric disorder**. The manner in which speech sounds/words are organized in the brain prior to saying them is intact. The disorder occurs as a result of the actual execution of speech. The motor system governing our speech articulators is thought to have its own "cognitive architecture" that is activated and monitored in part by the language system (Ballard et al., 2000). In the case of apraxia of speech this cognitive architecture is faulty.

ASSESSMENT OF NEUROGENIC COMMUNICATION DISORDERS

Dysarthria

Evaluation of the patient's speech clarity is a major component in the assessment of dysarthria. The examination includes evaluation of **speech intelligibility** at a variety of levels including: (a) individual speech sounds, (b) single word production, (c) reading aloud, and (4) conversational speech. Due to the obvious physical and motoric impairments associated with this condition, a number of neuromuscular features that may influence speech sound production are examined. These include assessments of oral-motor strength, speed of articulator movement, and accuracy and steadiness of voice pitch. If possible, SLPs may use various forms of equipment to assist in the assessment of dysarthria. For example, aerodynamic testing can be performed to examine the patient's respiratory abilities, in particular breath support for producing speech. Measurement of muscle activity through the use of **electromyographic** recording also can inform the SLP as to the role of various muscles in the production of speech.

Apraxia

There is no single factor or test that can be used to diagnose apraxia of speech. In addition, SLPs do not fully agree about which specific symptoms must exist for the diagnosis of an apraxia condition. The SLP looks for the presence of a group of symptoms, including those described above. Ruling out other contributing factors, such as muscle weakness or language-comprehension problems, also can help with the diagnosis. To diagnose acquired apraxia, the SLP may ask the person to perform speech tasks like repeating a particular word several times or repeating a list of words of increasing length (e.g., wreck, reckless, recklessly). The patient also may be asked to engage in conversation, during which time the SLP would note any inconsistent speech misarticulations. Aspects of nonspeech oral apraxia are also tested by having the patient perform volitional movements of the speech structures, such as whistling, coughing, or blowing. If available, use of instruments to directly image the brain are especially useful to help distinguish acquired apraxia of speech from other communication disorders in people who have experienced brain damage.

Aphasia

Assessment of aphasia is a problem-solving activity. The SLP must first determine whether the patient actually demonstrates aphasic symptoms. If so, the SLP will try to determine the nature or type of aphasia (e.g., fluent, nonfluent). Next, the SLP should appraise the patient's existing functional communication abilities. The assessment occurs in two stages. The first stage is the **initial assessment**, which happens at the patient's bedside while she or he is still a hospital inpatient. During this initial assessment, the SLP obtains a sample of the patient's spoken language and also assesses general language comprehension abilities. Within approximately 1 week following the initial assessment, the patient should have regained enough

strength to sit at a table and tolerate the demands of a more sustained interaction. The **primary assessment** occurs at this time and the patient's language expression and comprehension are fully evaluated, as well as reading and writing abilities.

A dilemma when performing a language assessment in a person with aphasia is that often there is no baseline record of the person's language abilities prior to the brain injury (i.e., the **premorbid state**). Information regarding the person's prior vocabulary and reading abilities, as well as general loquaciousness would be useful to the SLP in determining the severity of aphasia. The most logical source of this information would be to consider the person's prior vocation, educational background, or to simply ask the patient's family members. Those individuals closest to the patient may be at a loss as to how best to communicate with their loved one following a brain injury. Some common approaches to communication with people with aphasia have been developed by the National Aphasia Association and are shown in Table 9.4.

Cognitive-Communication Disorders

A cognitive-communication disorder encompasses difficulty with any aspect of communication that is affected by disruption of cognition (AHSA, 2004). Therefore, an assessment of this disorder should involve examination of all aspects of communication, particularly listening, speaking, gesturing, reading, and writing. The assessment also needs to include close inspection of the individual's cognitive abilities, including behaviors like attention, memory, and organization.

Table 9.4. Some Tips for Communicating With People Who Have Aphasia

- Praise and accept all attempts to speak.
- Avoid talking "down" to the person. Communicate to the person as an adult.
- Avoid speaking in the presence of excessive background noise.
- Allow time for the person to talk and permit a reasonable amount of time for the person to respond.
- Keep your communication simple so as ensure its understanding.
- Augment your speech with gestures and visual aids whenever possible.
- If needed, repeat a statement.
- Make sure you have the person's attention before communicating.

An important consideration in the evaluation of individuals who may have a cognitive-communication disorder is to consider the impact of the disorder on overall functioning. Therefore, the assessment incorporates observations of the individual in his or her home/daily environment and includes interviews with caregivers and other frequent communication partners (Hopper, 2005).

TREATMENT OF NEUROGENIC COMMUNICATION DISORDERS

Dysarthria

The treatment of dysarthria focuses on the improvement of speech clarity and speech naturalness. Specific goals for therapy are targeted toward altering speaking rate and increasing breath support, as well as muscle strengthening exercises designed to increase mouth, tongue, and lip movement. The SLP can help the person's caregivers or family learn to adapt to the environment so they can understand the person better. Among individuals with mild to moderate dysarthria, particularly those with Parkinson disease, a popular treatment approach known as the **Lee Silverman Voice Treatment** (LSVT) is in widespread use. The LSVT technique emphasizes high-effort loud phonation to improve respiratory, laryngeal, and articulatory functions during speech (Ramig et al., 2001) (see also Chapter 8).

In cases of severe dysarthria, such as those associated with advanced neurodegenerative disorders (e.g., ALS), it is unlikely the patient's speech clarity will improve with traditional treatment approaches. The SLP may recommend using somewhat nontraditional approaches to facilitate communication. In this case, **alternative** or **augmentative communication** (AAC) devices are considered. The construction of these devices and their use can range from basic to sophisticated. An example of a basic or low technology device would be an alphabet or picture board (Figure 9.14). The

FIGURE 9.14. Simplied example of an alternative communication device for use by individuals who are unable to use speech as a sole means of communication.

patient with dysarthria would simply point to letters or pictures on the board to express words and messages rather than attempting to verbally say the words. A sophisticated or high technology device might include a computer that has an artificial voice output. The theoretical physicist Stephen Hawking, who has ALS, uses an AAC device to communicate.

Apraxia

Treatment approaches for apraxia of speech depend on the severity of the impairment. In some cases, people with acquired apraxia of speech recover some or all of their speech abilities on their own. Individuals with mild apraxia might be taught strategies to help them correctly articulate multisyllabic words that tend to give them trouble. People with moderate to severe apraxia usually need frequent and intensive therapy sessions with a SLP. One approach to ther-

apy is to work on **sound-sequencing** skills. In this approach, a word to be spoken is dissected into individual consonants and vowels. The patient is asked to say the individual sounds in a controlled, deliberate fashion, while also thinking about how the lips and tongue should be placed in the mouth. Sometimes tapping or clapping out the rhythm of speech helps patients to speak more clearly. An alternative approach to having the patient produce individual speech sounds is to work on more complex forms of articulation first, such as two- and three-element consonant clusters (e.g., stop, street). The logic behind this approach is to help the patient gain control over more challenging forms of speech sound sequencing first, which will have a trickle-down effect of naturally stabilizing the articulation of less complex (individual) speech sounds (Maas et al., 2002). Patients with very severe apraxia may always experience difficulty with articulating speech sounds in a normal manner. In such cases, a decision may be made to use an AAC device, depending on the severity of the apraxia and communicative needs of the individual.

Aphasia

Patients who experience a brain injury resulting in aphasia may spontaneously recover their original communication abilities. Although some level of natural recovery might be expected in most patients with aphasia, speech-language therapy is still an important facet in the patient's recovery. The goal of therapy for patients with aphasia is to: (1) maximize recovery of impaired function, (2) assist in the development of communication strategies, and (3) help the patient adjust to the residual deficits of the brain injury. It is unlikely that any two patients with aphasia will experience an identical stroke, and patients do not come from identical backgrounds. So the treatment program for each patient is unique (Wambaugh et al., 2006).

Approaches to treating aphasia include: (1) stimulation, (2) memorization, and (3) inhibition. **Stimulation** involves encouraging the patient to use all modalities of communication to foster the return of language abilities that are impaired but appear to have the potential to be regained. For example, the patient may be asked to verbally "echo" language models provided by the SLP. The patient could be encouraged to read lips, attempt writing symbols/shapes, and read single words. In essence, the patient is asked to try everything in regards to expression of language.

Working on a patient's **memory** skills is thought to assist with the development of new neural pathways in the brain, which can lead to learning how to speak again. Memory tasks can include imitating/recalling motor sequences or repetition of phrases and sentences. Some individuals who have experienced a brain injury could show difficulty with **inhibiting** their emotion, especially those emotions that are generally suppressed. Patients might demonstrate uncontrollable laughing/crying or may become sexual aroused. This aspect of therapy attempts to assist the patient to recognize when these emotions are evident and to help extinguish them. For example, the SLP could ask the patient to purposely pretend to laugh uncontrollably and to have them halt doing so on the basis of a visual or verbal prompt.

Cognitive-Communication Disorders

Patients with this disorder typically have some level of intellectual impairment (e.g., dementia) that affects language, attention, memory, and personality. The goal of therapy is to assist patients in increasing their reliance on more intact cognitive abilities to compensate for those abilities that have become impaired. Hopper (2005) recommends a variety of treatment approaches to working with a patient with a cognitive-communication disorder. These approaches include: (1) validation therapy, (2) graphic cues, (3) Montessori techniques, and (4) caregiver training. **Validation therapy** is a technique used to confirm (through words and gestures) what the person with dementia says, regardless of accuracy or basis in fact, rather than correcting or re-orienting the person. **Graphic cuing** involves providing written factual information and/or familiar photographs to facilitate communication. This approach capitalizes on the patient's recognition memory and the ability to read aloud. **Montessori-based interventions** involve the development of structured activities which are appropriate to an individual's cognitive abilities that take place in the context of social interaction. Finally, when working with a patient with a cognitive-communication disorder, it is important to incorporate the patient's caregivers in the treatment program. Each letter in the acronym FOCUSED stands for a particular communication technique to be used by caregivers (Ripich & Ziol, 1998). The goal is to teach the patient a functional piece of information or behavior that can be used in everyday situations. A summary of the FOCUSED program is found in Table 9.5.

CULTURAL CONSIDERATIONS AND NEUROGENIC COMMUNICATION DISORDERS

A range of multicultural factors interact with neurogenic communication disorders. For example, **race** and **ethnicity** are predisposing factors for a number of neurological conditions that produce communicative impairments. In the United States, African Americans and Hispanics are at greater risk for dementia than other cultural groups (Qualls & Muñoz, 2005). African Americans, Hispanics, Native Americans, as well as Pacific Islanders are at particularly high risk for Type 2 (adult onset) diabetes,

Table 9.5. Summary of the FOCUSED Approach to Caregiver Training for Patients With Cognitive-Linguistic Impairments

F = Face	Face the person directly. Call his or her name. Touch the person. Maintain eye contact.
O = Orient	Orient the person to the topic by repeating key words. Repeat phrases. Use nouns and specific names.
C = Continue	Continue the same topic of conversation as long as possible. Restate the topic throughout the conversation.
U = Unstick	Help the person become "unstuck" when she or he uses a word incorrectly by suggesting the intended word.
S = Structured	Structure your questions so that the person can recognize and repeat a response. Provide two simple choices at a time. Use yes/no questions.
E = Exchange	Keep up the normal exchange of ideas used in everyday conversation. Give the person clues as to how to answer questions.
D = Direct	Keep sentences short, simple, and direct. Put the subject of the sentences first. Use hand signals, pictures, and facial expressions.

thus making these groups at greater risk for heart disease and stroke. Also, African Americans have the highest death rate from TBI, and long-term disability following TBI tends to be more severe for African Americans than other racial groups (Thurman et al., 1999).

The occurrence of various nervous system diseases, such as MS, differs according to **geographic region**. People living beyond the 40-degree latitude mark north or south of the equator are far more likely to develop MS than those living in warmer climates near the equator. This is especially true for people in North America, Europe, and New Zealand, whereas Asia continues to have a low incidence of MS. Caucasians are far more likely to develop MS than those of African heritage.

A person's **socioeconomic status** (SES) is also a consideration in neurogenic communication disorders. For example, **low SES** individuals are less likely to have access to appropriate health care than middle SES and high SES individuals. Lack of access to health care places these individuals at greater risk for later appearing conditions (e.g., hypertension, diabetes) that are precursors to some neurological conditions (e.g., stroke, dementia). Also, the diet of low SES individuals can lead to nutritional deficiencies that affect neurological growth and development, as well as the risk of and response to neurological impairment (Qualls & Muñoz, 2005).

The **bilingual speaker** who has experienced a brain injury resulting in language impairment presents a unique challenge for the SLP, not only from a multicultural perspective but from a neurologic perspective. The languages of a bilingual speaker are stored in the left hemispheres, similar to monolingual speakers; however, the languages may not completely overlap in cortical and subcortical regions in the brain (Roberts, 2001). This can result in quite different abilities in the two languages following the injury. It is important that the SLP recognize the likelihood of an uneven language profile in these patients.

CURRENT RESEARCH IN NEUROGENIC COMMUNICATION DISORDERS

Health Policy

Many individuals who demonstrate neurogenic communication disorders tend to be elderly who have experienced a medically based injury. Presumably, the government provides some level of financial support for the patient's overall rehabilitation. Yet, there is no universally agreed-on policy for provision of speech-language therapy services. Cost is a major factor in the provision of services, so it is important to consider the influence of **health and social policy** on provision of speech-language services. A small body of research is forming that is addressing the influence of government policy on the outcomes of individuals with neurogenic communication disorders (Worrall, 2000).

Deep Brain Stimulation

Medical advances in the treatment of various neurologic disorders may contribute to a concomitant reduction in communication disorders. Individuals with neurologic disorders such as Parkinson disease that affect muscle movement (including speech musculature) are often prescribed medications to help alleviate muscle stiffness and restricted range of movement. These drugs eventually prove to be ineffective as the severity of the disease progresses. However, there is innovative research that is designed to bypass the need for medications. Instead, treatment involves directly stimulating parts of the brain to help reduce disordered movement patterns. The procedure is referred to as **deep brain stimulation** (DBS) and involves inserting electrodes via a hair-thin wire through the skull into the area of the brain that controls movement (Figure 9.15). The patient is able to control the device with a neurotransmitter that sends electrical impulses down the wire into the brain. The person can turn the DBS on when needed, and turn it off during sleep (when the motor disturbance is minimal). Currently, there is controversy as to whether the use of DBS improves speech or has limited influence on speech clarity (Pinto et al., 2005).

ICF Framework

When considering assessment of neurogenic communication disorders, it is important to recognize that a brain injury can have a devastating, life-changing impact on a patient's everyday existence. Therefore, it is imperative to consider the patient's overall lifestyle and to take steps to reduce any barriers to everyday functioning. The **International Classification of Functioning** (ICF) framework was developed by the World Health Organization (WHO, 2001) as a model of practice for rehabilitation clinicians.

FIGURE 9.15. Illustration of deep brain stimulation.

The WHO ICF model shifts the concept of disability from one that focuses on impairments to one that focuses on the individual. Using an ICF perspective, a patient's disability can be assessed according to two factors: (1) **functioning and disability** and (2) **contextual factors**. Functioning and disability includes: (a) **body functions and structures**, which describes the actual anatomy/physiology and psychology of the human body, and (b) **activity and participation**, which describes the person's functional status, including communication, mobility, interpersonal interactions, self-care, learning, and applying knowledge. Contextual factors include: (a) **environmental factors**, which are those factors that are not within the person's control, such as family, work, government agencies, laws, and cultural beliefs, and (b) **personal factors**, which include race, gender, age, educational level, and coping styles. The characteristics of the ICF make it attractive to SLPs for the holistic treatment of patients with a communication disorder. Although the ICF is not a formal assessment tool, it provides a framework to identify the key issues that may impact a patient's overall rehabilitation. Research using the ICF is providing encouraging results for addressing various neurogenic communication disorders such as aphasia and TBI (Eden & Larkins, 2007).

Stem Cells

Stem cells are found in bone marrow and blood vessels in human embryos. They are the "starter" cells that have the ability to grow into adult tissue. Research has shown that stem cells, taken from embryos that are just a few days old can turn into any of the 300 different types of cells that make up the adult body (Wu et al., 2007). Although this research is still considered controversial and highly restrictive in some countries, the U.S. National Institute on Deafness and Other Communication Disorders (NIDCD) identifies the use of stem cells as a possible approach to improving communication disorders resulting from impaired or decreased nerve cells. Specific research of this nature has yet to be undertaken.

Management

Treatment of aphasia is varied and there is no agreed-on approach to managing this disorder. Attempts are underway to develop a coherent theory of therapy for aphasia that details not only *what* therapies work, but *why* they work, and with *whom*. At least two lines of research will likely contribute to this endeavor. The first line of research relates to the use of functional neuroimaging to study patterns of neural reorganization following brain injury. The second approach involves use of computational modeling of aphasia treatment (Beeson & Rapcsak, 2000). The hope is that through better understanding of the mechanisms involved in aphasia recovery, improved quality of treatment to aphasic patients will follow.

FYI

Advances in research are likely to lead to new ideas about the neurogenic bases of a variety of communication disorders, particularly those that currently have no identifiable cause, such as stuttering and specific language impairment (SLI).

speech: Theory, analysis, and treatment. *Aphasiology, 14,* 969–995.

Beeson, P., & Rapcsak, S. (2000). Toward a theory of therapy for aphasia. *Brain and Language, 71,* 22–25.

Cappa, S. (2000). Recovery from aphasia: Why and how? *Brain and Language, 71,* 39–41.

Duffy, J. (2005). *Motor speech disorders: Substrates, differential diagnosis, and management.* St. Louis, MO: Mosby.

Eden, D., & Larkins, B. (2007). The application of the International Classification of Functioning Disability and Health (ICF) in speech-language therapy: A case example of a client with aphasia following stroke. *New Zealand Journal of Speech-Language Therapy, 62,* 20–28.

Hopper, T. (2005, Nov. 8). Assessment and treatment of cognitive-communication disorders in individuals with dementia. *The ASHA Leader,* pp. 10–11.

Mass, E., Barlow, J., Robin, D., & Shapiro, L. (2002). Treatment of sound errors in aphasia and apraxia of speech: Effects of phonological complexity. *Aphasiology, 16,* 609–622.

Pinto, S., Gentil, M., Krack, P., Sauleau, P., Fraix, V., Benabid, A. L., & Pollak, P. (2005). Changes induced by levodopa and subthalamic nucleus stimulation on Parkinsonian speech. *Movement Disorders, 20,* 1507–1515.

Qualls, C. D., & Muñoz, M. L. (2005). Race-ethnicity, socioeconomic status, and cognitive-communicative functioning in individuals with neurogenic communication disorders: Clinical implications and research directions. *ECHO: E-Journal for Black and Other Ethnic Group Research and Practices in Communication Sciences and Disorders, 1*(1), 30–39.

Ramig, L. O., Sapir, S., Fox, C., & Countryman, S. (2001). Changes in vocal intensity following intensive voice treatment (LSVT) in individuals with Parkinson disease: A comparison with untreated patients and normal age-matched controls. *Movement Disorders, 16,* 79–83.

NEUROGENIC COMMUNICATION DISORDERS ON THE WORLD WIDE WEB

Listed below are Web sites that provide further information on the topic of neurogenic communication disorders. At the time of publication each Web site was freely accessible.

Aphasia Institute Videos
http://www.aphasia.ca/videos/aphasiavideo.html

Components of a Neurological Examination Video
http://www.neuroexam.com

Deep Brain Stimulation Video
http://www.webmd.com/video/early-parkinsons-surgery

Dysarthria Video
http://www.nle.nottingham.ac.uk/websites/stroke/videos/dysarthria2.html

Traumatic Brain Injury Video Library
http://www.traumaticbraininjury.com

REFERENCES

American Speech-Language-Hearing Association. (2004). Roles of speech-language pathologists in the identification, diagnosis, and treatment of individuals with cognitive-communication disorders. Practice guidelines and policies. *ASHA, Supplement 24.*

Ballard, K., Granier, J., & Robin, D. (2000). Understanding the nature of apraxia of

Ripich, D., & Ziol, E. (1998). Dementia: A review for the speech-language pathologist. In A. Johnson & B. Jacobson (Eds.), *Medical speech-langauge pathology: A practitioner's guide* (pp. 467–496). New York: Thieme.

Roberts, P. (2001). Aphasia assessment and treatment for bilingual and culturally diverse patients. In R. Chapey (Ed.), *Language intervention strategies in adult aphasia* (5th ed, pp. 208–232). Philadelphia: Lippincott Williams & Wilkins.

Thurman, D., Alverson, C., Dunn, K., Guerrero, J., & Sniezek, J. (1999). Traumatic brain injury in the United States: A public health perspective. *Journal of Head Trauma and Rehabilitation, 14*, 602–615.

Wambaugh, J. L., Duffy, J. R., McNeil, M. R., Robin, D. A., & Rogers, M. A. (2006). Treatment guidelines for acquired apraxia of speech: Treatment descriptions and recommendations. *Journal of Medical Speech-Language Pathology, 14*, 283–299.

World Health Organization. (2001). *International classification of functioning, disability, and health.* Geneva: Author.

Worrall, L. (2000). Future directions and research issues in functional communication assessment and treatment. In L. Worrall & C. Frattali (Eds.), *Neurogenic communication disorders: A functional approach* (pp. 331–344). New York: Thieme.

Wu, D. C., Boyd, A. S., & Wood, K. J. (2007). Embryonic stem cell transplantation: Potential applicability in cell replacement therapy and regenerative medicine. *Frontiers in Bioscience, 12*, 4525–4535.

DYSPHAGIA

OBJECTIVES

After reading this chapter, the student should be able to:

- Describe the basic anatomic and neuromuscular systems involved in swallowing.

- Demonstrate understanding of bedside methods of dysphagia assessment.

- Demonstrate understanding of instrumentation for the assessment and treatment of swallowing functions.

- Demonstrate knowledge of swallowing disorders including their etiologies.

- Describe current surgical techniques related to communicative and swallowing functions, and prosthetics.

- Describe various nonsurgical techniques related to the management of dysphagia.

- Describe multicultural considerations in the assessment and management of dysphagia.

INTRODUCTION

People swallow a thousand times or more each day. Swallowing begins at the lips and ends at the stomach. Swallowing is an activity that we tend to take for granted and perform easily. Yet the process of normal swallowing actually is a highly complex activity. Approximately 30 to 40 pairs of muscles, and at least six pairs of nerves, are involved in moving food from the lips to the stomach. To add to this complexity, these structures must perform in sequence with our breathing patterns to ensure the material being swallowed is directed toward the stomach rather than the lungs.

Among some disabled children and adults there is a breakdown in coordination of swallowing. This breakdown may be due to the person's: (1) wakefulness or awareness (2) brain functioning, and/or (3) muscular strength. The medical term for swallowing difficulty is called **dysphagia** ("dis fay ja" or "dis fah ja"). Dysphagia is one of the newest specialty areas in the SLP profession. Speech-language pathologists are called upon tens of thousands of times every day to evaluate swallowing in the estimated 18 million adults suffering from dysphagia in the United States and many millions more internationally. Dysphagia can severely affect an individual's quality of life and can also require a person to be dependent on others to be fed. Aside from these social issues, disordered swallowing may be life threatening. A person can run the risk of choking or having the airway blocked. Malnutrition, weight loss, and increased risk of dehydration are possible outcomes of prolonged periods of swallowing difficulties. Dysphagia also could pose a threat for respiratory infec-

---

FYI

Most people believe they chew their food thoroughly before swallowing but this may not be the case. It is recommended that, on average, we should chew food between 20 and 30 times before swallowing. The more we chew the more saliva we generate which helps break down food and facilitate the digestion process.

---

tions resulting from food entering the lungs rather than the stomach. What is generally considered an automatic and even pleasurable experience can be one of discomfort and worry.

TERMINOLOGY AND DEFINITIONS

There are a variety of terms associated with normal and disordered swallowing. To begin, the formal term used to describe the act of normal swallowing is **deglutition**. We swallow for two reasons. The first reason is maintenance. This type of swallowing is used to remove the natural buildup of saliva in the oral cavity. **Maintenance** swallowing tends to occur subconsciously and happens even when we sleep. Maintenance swallowing also has been observed in infants prior to birth. Although in most cases this type of swallowing occurs automatically, we also can swallow deliberately whenever we feel like clearing our throats. The second reason we swallow is for **ingestion**. This type of swallowing is for the consumption of liquids and foods. Ingestive swallowing of **per oral** (p.o.) nutrition (i.e., food taken by mouth) requires that we are awake and cognizant of the presence of food or fluid in the mouth. Typically, the process of swallowing food involves chewing. The technical term for chewing is **mastication**. When we chew, the food inside the mouth is turned into a soft mass referred to as a **bolus**. During deglutition, the bolus moves through the tubes of the digestive system in waves of alternating contraction and relaxation (i.e., snakelike movement) known as **peristalsis**.

The term dysphagia is a combination of the prefix *dys* (disordered) and the Greek word *phagein* (eat). Dysphagia can occur at locations anywhere from the lips to the stomach and is found in approximately 7% of the general population. Among people aged 50 years or older, the occurrence of dysphagia ranges anywhere from 15% to 30% and may be as high as 60% in acute hospital wards and nursing homes. The frequency of occurrence of dysphagia does not differ between females and males. A primary indicator of dysphagia is coughing moments after swallowing. This can lead to **aspiration**, which refers to the situation where food or liquid inadvertently enters the breathing airway (trachea) before, during, or after the swallow (Figure 10.1). Among individuals who experience a stroke, it is not uncommon for them to be susceptible to aspiration during the earliest days of recovery. A condition known as **reflux** is also indicative of dysphagia. Reflux is a backward flow of food or liquid. Esophageal reflux is a condition in

---

FYI

We swallow during our sleep; however, much less so compared to when we are awake. On average, we swallow approximately once per hour.

FIGURE 10.1. Illustration of aspiration.

Tongue

Aspiration to Airway

To Stomach

To Lungs

which the stomach contents flow backward into the esophagus.

Due to the obvious anatomic and physiologic processes underpinning swallowing behavior, it is important to be familiar with some of the primary physical structures involved in swallowing. Most of the key structures were covered in Chapter 3. A summary of these structures and their function in regard to swallowing is provided in Table 10.1. A corresponding illustration of the

Table 10.1. Primary Anatomic Structures Involved in Swallowing

Structure	Description
Oral Cavity	
Lips	Are responsible for sealing the oral cavity for preparation of swallow.
Tongue	Is responsible for pushing food toward the hard palate and back toward the pharynx.
Teeth	Are required for mastication (chewing).
Saliva	A special digestive enzyme for softening and moistening food. Glands are located in the cheeks, the underside of tongue, and the underside of mandible.
Nasal Cavity	
Velum	The soft palate muscles that rise during swallowing to close off the nasal cavity from the oral cavity.
Pharynx	
Muscles	A series of overlapping muscles in the throat cavity. The cavity extends from the back of the nasal cavity to the top of the larynx.
Epiglottis	A leaf-shaped cartilage which protects the vocal folds from collecting foreign matter and diverts the bolus around the airway.
Valleculae	The space between the base of the tongue and the epiglottis. The collection of residue in this space indicates a problem with tongue movement during swallowing.
Upper Esophageal Sphincter	A specialized muscle that separates the pharyngeal and esophageal cavities.
Trachea	
Cartilage	A series of cartilaginous rings that form the wind pipe. The trachea branches off from the base of the pharynx and leads to a series of smaller tubes comprising the lungs.
Esophagus	
Muscle	A long muscular tube that branches off from the pharynx and sits behind the trachea. This is the "food tube" that serves as the conduit to the stomach. The esophagus normally is collapsed and only opens during swallowing.

major structures used for swallowing and their anatomic location is provided in Figure 10.2.

From start to finish, normal swallowing is almost instantaneous activity, taking around 2 minutes to accomplish. Although swallowing is relatively quick and automatic, the process of moving liquid or food towards the stomach is extremely complicated. To conceptualize swallowing, it is useful to think of the process of swallowing as occurring in a series of three sequential stages: (1) oral, (2) pharyngeal, and (3) esophageal. Each stage represents specific physiologic activity in the progression of moving material from the mouth to the stomach. These three stages are illustrated in Figure 10.3.

FIGURE 10.3. The three stages of swallowing, including the oral (transfer), pharyngeal (transport), and esophageal (entrance) stages.

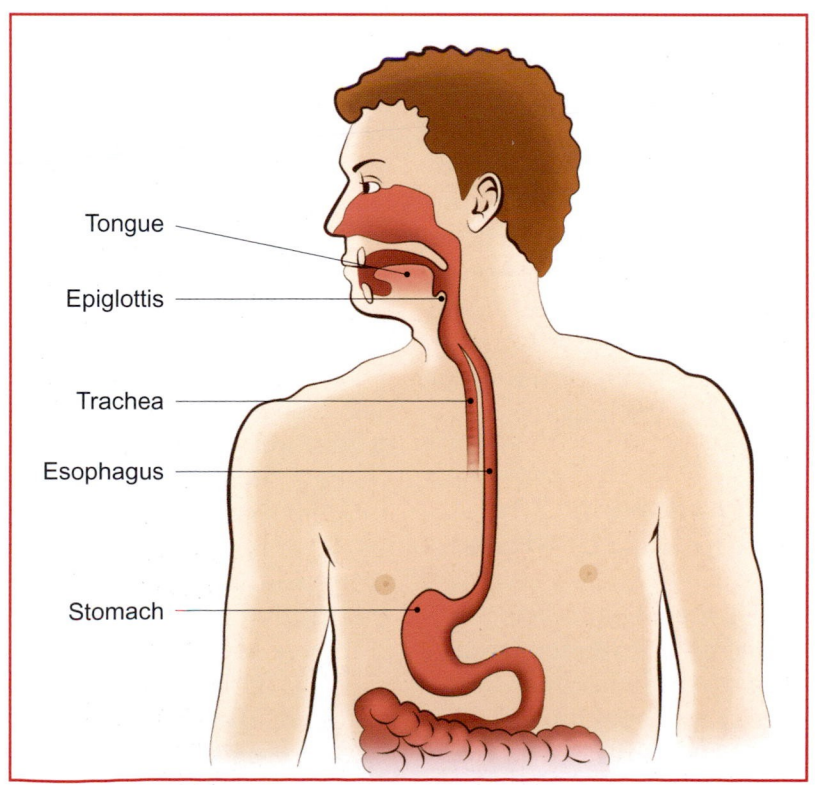

FIGURE 10.2. Swallowing anatomy.

Stage 1 of Swallowing: The Oral (Transfer) Stage

The **oral stage** begins when we take food or drink into our mouths. Once material is placed in the mouth, the lips are sealed. The tongue then moves the material around the mouth for mastication. Saliva helps to soften and moisten food to create a bolus that is easy to swallow. This stage is one of preparation for swallowing by transferring the food or drink to the back of the mouth. We maintain normal nasal breathing during this stage.

Stage 2 of Swallowing: The Pharyngeal (Transport) Stage

The **pharyngeal stage** begins once the tongue transfers the food or liquid bolus to the back of the throat. Once the bolus reaches the back of the mouth, a reflex automatically occurs that transports the bolus through the pharynx. During this stage of the swallow, the nasal cavity is closed off from the oral cavity to prevent food from going through the nose. Muscles of the throat serve to shorten the pharynx and push the food toward the esophagus. The larynx closes tightly and breathing stops to prevent food or liquid from entering the lungs.

Stage 3 of Swallowing: The Esophageal (Entrance) Stage

The **esophageal stage** begins when the bolus is directed away from the trachea and enters the esophagus, which is the canal that carries food and liquid to the stomach. The esophagus is separated from the pharynx by a sphincter muscle which relaxes and is pulled open by muscles of the throat. After the bolus

exits the pharynx, the normally collapsed esophagus is pushed open by the propelling bolus. During this process of the swallow, peristalsis occurs to move the bolus through the esophagus into the stomach. Once the bolus is fully in the esophagus and the sphincter is again closed, the airway is re-opened and normal breathing resumes.

HISTORIC ASPECTS OF DYSPHAGIA

To an outsider, an SLP may not seem to be the most qualified individual to deal with swallowing difficulties. By the very nature of their professional title, an SLP supposedly works exclusively with speech and language problems. Yet some SLPs have been indirectly treating aspects of dysphagia since the early 1930s. This early work was focused primarily on young children with oral-motor disorders such as cerebral palsy, as well as head and neck surgery patients. One of the core features in the educational curriculum of an SLP student has always been knowledge of the anatomy and physiology of the head, neck, and respiratory system. This coursework, along with extensive clinical education with clients who have disordered function of the oral, pharyngeal, and laryngeal systems, made SLPs the prime candidates for assessing and treating dysphagia. Prior to the involvement by the SLP profession, no other health professions specifically included dysphagia as part of their scope of practice.

Two individuals from the United States are often given credit for advancing the profession in regard to helping people with swallowing problems. The first is **George L. Larsen**, who in the early 1960s developed the SLP program

One of the pioneers of speech-language pathology, Dr. Grant Fairbanks (1910–1964) died by asphyxiation as a result of choking on a piece of food that had lodged in his throat. Dr. Fairbanks died tragically while onboard an airplane in 1964 traveling from San Francisco to Chicago (see also Chapter 5).

would be expected that improvements in speech production would follow. Although this was not found to be the case, Larsen is credited with establishing a range of therapeutic techniques to help individuals regain the ability to swallow. His approach to the evaluation, management, and treatment of swallowing difficulties was considered artistic and intuitive (Miller & Groher, 1993).

The next major advancement in dysphagia was made by **Jeri A. Logemann** who completed a PhD from the Department of Communication Disorders at Northwestern University (Illinois) in the early 1970s with particular emphasis in dysphagia (Figure 10.4). Logemann applied a more rigorous scientific methodology to assessing and treating dysphagia compared to Larsen by undertaking controlled examinations of swallowing physiology and treatment efficacy. Logemann also made major contributions in regard to outlining the

at the Seattle Veterans Administration Hospital. Due to Larsen's employment in a hospital setting, he was aware of a large number of people who experienced difficulties with both speech and swallowing. To his dismay, he found that most SLPs tended to address only speech difficulties, leaving the swallowing difficulties to either go unaddressed or be dealt with by some other health profession (e.g., neurologist, otolaryngologist, nurse, physiotherapist, occupational therapist). Larsen believed that a patient who showed both speech and swallowing problems was the result of a similar nervous system disturbance. Therefore, by working on swallowing it

FIGURE 10.4. Jerilyn A. Logemann has made important clinical contributions to the field of dysphagia. Permission granted by J. Logemann.

essential educational and clinical training required of SLPs dealing with dysphagia. Education in dysphagia is now a standard component among all SLP university programs worldwide.

It is important for SLPs to recognize that due to the complex medical issues involved in management of the dysphagic patient, this area of clinical practice is by necessity and design an interdisciplinary clinical field. Appropriate management includes input from a variety of health professionals, including but not limited to neurology, otolaryngology, radiology, and dietetics. Indeed substantial research that guides our understanding of swallowing comes from outside of speech language pathology. One such example involves the research of the French physiologist **Andre Jean** (Figure 10.5). Over the past 20 years, Professor Jean has been instrumental in defining the role of the brainstem in normal and disordered swallowing.

The past 20 have witnessed a dramatic growth of involvement by SLPs in the field of dysphagia both in regard to service delivery and research. More than one-third of present day SLPs deal with dysphagia as part of their annual caseload. For SLPs working in a health care setting, dysphagia can often exceed 80% of the total caseload. In 1986, a research journal entitled *Dysphagia* was created. This is an interdisciplinary journal dedicated exclusively to the many aspects of normal and disordered swallowing.

TYPES OF DYSPHAGIA

There are three generally agreed-on types of dysphagia: (1) **oropharyngeal dysphagia**, (2) **esophageal dysphagia**, and (3) **functional dysphagia**. The first two types are related to known anatomic or physiologic difficulties with swallowing. The third type is a form of dysphagia with no known causal factors.

Oropharyngeal Dysphagia

This is the most common type of dysphagia. The anatomical description of this form of dysphagia indicates that the condition affects the transfer of liquid or food from the mouth and pharynx into the esophagus. This type of dysphagia results from abnormalities of muscles, nerves, or structures of the oral cavity and pharynx. Attempts to swallow food may be misdirected upward toward the nasal cavity. Many patients choke or cough when swallowing and may have

FIGURE 10.5. Andre Jean has examined the role of the brainstem in normal and disordered swallowing. Permission granted by A. Jean.

food or fluids enter the trachea instead of the esophagus. This can allow harmful bacteria to grow in the lungs or bronchial tubes, resulting in a condition known as **aspiration pneumonia** (Figure 10.6). Patients often complain of difficulty chewing and swallowing both liquids and foods. They appear to have a hoarse or wet-sounding voice which may be accompanied by bad breath.

Esophageal Dysphagia

This type of dysphagia is less common than oropharyngeal dysphagia and arises during the latter stages of the swallowing sequence. Patients with esophageal dysphagia have difficulty passing a bolus of food from the esophagus to the stomach. Patients usually complain of swallowing solid foods, as opposed to both solid foods and liquids. Their swallowing difficulty is due to either an obstruction or stricture (i.e., narrowing) of the esophagus or else problems with peristalsis (i.e., a motility problem). Patients report that it feels like food is stuck in the base of their throat or in the chest. Patients generally point to their neck as the primary region of the problem, indicating that the site is at or below this region.

Functional Dysphagia

The least frequently occurring type of dysphagia is known as **functional dysphagia**. This form of dysphagia is poorly understood, primarily because there is no identifiable anatomic cause. Examples of functional dysphagia include difficulty in swallowing pills and

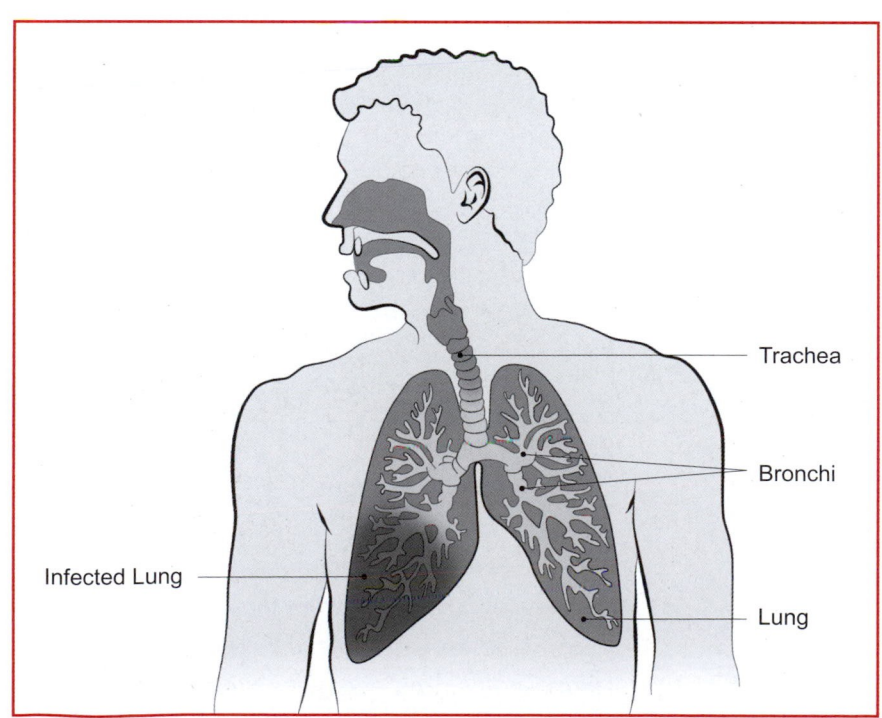

FIGURE 10.6. Illustration of lung infection that can result from aspiration.

a condition known as **globus**, which is the sensation of having a lump in one's throat. The International Foundation for Gastrointestinal Disorders defines functional dysphagia as the sensation of solid and/or liquid foods sticking, lodging, or passing abnormally through the esophagus. Functional dysphagia is diagnosed based on symptoms present for at least 3 months and not associated with anatomic abnormalities such as reflux (Galmiche et al., 2006).

CAUSES OF DYSPHAGIA

Although there are three primary types of dysphagia, the causes of dysphagia are numerous. Swallowing requires healthy functioning of many different oral structures, muscles, and nerves, so a wide range of medical and even dental conditions can cause dysphagia. Dysphagia actually is a symptom of an underlying condition. A list of likely causes associated with the three types of dysphagia is provided in Table 10.2. A common cause of oropharyngeal dysphagia is a **cerebrovascular accident** (i.e., stroke). Dysphagia can result from strokes that affect the area of the brain that controls motor actions, particularly the frontal lobes of the cerebrum. Strokes that affect the area of the brain that houses the **swallowing center** also can lead to dysphagia. The swallowing center is made up of a network of neurons in the brainstem that are responsible for the reflexive act of swallowing. About half of all stroke victims experience some degree of dysphagia during the earliest days following the stroke. In most cases, normal or near-normal swallowing function returns within 1 week poststroke,

Table 10.2. Some Likely Causes of Various Types of Dysphagia	
Type	**Cause**
Oropharyngeal dysphagia	Stroke
	Parkinson disease
	Muscular dystrophy
	Cleft palate
	Tumors of mouth or pharynx
	Drug/radiation-induced dry mouth (xerostomia)
Esophageal dysphagia	Esophageal spasms
	Tumors of the esophagus
	Age-related changes of motor function of esophagus
	Lack of involuntary esophageal peristalsis (achalasia)
	Pill-induced inflammation of the esophagus
	Esophagitis due to gastroesophageal reflux disease (GERD)
	Narrowing of lower esophageal ring (Schatzki's ring)
Functional dysphagia	Stress

although dysphagia and aspiration will persist in some. Additionally, people with disorders of the nervous system, such as cerebral palsy or Parkinson disease, could experience oropharyngeal dysphagia. Traumatic brain injury and progressive neurologic diseases like multiple sclerosis (MS) and motor neuron disease (amyotrophic lateral sclerosis—ALS) may cause oropharyngeal dysphagia. Any number of cancers affecting the head and neck also can lead to oropharyngeal dysphagia. These various conditions may affect the coordination of the swallowing muscles or limit sensation in the mouth and throat. To compound matters, sometimes the preferred treatment for various types of cancers (e.g., radiation or drugs) has side effects that can cause dysphagia.

A frequent cause of esophageal dysphagia is a structural problem that creates a blockage within the esophagus. The blockage prevents food and liquid from moving towards the stomach. The most common structural problems are esophageal cancer, strictures, and narrowing of the lower region of the esophagus (called Schatzki's rings). An infection or irritation can also cause narrowing of the esophagus, resulting in a condition known as **esophagitis**. One type of irritation is gastroesophageal reflux disease (GERD). **GERD** (or acid reflux), is a condition in which acid, bile, and partially digested food in the stomach back up into the esophagus. Partially digested food contains a strong acid that can inflame and damage the lining of the esophagus. Many people think that heartburn (or acid indigestion) is a separate disease. It actually is one symptom of GERD. Heartburn is an unpleasant burning sensation behind the breastbone that usually occurs after a meal.

FYI

The term **odynophagia** refers to the feeling of pain or a burning sensation upon swallowing. Such pain may be a symptom of a serious medical condition.

The absence of a clear anatomical reason for the occurrence of functional dysphagia leads most experts to speculate that the cause of this condition is a combination of physiologic and psychosocial problems (Galmiche et al., 2006). Anecdotal information has been reported that individuals who show functional dysphagia may show significantly higher instances of anxiety and depression compared to those who do not have this form of dysphagia (Clouse et al., 1999).

Finally, dysphagia is not limited to adults. Young children can experience difficulties with swallowing. **Pediatric dysphagia** is not simply an adult problem on a smaller scale. As previously pointed out in Chapter 3, the anatomic configuration of a young child's vocal tract is quite different from a fully grown adult vocal tract. These developmental differences in pharyngeal and laryngeal anatomy also can influence the manner of swallowing in children compared to adults. Normal adult swallowing is a complicated process but because the underlying swallowing anatomy is fully mature, the process of swallowing is quite stable. In children, ongoing physical growth and development of motor coordination create a situation whereby swallowing behavior changes "in step" with anatomic changes (Kramer & Eicher, 1993). In pediatric populations, dysphagia may be present in babies who are

---

FYI

The developing fetus begins to swallow as early as 10-weeks gestation. During the last trimester, the fetus swallows up to a liter of amniotic fluid per day.

Table 10.3. Some Warning Signs of Dysphagia

- Coughing
- Drooling
- Choking
- Food of fluid coming out of the nose
- Gurgly voice quality
- Wet-sounding breathing
- Spillage of food or liquid from the mouth
- Frequent throat clearing
- Low grade fever
- Progressively slower rate of food intake
- Difficulty initiating a swallow
- Pain upon swallowing
- Food or liquid left in the mouth after a swallow
- Difficulty manipulating food or liquid in the mouth
- Weight loss

---

born prematurely, who have genetic syndromes (e.g., Down syndrome), or maxillofacial deformities. Infants who are born with a cleft lip and palate are unable to suck properly, which complicates nursing and drinking from a regular baby bottle. Swallowing difficulties have been reported to occur in as many as 25% of all children, with greater prevalence in children with physical disabilities, medical illness, and prematurity (Manikam & Perman, 2000).

ASSESSMENT OF DYSPHAGIA

All of us at some time have experienced difficulty swallowing. Perhaps it was that time when you were taking a drink and someone made you laugh so hard that fluid went through your nose. Or perhaps you once choked on a piece of food. For most of us, these events are fleeting; however, for some individuals, swallowing difficulties occur more often. There are a number of symptoms that require evaluation for a possible swallowing problem. A list of some of the warning signs for dysphagia is provided in Table 10.3.

The procedures used for assessing the presence of dysphagia fall into two general categories: (1) **clinical assessment** and (2) **instrumental assessment**.

Clinical assessment is an approach commonly used for the initial screening of swallowing dysfunction, and as the term suggests, typically occurs while a patient is in a clinic setting. Sometimes this may involve assessing a patient sitting upright in a hospital bed. The approach is designed to determine a patient's cognitive abilities, language abilities, and readiness to eat or swallow (Sitoh et al., 2000). Clinical assessments have been criticized for being too general and lacking in necessary precision to detect pharyngeal pathophysiology or moments of aspiration. Yet most SLPs would agree there is a need for a simple bedside assessment that would at least identify patients who are "at risk" for aspiration. Detection of dysphagia at a patient's beside mandates the SLP to be highly suspicious of swallowing difficulties, and have a clear understanding of the mechanisms of swallowing. An important feature of a bedside assessment requires the patient to ingest fluids and foods of different textures when seated in an upright position. While the patient is swallowing, the SLP observes whether: (1) swallowing occurred in a natural, automatic fashion, (2) there was drooling during the swallow, (3) the patient coughed during swallowing, and (4) the patient's voice sounded hoarse. Based on the bedside swallowing assessment, a patient would be diagnosed by the SLP to have *possible* dysphagia if any one of these four observations were present.

Another rather novel bedside approach to evaluating normal swallowing involves a procedure known as **cervical** (neck) **auscultation**. The process of auscultation is the diagnostic listening of sounds. Physicians perform this diagnostic test frequently by using a stethoscope to listen to heart and lung sounds. In the case of cervical auscultation, a stethoscope is placed in the region of the neck and the patient is asked to swallow. Based on listening to the swallow, the SLP makes a perceptual judgment as to the functioning of the swallow based on the perceived "crispness" of the signal. Some experts believe there is a distinct acoustic pattern of normal swallowing that can be used as a backdrop to evaluate disordered swallowing (Huckabee et al., 2005); however, application of cervical auscultation as a standard clinical measure has not received widespread support.

Use of instrumentation to determine the existence of dysphagia provides a more in-depth form of assessment compared to the bedside approach. In most cases, the instruments employed by the SLP allow for visualization of the various stages of swallowing. Although this may seem the logical choice for determining the existence of swallowing difficulties, there are drawbacks associated with the various instrumental techniques. Some of the most common instrumental assessment techniques are: (1) **videofluoroscopic swallowing study (VSS)**, (2) **fiberoptic endoscopic evaluation of swallow** (FEES), (3) **ultrasound**, and (4) **electromyography** (EMG).

Videofluoroscopic Swallowing Study

The VSS approach to determining the existence of dysphagia involves an imaging technique known as **videofluoroscopy**. Fluoroscopy is a procedure that allows for a dynamic x-ray to be taken of a person's bodily organs as they are actually moving. Because swallowing is a form of bodily movement, fluoroscopy is amenable to the visualization of swallowing. The most common anatomic view is a cross-section (side view) of the entire vocal tract to allow for examination of swallowing from start to finish. A typical fluoroscopic image of the vocal tract is shown in Figure 10.7. The VSS procedure is usually completed under the direction of an SLP, while working with a radiologist. The radiologist operates the videofluoroscopy equipment and, along with the SLP, provides an interpretation of the radiographic images. To visualize swallowing behavior, the patient is required to swallow a radiopaque substance known as **barium**, which can easily be detected using an x-ray. As the patient swallows the barium substance, the various movements of the swallow are video-recorded

A

B

FIGURE 10.7. Fluoroscopic examination of swallowing. (**A**) The general procedures of the examination are shown. (**B**) The resultant image of the vocal tract is shown. The white substance in the vocal tract is a radiopaque substance known as barium.

Labels on figure A: Fluoroscopy Tube, Fluoroscopy Table

for later analysis. This x-ray helps the SLP determine what types of food and drink are safe to swallow and what type of dysphagia therapy might be appropriate. A primary drawback with the VSS approach is that the x-ray beams directed into the body for visualization expose the patient to mild levels of radiation. Such radiation is cumulative on the body and is not dissipated. Therefore, it is advisable to perform this procedure as infrequently as possible. The use of VSS has proven to be an effective instrumental approach to evaluating swallowing function and will likely continue to be performed regularly for years to come.

FEES

Although use of VSS is widely considered the "gold standard" examination for oral and pharyngeal dysphagia, another instrumental approach known as fiberoptic endoscopic evaluation of swallowing (FEES) is gaining widespread appeal. The FEES procedure involves use of a flexible endoscope to visualize the pharyngeal and laryngeal structures involved in swallowing. An endoscope is a thin, flexible tube that contains both a light source and a camera lens that provides an image on a computer monitor. This tube can be inserted into bodily orifices that are typically difficult to visually examine (stomach, larynx, ear canal), thus providing an opportunity to assess both structure and function. Langmore, Schatz, and Olsen (1988) were the first group of researchers to describe the FEES technique for evaluating oropharyngeal dysphagia. FEES originally was conceived to be used as a backup, or secondary procedure, performed only when VSS was not available or conven-

ient. For example, use of VSS is not feasible for patients in an intensive care unit (ICU), or in a nursing home, or for patients who are extremely obese. The FEES procedure involves the insertion of a flexible endoscope into the nose to visualize the pharynx and larynx immediately before and after eating and drinking foods and liquids of different consistencies (Figure 10.8). Depending on the laws established for various countries (and states) the approach can be done exclusively by the SLP or may require additional medical personnel. During the actual swallow, the video image on the computer monitor becomes momentarily obliterated (i.e., a whiteout). The image is restored upon completion of the swallow. A telltale sign of dysphagia is the observation of any pooling of fluid that accumulates in the valleculae or piriform sinuses in the pharynx either before or after the swallow. Although the view provided by FEES is not as dynamic as VSS, it is far less damaging to the patient. The patient does not need to ingest barium but rather food (milk, pudding) that is dyed either blue or green to make for better visualization. FEES has the advantage of being free from radiation, so patients undergoing this test can be examined for longer time intervals or at repeated intervals. A disadvantage of FEES is that aspiration may not be noted as reliably as VSS, as the whiteout phenomenon at the height of the swallowing is often when aspiration occurs.

Ultrasound

Ultrasound has been used to image the human body for at least 50 years. It is one of the most widely used diagnostic

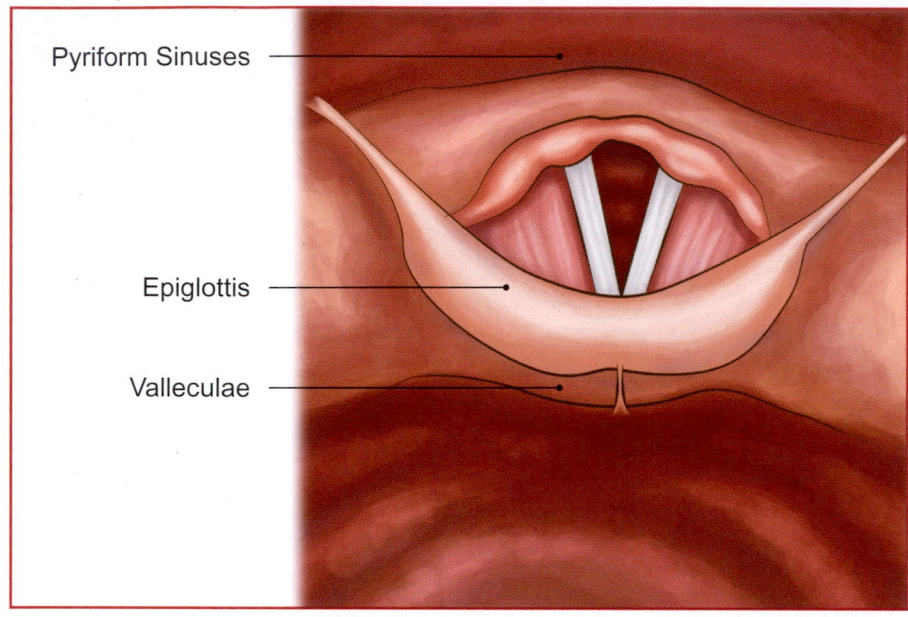

A

B

FIGURE 10.8. View of pharyngeal area during a fiberoptic endoscopic examination of swallowing (FEES) procedure. (**A**) reflects a normal swallow. (**B**) shows a disordered swallow as indicated by pooling of fluid in the valleculae.

tools in modern medicine. Health care professionals use ultrasound to view the heart, blood vessels, kidneys, liver, and other organs. Ultrasound is commonly used during pregnancy to examine the developing fetus (see also Chapter 11).

During an ultrasound test, a special technician or doctor moves a device called a transducer over a specific body part. The transducer sends out high-frequency sound waves, which bounce off the tissues inside the body and the same transducer captures the sound waves that bounce back. These sound waves are then translated and assembled into a visual image on a computer monitor. This same technology can be used to track tongue movement during a swallow. The procedure works by holding a transducer under the patient's chin and high-frequency sound waves travel through the tissues in the neck and are reflected off the tongue to create an image. Because the approach is exclusive to the tongue's role in swallowing, only the oral stage of swallowing can be evaluated; however, the approach is far less invasive than the VSS and FEES approaches. An example of the ultrasound approach to evaluating swallowing is shown in Figure 10.9.

FIGURE 10.9. Illustration of ultrasound examination of the tongue during the oral stage of swallowing.

EMG

When a muscle is used (i.e., contracts) it generates a very small electrical signal, which can be detected with an antenna (i.e., an electrode). This instrumental procedure is known as EMG. When a very thin wire electrode is inserted directly into a muscle, the activity of the muscle can be viewed and recorded. There also are less invasive disc electrodes that can simply be taped to the surface of the skin. In regard to swallowing, a variety of muscles in the region of the mouth, larynx, and pharynx can be examined using the EMG approach. A muscle that is not working correctly will emit an electrical signal that is different from a normal functioning muscle. In an extreme case where a muscle is paralyzed, it is possible that no electrical activity would be emitted. Examples of EMG signals found in normal and disordered swallowing are presented in Figure 10.10. A drawback with this approach is that the procedure can be highly invasive, requiring insertion of an electrode directly into the muscle. The use of a surface electrode may also be problematic because these electrodes are attached to the surface of the skin and the EMG signal can be obscured due to multiple muscles overlapping. This form of instrumental swallowing assessment is not routinely used in a clinical setting. Rather, it is used more often in research settings (Perlman, 1993).

TREATMENT OF DYSPHAGIA

Successful management of dysphagia requires a team of various health specialists such as the SLP, occupational and physical therapy, otolaryngologist,

A

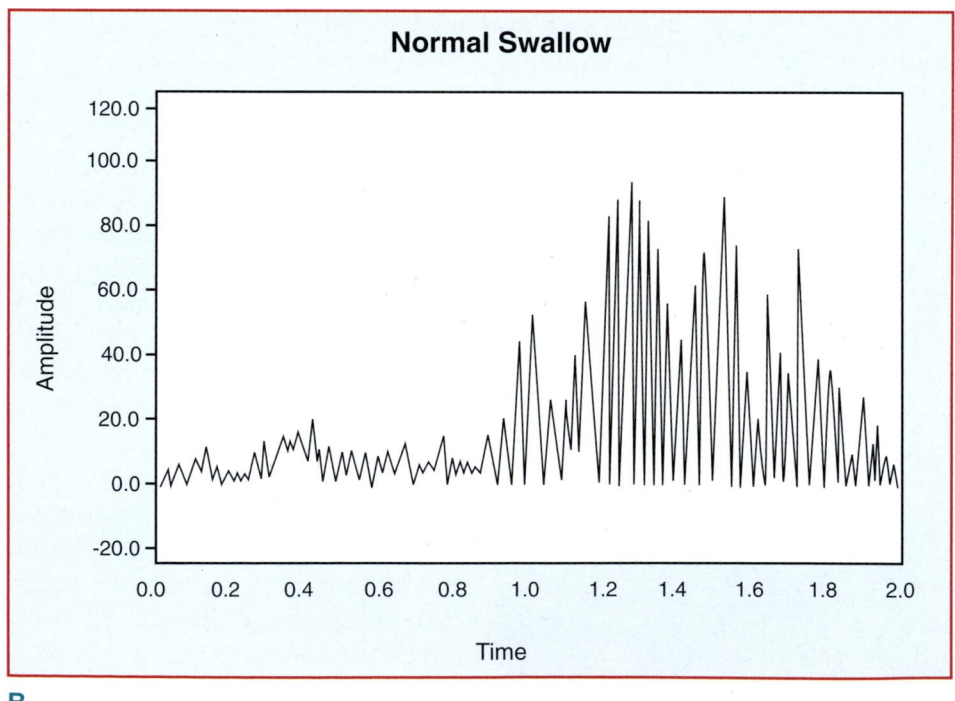

B

FIGURE 10.10. (**A**) provides an illustration showing surface electrode placement for electromyographic (EMG) recording of swallowing. (**B**) is an idealized EMG recording reflecting normal muscle functioning during a swallow. *continues*

neurologists, gastroenterologist, as well as a dietician. Once the cause of the dysphagia is found, there are a number of treatment approaches to consider, including: (1) swallowing therapy, (2) lifestyle changes, (3) drugs, and (4) surgery.

C

FIGURE 10.10. *continued* (**C**) reflects impaired muscle functioning during a swallow.

Swallowing Therapy

The SLP could be called on to test the person's ability to eat and drink and may teach the person new ways to swallow. The therapy program established for the patient is tailored to suit her or his medical condition. Treatment may involve rehabilitation exercises to strengthen weak oral and pharyngeal muscles or to improve coordination of the overall swallowing musculature. For others, treatment may involve learning compensatory swallowing strategies. For example, some people might have to eat and drink with their head turned to one side or looking straight ahead. Preparing food in a certain way or avoiding certain foods can help other people. Some fluids which might normally be easily aspirated can be altered by adding a thickening agent. The patient may be discouraged from swallowing hot or cold items if they are particularly sensitive to reflux.

FYI

Acid reflux is a warning sign of dysphagia. In addition, acid reflux can serve to impair our speaking voice. In extreme cases of reflux, acidic juices may back up from the stomach and irritate the laryngeal mechanism, including the vocal folds.

Lifestyle Changes

As noted earlier, acid reflux is a dysphagic condition that can have serious consequences on health and quality of life. There are a number of steps people can take to greatly reduce the likelihood of reflux disease. These steps involve changes in lifestyle such as increased exercise and diet modification. Some common recommendations include:

- Eat smaller, more frequent meals
- Eat a bland diet
- Avoid alcohol and caffeine
- Lose weight
- Reduce stress
- Avoid eating 3 hours before bedtime
- Slightly elevate your head while sleeping

Drugs

The prescription of drugs to treat dysphagia typically has been dictated on the basis of the particular medical condition contributing to the disorder. Due to the wide range of causes that could contribute to dysphagia, there presently is no "magic pill" that can cure dysphagia. In many cases, drugs serve to relieve some of the symptoms of dysphagia, primarily those associated with esophageal dysphagia. The types of medications found to be useful include over-the-counter antacids that are taken before or after eating. There also are prescription medications known as proton-pump inhibitors, which substantially reduce acid production in the stomach.

Surgery

A typical surgical treatment of dysphagia involves muscle incisions to release muscle tension or to stretch/dilate an unusually narrow stricture. For some, however, consuming foods and liquids by mouth may not be possible in the immediate future. These individuals must use other methods to nourish their bodies. Usually this involves surgical intervention to create a new feeding system, such as a **feeding tube**, that bypasses the part of the swallowing mechanism that is not working normally. It is common to have a feeding tube inserted during the early stages of severe dysphagia to reduce the risk of aspiration pneumonia. The tube also helps ensure that the person's nutrition and hydration is adequate. These tubes can be easily removed if and/or when the dysphagia diminishes. Two main types of feeding tubes are used: (1) paraenteral tubes and (2) enteral tubes.

A **parenteral tube** (or IV tube) is administered through either a central or peripheral heart vein (Figure 10.11). The tube is essentially a catheter that provides micronutrients directly into the blood stream. It is only appropriate for individuals whose stomach and intestines are not working properly. The tube allows for the digestive tract to heal after surgery to the stomach or bowel and is kept in place with a stitch. Use of a parenteral tube typically is a very costly surgical procedure.

Enteral tubes involve providing nutrition directly into the stomach or small intestine. There at two general types of enteral tubes: (1) nasogastric and (2) gastrostomy. A **nasogastric tube** (or NG tube) is used on a short-term basis and entails passing a tube through the nose, pharynx, and esophagus directly into the stomach. Once the tube is correctly positioned, it is taped to the patient's nose or cheek to keep it in place. Food passes through it into the stomach.

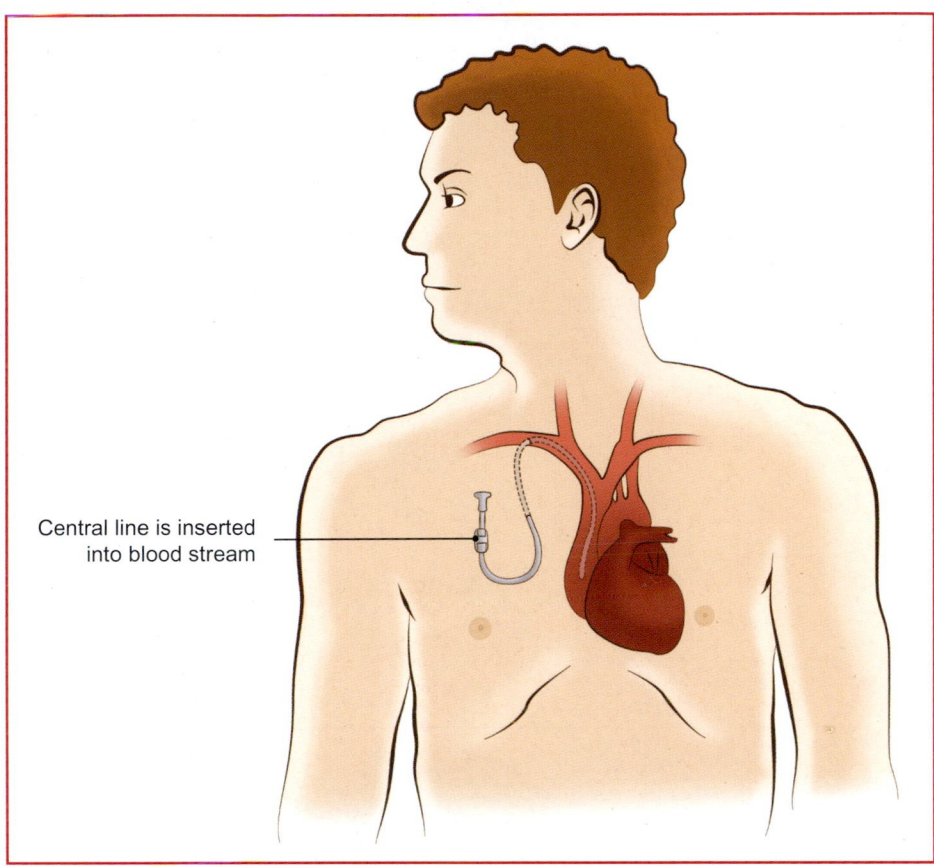

Central line is inserted
into blood stream

FIGURE 10.11. Parenteral tube. Nutrients are delivered directly into the blood stream for patients who are unable to swallow.

A **gastronomy tube** (or percutaneous endoscopic gastrostomy—PEG tube) is used on a longer term basis or for indefinite time periods. Like an NG tube, food passes through it into the stomach, but unlike an NG tube, an external opening is made in the abdomen and the tube is placed directly into the stomach. The feeding tube is held in place with either a stitch, a small inflated balloon around the tube just under the skin, or a flange around the tube just under the skin. This form of enteral feeding is more invasive than NG tubes. Examples of the two types of enteral feeding tubes are shown in Figure 10.12.

CULTURAL CONSIDERATIONS AND DYSPHAGIA

The SLP who works with patients who have dysphagia may encounter a unique set of social and cultural issues that need to be considered as part of the overall treatment plan. Riquelme (2007) has identified four particular factors that, if not considered, may hinder the SLPs effectiveness in treating dysphagia. These factors include: (1) language barriers, (2) physical space, (3) ageism, and (4) food and nutrition.

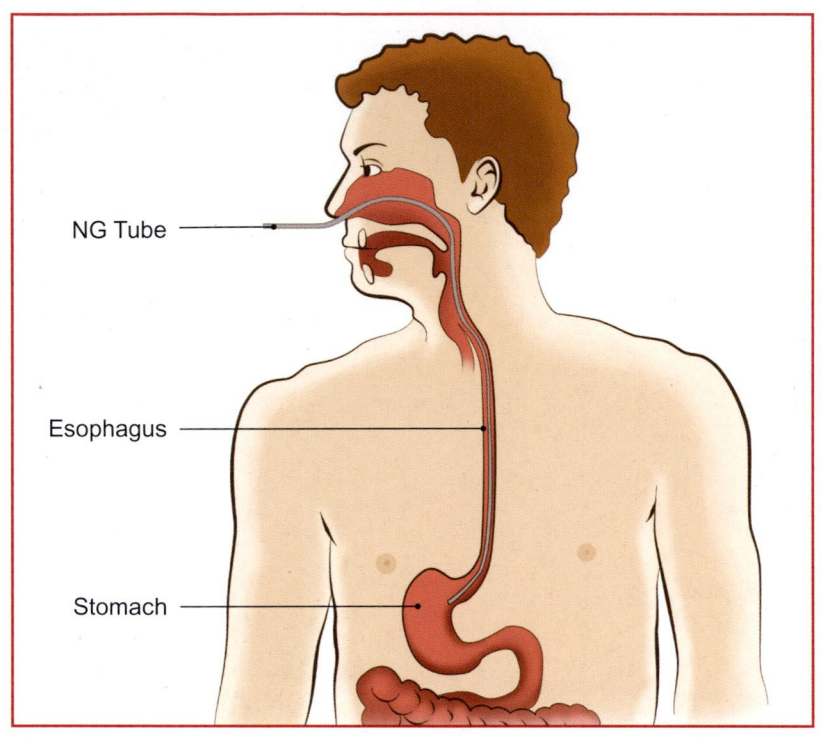

A

B

FIGURE 10.12. Examples of enteral tubes for patients to consume food and liquid if unable to swallow. A nasogastric (NG) tube, gastronomy tube is shown in (**A**) and a percutaneous endoscopic gastrostomy (PEG) tube is shown in (**B**).

Language Barriers

Based on the introductory material presented in this chapter, it is evident that a large and unique vocabulary is used when dealing with the disorder of dysphagia. These terms are, in many cases, quite foreign even for someone who may speak the same language as the SLP, so speaking the same language may not ensure there is a cultural connection between the clinician and client. In cases where the client speaks English as a second language, the SLP may need to use an interpreter to communicate with the patient, and if so, great care should be taken in monitoring how the translated information is presented. Sensitivity to a patient's knowledge of medical terminology is important. Not everyone understands terms such as NPO (no foods per oral/mouth), aspiration, or reflux.

Physical Space

One aspect of assessing and treating dysphagia that is not found in most areas of speech-language pathology is the literal "hands on" approach to assisting the patient. Any sort of touching used by the SLP needs to be clarified with the patient beforehand. There may be times when adjusting the patient's posture or palpating the patient's throat during swallowing could be inappropriate. The SLP should not assume the patient understands all of the procedures involved in an examination and subsequent treatment. In addition to matters concerning physical proximity, the clinical setting may also need to be considered when dealing with dysphagia. Lyon (1997) recommends that working in the patient's home is the best environment for working on dysphagia because it is the most natural setting for the patient. By doing so, there is a greater likelihood of patient compliance and carryover of treatment recommendations.

Ageism

In most cases, the dysphagic patient is elderly and the SLP is not. The age difference between client and clinician can impact overall interactions and patient compliance, both of which are critical to effective treatment outcomes (Riquelme, 2007). For many ethnic groups, elderly people are treated with great overt respect and these individuals hold high social status within the immediate and extended family. This needs to be acknowledged during clinical interactions. The SLP-patient relationship needs to be equalized or at least balanced to effectively provide culturally competent care.

Food and Nutrition

Issues concerning food and nutrition for the dysphagic patient can be particularly challenging in a multicultural population. Eating a meal with others is an enjoyable and highly social activity, and in some cultures, eating implies a sense of community. The American holiday of Thanksgiving is just one example how food can be linked to culture. If the patient with dysphagia has difficulty partaking in food consumption, yet his or her culture places high importance on food, steps need to be taken to ensure that a balance between food and culture is maintained. When selecting types of foods, the SLP may encounter difficulty with the patient due to their prior history and culture of eating. Therefore, it is important to seek input from a nutritionist. For example, when establishing a diet that does not recommend solid foods (due to increased risk of aspiration), some patients may report they *are not able to do without fish.* So when selecting specific foods, it is important to provide a patient with choices that reflect cultural preferences. For instance, the choice of pureed plantains versus potatoes may be quite important to a Latino patient who normally does not have potatoes in his or her diet (Riquelme, 2007).

CURRENT RESEARCH IN DYSPHAGIA

Scientists are conducting research that is designed to improve the ability of physicians and SLPs to evaluate and treat swallowing disorders. Much of this research focuses on the various stages of the swallowing process. Research involves examining people of all ages, including those who do not have dysphagia. Some of the current areas of rehabilitation research being explored are: (1) **EMG feedback**, (2) **electrical stimulation**, and (3) **neural plasticity**.

EMG Feedback

One exploratory method to treating dysphagia involves use of EMG as a form of **biofeedback**. Biofeedback refers to the use of equipment to measure body functions that are not monitored consciously. These measurements are typically converted to electrical signals that are displayed on a computer monitor. The patient learns to manipulate the signal pattern by controlling specific body functions that correspond to the signal. Current research has shown that patients with dysphagia can show improvement in their swallowing when provided with visual patterns of surface EMG recordings collected in the face and neck region (Huckabee & Cannito, 1999).

Electrical Stimulation

The use of neuromuscular electrical stimulation (E-stim) is not uncommon in rehabilitative medicine. The general theory behind E-stim is that an electrical current is used to simulate the same electrical impulses that are activated during normal exercise. By passively activating the muscle, the body responds in much the same way as during normal exercise. When placing a pair of skin surface electrodes on the target muscle or muscle group and sending electrical impulses through the skin to underlying nerves, contraction and relaxation of the muscle occurs in a rhythmic pattern that is similar to daily exercise (Leelamanit et al., 2002). Electrical stimulation of swallowing musculature for the treatment of dysphagia recently has been trialed in a number of studies (e.g., Sabet et al., 2005). The U.S. government (Federal Drug Administration) has approved E-stim as a treatment of adult and pediatric dysphagia, although there is controversy surrounding its standard use in clinical settings. At present there is insufficient empirical research supporting its effectiveness in both children and adults.

Neural Plasticity

Dysphagia rehabilitation historically has focused on teaching the patient alternative ways of swallowing to prevent aspiration and improve swallowing efficiency. The patient also is provided with strengthening exercises to improve overall swallowing behavior. However, there is little documented evidence as to the best approach (or exercises) to improve swallowing. Recently, there has been research exploring the role of **neural plasticity** and dysphagia (Robbins et al., 2008). Neural plasticity refers to the ability of the brain and/or certain parts of the nervous system to change in order to adapt to new conditions, such as an injury (see also Chapter 9). In many ways, the rehabilitative techniques used by physiotherapists rely heavily on the notion of neural plasticity. These therapists will not simply tell a stroke patient to stand up and walk—they first work on strengthening muscles of interest and discrete movements until patients can stand and take a few steps. They start with the components of a movement and then ultimately train the movement of interest, which in this case would be walking. By working on discrete physical movements, the therapist is working to strengthen the overall neuromuscular patterns associated with walking. The same logic is now being applied to the treatment of dysphagia. By starting with the first stage of the swallowing process, the patient is taught to consciously move toward task-specific exercises and more challenging levels of swallowing (Burkhead, Sapienza, & Rosenbek, 2007). As research progresses in this area, the most optimum approaches to treating dysphagia may be discovered.

DYSPHAGIA ON THE WORLD WIDE WEB

Listed below are Web sites that provide further information on the topic of dysphagia. At the time of publication each Web site was freely accessible.

A Look Inside Swallowing Disorders Video
http://www.webmd.com/video/swallowing-disorders

Dysphagia Online
http://www.dysphagiaonline.com

Dysphagia Resource Center
http://dysphagia.com/

Oropharyngeal Dysphagia Video
http://www.nature.com/gimo/contents/pt1/fig_tab/gimo82_V1.html

The Voice and Swallowing Center Videos
http://www.voiceandswallowing.com/

REFERENCES

Burkhead, L., Sapienza, C., & Rosenbek, J. (2007). Strength-training exercise in dysphagia rehabilitation: Principles, procedures, and directions for future research. *Dysphagia, 22,* 251–265.

Clouse, R., Richter, J., Heading, R., Janssens, J., & Wilson, J. (1999). Functional esophageal disorders. *Gut, 45*(Suppl.), II31–II36.

Galmiche, J., Clouse, R., Balint, A., Cook, I., Kahrilas, P., Paterson, W., & Smout, A. (2006). Functional esophageal disorders. *Gastroenterology, 130,* 1459–1465.

Huckabee, M. L., & Cannito, M. P. (1999). Outcomes of swallowing rehabilitation in chronic brainstem dysphagia: A retrospective evaluation. *Dysphagia, 14,* 93–109.

Huckabee, M. L., Coombe, T., & Robb, M. (2005). Repeatability of the acoustic swallowing pattern in normal adults. *Journal of Medical Speech-Language Pathology, 13,* 213–221.

Kramer, S., & Eicher, P. (1993). The evaluation of pediatric feeding abnormalities. *Dysphagia, 8,* 215–224.

Langmore, S. E., Schatz, K., & Olsen, N. (1988). Fiberoptic endoscopic examination of swallowing safety: A new procedure. *Dysphagia, 2,* 216–219.

Leelamanit, V., Limsakul, C., & Geater, A. (2002). Synchronized electrical stimulation in treating pharyngeal dysphagia. *Laryngoscope, 112,* 2204–2210.

Lyon, J. (1997). Optimizing communication and participation in life for aphasic adults and their prime care givers. In G. Wallace (Ed.), *Multicultural neurogenics* (pp. 137–159). San Antonio, TX: Communication Skill Builders.

Manikam, R., & Perman, J. A. (2000). Pediatric feeding disorders. *Journal of Clinical Gastroenterology, 30,* 34–46.

Miller, R., & Groher, M. (1993). Speech-language pathology and dysphagia: A brief historical perspective. *Dysphagia, 8,* 180–184.

Perlman, A. (1993). Electromyography and the study of oropharyngeal swallowing. *Dysphagia, 8,* 351–355.

Riquelme, L. (2007). The role of cultural competence in providing services to persons with dysphagia. *Topics in Geriatric Rehabilitation, 23,* 228–239.

Robbins, J., Butler, S., Daniels, S., Gross, R., Langmore, S., Lazarus, C. L., . . . Rosenbek, J. (2008). Swallowing and dysphagia rehabilitation: Translating principles of neural plasticity into clinically oriented evidence. *Journal of Speech, Language, and Hearing Research, 51,* S276–S300.

Sabet, F., Williams, J., & Tolat, R. (2005). Electrical stimulation for dysphagia: A case study and review. *American Journal of Physical Medicine and Rehabilitation, 84*(3), 231.

Sitoh, Y., Lee, A., Phua, S., Lieu, P., & Chan, S. (2000). Bedside assessment of swallowing: A useful screening tool for dysphagia in an acute geriatric ward. *Singapore Medical Journal, 41,* 376–381.

GENETICS AND SYNDROMES

OBJECTIVES

After reading this chapter, the student should be able to demonstrate:

- Knowledge of the biological aspects of genetics that impact the process of normal human development.

- Knowledge of the terminology pertaining to genetics.

- Understanding of the historical aspects of genetics.

- Knowledge of various genetic and chromosomal syndromes and the respective impacts on various aspects of hearing and speech-language development.

- Knowledge related to genetic counseling and genetic testing.

- Knowledge of various forms of treatment for genetic conditions.

- Understanding of the relationship between ethnicity and genetic disorders.

INTRODUCTION

Genetics refers to "life" or the "beginning." The field of human genetics is concerned with inheritance of traits. We often see family traits in various generations of family, such as facial features or body shape and size. By closely studying these traits, particularly those that may impact normal healthy functioning, we are able to answer questions about human nature, understand various diseases, and develop effective treatments for diseases. Aside from disorders resulting from physical injury, most communication disorders are genetically based. Many functional (or idiopathic) communication disorders are thought to have some form of genetic basis. Most hearing impairments have a genetic origin and approximately 50% of all cases of newborn deafness are due to faulty genetics. It is important for audiologists and speech-language pathologists to understand the rules of inheritance and the means of preventing genetic disorders (Gerber, 1990).

A **syndrome** refers to a distinct group of symptoms that together are characteristic of a specific disorder or disease. For example, the common cold is a familiar syndrome, having symptoms such as a runny nose, cough, and fever (Gerber, 1990). A wide range of syndromes have a communication disorder as a prevailing symptom. These syndromes are linked to a genetic abnormality. Although speech-language pathologists and audiologists are not qualified to render a genetic diagnosis, they are required to diagnose the type of speech problem or exact nature of hearing loss. Therefore, these professionals need to be aware of the manner in which various genetic conditions can affect features of speech and hearing. The purpose of this chapter is to provide an introduction to the field of genetics and the influence of genetic-based syndromes on communication disorders. A long list of syndromes show speech, language, hearing, and cognitive impairments, some of which are quite rare. The focus of this chapter is on syndromes that an audiologist or speech-language pathologist may encounter during their professional careers.

TERMINOLOGY AND DEFINITIONS

Prior to presenting features of various syndromes, it is necessary to provide a refresher on the terms and concepts related to human genetics. Life begins with a **cell**, which is the smallest unit of living matter. The human body is composed of 100 trillion cells in many shapes and sizes. Inside the body of the cell sits the **nucleus**, which is a vast storehouse of biochemical information. Within the nucleus reside **chromosomes**. The term chromosome means "colored body from *chroma* (meaning color) and *soma* (meaning body). The term originated from the observation by the German anatomist, **Wilhelm Waldeyer** (1836–1921) who in 1888, found that the material comprising chromosomes could be observed in clear detail following staining for microscopic examination (Figure 11.1). Chromosomes are found in every cell of the body except for red blood cells. Each chromosome contains two very long coiled strings of **DNA** (deoxyribonucleic acid). **Genes** are located on these DNA strings. They are the functional units of heredity that occupy a very specific place on a chromosome and have two functions: (1) they contain the basic set of instructions for putting together an organism, and (2) they regulate the function, growth, and development of an organism after birth. Genes carry information for making all the proteins required by all organisms. These proteins determine, among other things, how the organism looks, how well its

FIGURE 11.1. Wilhelm Waldeyer. German anatomist who discovered chromosomes.

body metabolizes food or fights infection, and sometimes even how it behaves. There are approximately 30,000 genes distributed among the chromosomes of the human body. Amazingly, only 2% of the DNA string contains genes. The remaining 98% of the material comprising the string was once referred to as "junk DNA" because it appeared to consist of meaningless sequences. However, research is slowly unraveling the function of this remaining DNA. The basic genetic template of a cell is shown in Figure 11.2.

Normal human cells contain 46 chromosomes that exist in 23 pairs. Not all species have the same number of chromosomes. For example, cats have 38 chromosomes and fish have 78 chromosomes. Among the 46 chromosomes found in humans, 23 chromosomes are received from each parent. The number assigned to the first 22 pairs is related to chromosome length. Chromosome pair 1 is longest and contains the most genetic material. Chromosome pair 22 is the shortest. Chromosome 23 designates sex. Among females, the 23rd chromosome pairing is known as XX. The male body contains two types of sex chromosomes known as XY. The Y chromosome of the 23rd chromosome, while designating the male sex, is also found to contain the

| Cell | Nucleus | Chromosomes | DNA/Genes |

FIGURE 11.2. Genetic template of a cell.

FYI

The number of chromosomes varies considerably across living organisms. Among animals, the mosquito is low on the list with 6 in total, whereas the hermit crab tops in at 254. Among plants, hawkweed has 8 chromosomes per cell and ferns have 1,200 chromosomes.

---

least amount of genetic material across the entire set of 46 chromosomes. Males produce both X- and Y-bearing sperm. Sex is determined by the father, depending on whether an X-bearing sperm or Y-bearing sperm joins with the female X chromosome.

Each chromosome consists of two strands that resemble an "X" in structural appearance. The point at which the two strands cross is called the **centromere**. An individual chromosome can be further described with regard to the location of the centromere: a **metacentric** chromosome has a centromere in the approximate center, a **submetacentric** chromosome has a centromere that is slightly off center, and an **acrocentric** chromosome has a centromere that is near the tip of the chromosome. The top two arms of each chromosome are called the short arms; the lower two arms are called the long arms. Examples of various chromosome shapes are displayed in Figure 11.3.

The entire DNA of an organism, including its genes, is called the **genome**. Knowledge about the effects of DNA variations among individuals can lead to new ways to diagnose, treat, and even prevent thousands of genetic disorders. Begun formally in 1990, the **Human Genome Project** (HGP) was a 13-year effort coordinated by the U.S. Department of Energy and the National Institutes of Health. Additional contributions to the HGP came from China, England, France, Germany, and Japan. The international effort to sequence the 3 billion DNA letters in the human genome is considered by many to have been the most ambitious scientific undertaking of all time, even compared

Metacentric   Sub-metacentric   Acrocentric

FIGURE 11.3. The various shapes of chromosomes.

to splitting the atom or landing on the moon. The project was expected to take 15 years to complete, but rapid technological advances pushed forward the completion date to 2003. The goal of the project was to identify all of the genes in human DNA. Originally, it was assumed the human body consisted of 60,000 to 100,000 genes. It was discovered that humans are made up of approximately 30,000 genes. In the years since completion of the HGP, the human genome database has enabled identification of a number of genes that are associated with disease. As a result, more objective and accurate diagnoses are being made for various genetic conditions even before overt clinical symptoms are observed.

Heredity is the genetic transmission of characteristics from parent to offspring. The term **genotype** refers to the genetic variation which separates one individual from another. No two individuals have the exact same genotype. But, you might ask, do identical twins have the same genotype? The answer is a resounding yes and no. The answer is yes, if we consider that identical twins have the same DNA because they came from a fertilized egg cell (zygote) that gets split in half. But the answer is also no, because even though identical twins may have the same DNA, their genes are in different bodies. Alone, DNA does nothing—it is like a book sitting on a shelf. It sits there until someone (or something, like a protein) comes along to read it and assemble the information (i.e., to create a person). The way a protein interprets the gene can vary, which is why identical twins may have different fingerprints, and even look different. This is because their bodies are taking the same DNA and using it in different ways. The physical expression of genetic variation (i.e., traits) is referred to as **phenotype**. The complete set of chromosomes for an individual is referred to as the **karyotype**. An example of the karyotype for a female and male is provided in Figure 11.4. Note that the most obvious difference in karyotype is in regard to chromosome 23, which is the sex chromosome.

HISTORIC ASPECTS OF GENETICS

A time line of some of the major events that shaped the field of genetics is displayed in Table 11.1. Some of the more profound events are detailed below. From the earliest recorded history, ancient civilizations observed patterns in reproduction. Animals bore offspring of the same species, children resembled their parents, and plants gave rise to similar plants. Some of the earliest ideas about reproduction, heredity, and the transmission of information from parent to child were the **particulate theories** developed in ancient Greece during the fourth century BC. These theories posited that information from each part of the parent had to be somehow transmitted to create the corresponding body part in the offspring. For example, the particulate theories held that information from the parent's heart, lungs, and limbs was transmitted directly from these body parts to create the offspring's heart, lungs, and limbs.

One reason particulate theories were inaccurate was that they relied on observations unaided by the microscope. The microscope was invented around 1600 by a Dutch spectacle maker, **Zacharias Janssen** (1580–1538). The English naturalist **Robert Hooke** (1635–1703)

A

B

FIGURE 11.4. Female (**A**) and male (**B**) karyotype. Note the obvious difference in regard to pairing of the 23rd (sex) chromosomes.

Table 11.1. Some Milestones in the Field of Genetics	
Year	*Event*
1590	The microscope is invented by Zacharias Janssen.
1858	Charles Darwin announces the theory of natural selection.
1863	Studying peas, Gregor Mendel discovers that traits are transmitted from parents to progeny by discrete, independent units, later known as genes. His observations lay the groundwork for the field of genetics.
1869	Johann Friedrich Miescher discovers **DNA** in human white blood cells and in the sperm of trout.
1879	Walther Fleming discovers chromatin, the rodlike structures inside the cell nucleus that are later named chromosomes.
1905	Nettie Stevens and Edmund Wilson independently describe the behavior of sex chromosomes.
1907	Thomas Hunt Morgan work on *Drosophila* (i.e., the fruit fly) leads to further understanding of genetics.
1953	James Watson and Francis Crick publish their findings describing the double helical structure of DNA, marking the beginning of the modern era of genetics.
1972	The DNA composition of humans is found to be 99% similar to that of chimpanzees and gorillas.
1983	The first artificial chromosome is synthesized.
1983	James Gusella uses blood samples to demonstrate that the Huntington disease gene is on chromosome 4.
1984	The DNA fingerprinting technique is developed.
1990	The first federally approved gene therapy treatment is performed on a 4-year-old girl with an immune disorder.
1996	Discovery of a gene associated with Parkinson disease provides insight as to its cause and potential treatment.
1997	Scottish scientists report cloning a sheep, named Dolly, using DNA from adult sheep cells.
2000	The Human Genome Project presents its preliminary results.

was the first to use this device to identify plant cells, specifically the cell walls in cork tissue. Hooke coined the term *cells*. The boxlike shape of cells in cork reminded him of the cells of a monastery. Over the next century, improvements in microscopy and the increasing study of cytology (i.e., the formation, structure, and function of cells) enabled scientists to identify parts of the cell.

One of the most important developments in the study of hereditary processes came in 1858, when **Charles Darwin** (1809–1882) and **Alfred Wallace** (1823–1913) announced the theory of natural selection (see also Chapter 1). The premise of this theory was that members of a population who are better adapted to their environment will be the ones most likely to survive and pass their traits on to the next generation. Darwin published this theory in 1859 in the classic text, *On the Origin of Species by Means of Natural Selection*. At the time of publication, Darwin's work was not viewed favorably. Religious leaders believed the theory refuted the biblical interpretation of how life on Earth began. To this day, debate continues regarding evolution and creationism.

During the period of 1856 to 1863 the Austrian **Gregor Mendel** (1822–1884) conducted carefully designed genetic experiments with nearly 30,000 pea plants (Figure 11.5). Mendel was an Augustinian monk who taught natural science to high school students. He cultivated pea plants in the monastery garden and chose to study them because they had distinct, identifiable characteristics that could not be confused. His experiments were designed to test the inheritance of a specific trait from one generation to the next. For example, to test inheritance of the characteristic of plant height, Mendel self-pollinated by hand several short pea plants, and the seeds they produced grew into short plants.

In 1907, the American **Thomas Hunt Morgan** (1866–1945) studied *drosophila* (i.e., the fruit fly) as a means of understanding genetic traits (Figure 11.6). This research revolutionized the study

FIGURE 11.5. Gregor Mendel. His genetic experiments with pea plants were designed to test the inheritance of specific traits.

FIGURE 11.6. Thomas Hunt Morgan. Studied fruit flies as a means of understanding genetic traits.

of genetics because the fly's rapid life cycle and minute size enabled Morgan to undertake a large number of experiments over a short period of time. Contrast the whole year required between generations of peas with the 2 weeks needed for the lifespan of a fruit fly. Morgan was able to study hundreds of fruit fly characteristics. In addition, he identified gene mutations, such as discovery of some fruit flies having a white-eyed mutation.

Nettie Maria Stevens (1861–1912) was an American biologist and geneticist who studied under the guidance of Thomas Hunt Morgan (Figure 11.7). Based on research with beetles, she helped prove that chromosomes determine the sex of an organism. Prior to this discovery, researchers assumed that the sex of an organism was influenced by food and temperature conditions during the early stages of an organism's development.

The discovery in 1953 of the double-helix structure of DNA marked the

beginning of the modern era of genetics. The American anthropologist **James Watson** (b. 1928) and British physicist **Francis Crick** (1916–2004) worked together at the University of Cambridge (Figure 11.8). Many of their findings

FIGURE 11.7. Nettie Maria Stevens. American biologist who helped proved that chromosomes determine the sex of an organism.

FIGURE 11.8. James Watson and Francis Crick. Discoverers of the double-helix structure of DNA.

were based on examination of x-ray diffraction photographs. In 1988, Watson was later appointed as head of the Human Genome Project (HGP) at the National Institutes of Health.

TYPES OF SYNDROMES

Use of the term birth defect is a generalized description of any genetic or non-genetic condition that occurs at birth. The term is not entirely accurate because: (1) some abnormalities may not be present at birth and are evident only after the child begins to mature (such as dentition), and (2) the term does not take into account abnormalities of behavior. A more accurate description of these conditions is a **congenital anomaly**. An example in which both physical and behavioral anomalies surface later in a child's development is fetal alcohol syndrome (FAS). The characteristics of FAS are described later in this chapter.

Syndromes can be broadly classified into two types: (1) **chromosomal syndromes** and (2) **genetic syndromes**. Chromosomal syndromes involve visible changes in the chromosomal structure (i.e., karyotype) of the individual. These types of syndromes typically result in rather severe anomalies such as

---

FYI

Gene splicing is a technique used to join segments of DNA (often from different individuals or species) to form a new genetic combination called recombinant DNA. This is one of the techniques used in genetic engineering.

---

physical abnormalities, cognitive impairments, and communication disorders. The reason for the severe anomalies is that impairment of chromosomal structure tends to affect a large number of genes. On the other hand, genetic syndromes often involve a single affected gene. The outward appearance of chromosomes may appear fine. It is a specific gene that is abnormal. The problems arising from a genetic syndrome can range from mild to severe, depending on the specific gene that is affected.

Chromosomal Syndromes

Approximately 7 out of every 1,000 births will be affected by a chromosomal disorder. These disorders account for approximately half of all spontaneous abortions that occur during the first trimester of pregnancy (Gerber, 1990). There are five basic abnormalities that can occur in chromosomal structure: (1) deletion of whole chromosomes, (2) deletion of parts of a chromosome, (3) addition of whole chromosomes, (4) addition of parts of chromosomes, and (5) restructuring (or rearranging) of chromosomes. Most people who have a chromosomal syndrome exhibit the chromosomal abnormality in every cell in the body. However, there are rare cases in which only a portion of the body's cells are affected. This condition is referred to as **mosaicism**. Individuals with mosaicism generally show less severe abnormalities than if all cells were affected. The chromosomal syndromes of: (1) Down syndrome, (2) Cri du Chat syndrome, and (3) Turner syndrome are profiled below.

Down Syndrome

This is the most frequently occurring human chromosomal disorder. In this particular condition, the karyotype is characterized by a chromosomal addition to the 21st chromosome. The condition is referred to as trisomy 21, indicating the particular karyotype (Figure 11.9). The condition was named after **John**

A

B

FIGURE 11.9. Down syndrome karyotype (**A**) and a photograph of a boy with Down syndrome (**B**). (From Vanellus at Wikimedia Commons.)

Langon Down (1828–1896), an English physician who published *Observations of an Ethnic Classification of Idiots* in 1866. He identified a group of patients with similar features and called them mongoloid idiots. The term "idiot" was in common use at the time to describe intellectual impairment, "mongoloid" was in reference to the supposed similarity in appearance to people of east Asia. These days, neither term is socially acceptable. Although Down is credited with identifying the syndrome, the precise chromosomal structure of trisomy 21 was not identified until nearly 100 years later by **Jerome Lejeune** (1926–1994). Down syndrome is found to occur in approximately 1 out of every 800 births. Down syndrome is a chromosomal disorder caused by an error in cell division and the likelihood of such an error increases with maternal age (Hook et al., 1983), meaning that an older female is more prone to give birth to a child with Down syndrome. The occurrence dramatically increases to 1 out of every 25 births among women over the age of 45 years (Table 11.2). The average life expectancy of an individual with Down syndrome is 55 years of age.

The phenotype of Down syndrome is provided in Table 11.3. Included among these characteristics are heart anomalies, dry skin, fine soft hair, hypotonia (i.e., reduced muscle tone), brachycephaly (i.e., a widening of the skull with a flat back of head), Class III malocclusion, protruding tongue, and intellectual disability that is very rarely severe. Males with Down syndrome may also have hypogonadism—a defect of the reproductive system that results in lack of function of the gonads (i.e., sterility) in males. The communication disorder often found in Down syndrome is delayed onset of language. Although

Table 11.2. Approximate Occurrence of Down Syndrome Births According to the Mother's Age

Age of Mother (Years)	Frequency of Down Syndrome (Per Births)
15–19	1/1,250
20–24	1/1,400
25–29	1/1,100
30–32	1/875
33–35	1/500
36–38	1/225
39–41	1/100
42–44	1/50
45+	1/25

these children eventually will develop communication skills, the length of utterance and size of vocabulary is reduced and dependent primarily on the severity of intellectual disability. Children with Down syndrome also may show speech articulation difficulties resulting from reduced muscle tone in the oral cavity, combined with dentition irregularities. The hearing abilities of individuals with Down syndrome usually are normal, although children can experience higher than average bouts of otitis media.

Cri du Chat Syndrome

Jerome Lejeune (1926–1994) first described Cri du Chat syndrome in 1963. Legeune was a French pediatrician and geneticist who was also the first to identify the precise chromosomal structure of Down syndrome. Cri du Chat (mean-

Table 11.3. Phenotype of Some Chromosomal Syndromes

Chromosomal Syndrome	Phenotype
Down syndrome	Hyptonia
	Protruding tongue
	Brachycephaly
	Heart anomaly
	Dry skin
	Fine soft hair
	Hypogonadism
	Obesity
	Short fifth finger
	Class III malocclusion
	Cognitive impairment
Cri du Chat syndrome	High-pitched voice
	Hypotonia
	Microcephaly
	Orbital hypertelorisim
	Down-slanting eyes
	Ear tags
	Small stature
	Occasional cleft palate
	Severe cognitive impairment
Turner syndrome	Short stature
	Short webbed neck
	Heart anomalies
	Renal anomalies
	Lack of sexual development
	Low-set ears
	Low hairline
	Shield-shaped chest
	Occasional cleft palate
	Puffy hands and feet
	Hearing loss

ing "cat's cry" in French) syndrome is named for the catlike cry made by infants with this chromosomal disorder, which is caused by an abnormally small larynx. Cri du chat syndrome is also called 5p minus (5p–) syndrome because it is caused by a partial deletion of the short or "p" arm of chromosome 5 (Figure 11.10). The syndrome has been estimated to occur in 1 of every 50,000 live births. It accounts for 1 in every 500 cases of intellectual disability. Approximately 50 to 60 children are born with Cri du Chat syndrome in the United States each year. The syndrome is found to occur in all races and in both sexes. There is a

A

B

FIGURE 11.10. Karyotype of Cri du Chat syndrome (**A**) and photograph of Ariella at age 6 years (**B**). (Photograph used with permission of the Cri du Chat Support Group of Australia.)

slight female predominance with the ratio of occurrence estimated to be 3 girls to 2 boys. At birth, these children may show a failure to thrive because of feeding difficulties; however, those who do survive have a normal life expectancy. Individuals with Cri du Chat tend to be loving and highly social.

The phenotype of Cri du Chat syndrome is provided in Table 11.3. Individuals with this syndrome have unusual facial features such as down-slanting eyes, ear tags, small head size (i.e., microcephaly), small jaw size (i.e., micrognathia), and a large distance between the eyes (i.e., hypertelorism). The children also demonstrate hypotonia, and may be born with a cleft palate. A severe intellectual impairment occurs because of the large deletion of genetic material from the chromosome. In addition to the classic feature of a catlike cry or high-pitched voice, the voice also may have a nasal quality if the child was born with a cleft palate. As a result of the severe intellectual impairments, development of oral language can be a challenge. A small number of children never learn to speak; however, most are able to speak and make themselves understood to some degree, which they supplement with both formal and informal gestures. A conductive hearing loss may be present, resulting from persistent otitis media.

Turner Syndrome

Turner syndrome is named after the American physician **Henry Turner** (1892–1970), who first described the condition in 1938. Turner syndrome affects only women and is caused by a total absence of one of the sex (23rd) chromosomes in some or all cells throughout the body (Figure 11.11). About 1% of all female conceptions have a missing X chromosome. Of these, the majority (99%) spontaneously abort, usually during the first trimester of pregnancy. Turner syndrome affects around 1 out of every 2,500 live female births. Most women with Turner syndrome can live relatively normal lives. The prognosis for a person with Turner syndrome is dependent on other conditions that may be present. For example, there is a tendency toward heart or kidney defects, which may significantly impact the quality of life.

The phenotype of Turner syndrome is provided in Table 11.3. Individuals with this syndrome show short stature, a shieldlike chest, stocky build, and puffy hands and feet. The neck is short and wide (web neck), and the ears are low-set. There is a lack of sexual development. Otitis media is common. There is no greater propensity to intellectual impairments than the general population. The phenotype of Turner syndrome is not easy to identify at birth. Many are identified around the time they enter school (due to their short stature) or around the time of puberty (due to lack of sexual development). The primary communication disorder in Turner syndrome is hearing impairment. A sensorineural hearing loss has been found to occur in as many as 65% of all cases and 10% of these individuals are deaf. Usually, language abilities are normal. Speech articulation difficulties may occur as a result of over crowding of the teeth and a high arched palate.

Genetic Syndromes

Although genetic syndromes are chromosome based, they are categorized separately. These are conditions that do not have a visible cellular abnormality.

unable to breast feed. As the children grow, they develop better muscle tone and strength. Motor milestones such as standing, walking, and running are achieved but delayed in comparison to same-age peers. Stage 2 of PWS occurs during the age range of 2 to 6 years. This stage is characterized by an insatiable appetite. During this time frame, children with PWS are likely to exhibit intellectual disabilities, with IQs ranging from low-normal to moderate mental impairment. Disordered speech and language often is observed among individuals with PWS that is associated with the child's overall level of cognitive functioning. The communication impairment found in PWS includes delayed speech and language development that parallels that found for achieving basic motor milestones. Children with PWS also may show hypernasal speech early in life that is linked to poor muscle tone. The hypernasality generally decreases as the child's strength and muscle tone improves.

Fetal Alcohol Syndrome

An infant born to a mother who drinks alcohol during her pregnancy, even in modest amounts, may be born with FAS. The condition of FAS results in growth retardation, unusual physical and facial features, and intellectual impairment. Children have suffered the consequences of their mothers' alcohol consumption since people began to drink alcohol. In 1973, the term FAS was coined by Kenneth Jones and David Smith, two pediatric dysmorphologists, who described the signs of alcohol exposure in infants at birth and early childhood. FAS is a teratogenic disorder that causes gene mutation. On average, three out of five women drink alcohol. A woman's body metabolizes alcohol more quickly than a man's and thus, they become intoxicated more easily. When pregnant women drink, the developing fetus receives a strong dose of alcohol. The internationally recognized rate of occurrence of FAS is 1 to 3 out of every 1,000 births. In 9 out of every 1,000 births, infants will show some (but not all) signs of alcohol exposure. This condition is referred to as alcohol-related neurodevelopmental disorder (ARND) or fetal alcohol effects (FAE). It is estimated that 25 to 45% of women with chronic alcoholism will give birth to children with FAS if they drink heavily during pregnancy (Table 11.5).

It is difficult to pinpoint the exact gene (or genes) that are mutated because the mutation is linked to: (1) the amount of alcohol consumed by the mother, (2) the time of pregnancy during which alcohol was consumed, and (3) the likely

---

FYI

In early 2001, a discovery was made claiming that a specific gene, *FOXP2* (located on chromosome 7), was the primary gene for learning to acquire language. This conclusion was based on genetic examination of a family with a long history of communication disorders. Members of the family showed a mutation of this particular gene. We now know that this particular gene, although contributing a major role to communication, is likely one of many genes necessary for regulating speech and language.

interaction of alcohol consumption with other drugs. The early months of fetal growth involve development of the face, limbs, heart, and brain. Therefore, mothers who drink during the first trimester of pregnancy give birth to children with the most severe problems because the alcohol abuse occurs during the period when many physical features of the child are developing. This is also a time when many women may not even realize they are pregnant. Women who abstain from alcohol in early pregnancy may feel comfortable drinking during the final months of the pregnancy. Yet it is during the last trimester of pregnancy that some of the most complex features of brain development take place. Even moderate alcohol intake, and especially periodic binge drinking, can seriously damage the developing nervous system of the fetus.

A list of the phenotype of FAS is provided in Figure 11.15. The phenotype found in 50% (or more) of the cases of FAS include: (1) below average height and weight, (2) microcephaly, (3) micrognathia, (4) thin upper lip, (5) hyperactivity, and (6) intellectual impairment. Problems associated with FAS tend to intensify as children move into adulthood. These can include mental health problems, troubles with the law, and the inability to live independently. The

Table 11.5. Some Facts About Alcohol Consumption

- A "drink" is defined as a 12-oz. beer, 1.5-oz. shot of 80-proof liquor, or 4-oz. glass of table wine.

- Legally intoxicated is defined as a blood alcohol level (BAL) of .08%.

- Permanent brain cell damage begins at a BAL of .07%.

- A 100-lb (45 kg) female consuming 5 standard drinks will reach a BAL of .25%, which is three times the legal BAL limit.

- BAL decreases .01% per hour.

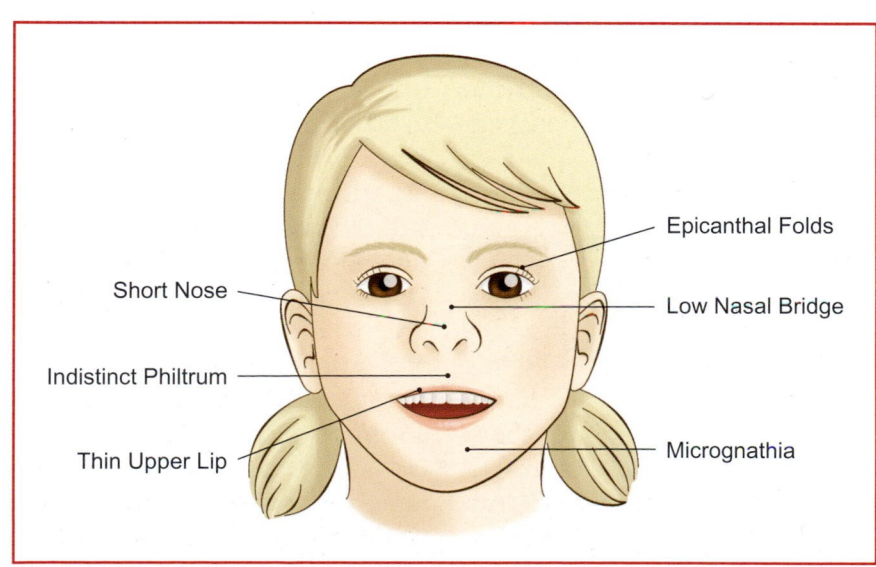

FIGURE 11.15. Phenotype of fetal alcohol syndrome.

FYI

There is genetic evidence that suggests some people were "born to smoke." In 1999, researchers found that people who carry the gene SLC6A3-9, located on chromosome 5, were less likely to become addicted to cigarette smoking than those without the gene. The particular gene is found to be important for the transfer of the neurotransmitter dopamine, which is a natural stimulant created in the brain. Those without the gene may be more vulnerable to the addictive (i.e., stimulating) effects of tobacco.

communication problems found in FAS include a general overall delay in speech and language development. The child with FAS also may show speech articulation problems and swallowing problems due to poor motor coordination. If a child with FAS has an intellectual impairment, there is likely to be an associated language impairment, the severity of which is dependent on the severity of the intellectual disability. The condition of FAS, and all damage caused by prenatal alcohol exposure, is 100% preventable by simply choosing not to drink alcohol. FAS cannot be cured, but the effects of the disabilities can be managed.

ASSESSMENT OF GENETICS AND SYNDROMES

We are continually learning more about the genetics of various diseases and syndromes and how these conditions run in families. Two forms of assessment are: (1) genetic counseling and (2) prenatal diagnosis. **Genetic counseling** is designed to help a person or family understand their risk for genetic conditions (such as Down syndrome), to educate the person or family about the condition, and assess the risk of passing the condition on to children. Traditionally, a genetic counselor has a master's degree in genetic counseling and has studied genetic diseases and how they run in families. Table 11.6 provides a list of situations whereby a person may wish to seek genetic counseling.

As the term suggests, **prenatal diagnosis** involves assessing the fetus prior to birth. Two forms of prenatal testing used routinely on pregnant women are: (1) maternal blood sampling and (2) ultrasound scanning. Between 15 and 19 weeks of pregnancy, women are offered a **blood test**. A pregnancy blood test measures the exact amount of the pregnancy hormone called human chorionic gonadotropin (hCG) in the bloodstream. This measurement can help give a rough estimate of the age of the fetus. It also can help determine if the pregnancy is progressing normally.

Ultrasound scans are performed on most pregnant women between 16 and 19 weeks of pregnancy. The process of

> **Table 11.6.** Situations Where it is Advisable to Seek Genetic Counseling
>
> - Individuals who are concerned they might have an inherited disorder.
> - Women who are pregnant or planning to be after the age of 35.
> - Couples who already have a child with an inherited disorder.
> - Women who have had three or more miscarriages.
> - People concerned that their jobs, lifestyles, or medical history may pose a risk to the outcome of pregnancy. Common causes of concern include exposure to radiation, medications, illegal drugs, chemicals, or infections.
> - Couples who would like testing or more information about genetic conditions that occur frequently in their ethnic group.
> - Couples who are first cousins or other close blood relatives.
> - Pregnant women whose ultrasound examinations or blood testing indicate that their pregnancy may be at increased risk for certain complications.

fetal **ultrasound** testing was developed in the late 1960s and involves applying a clear, water-based conduction gel to the surface of the pregnant woman's abdomen that helps with the transmission of sound waves. A hand-held probe called a transducer is then moved over the area and delivers a series of sound waves that bounce off the curves and variations inside the body, including the fetus (Figure 11.16). These sound waves are translated into a pattern of light and dark areas that create an image of the fetus on a monitor. The procedure is noninvasive, safe, and painless for the mother and fetus. Generally, an obstetrician performs an ultrasound test to determine if a woman is pregnant and whether there is more than one fetus. An ultrasound test also can be used to detect abnormalities in the development of the fetus such as growth retardation, heart and kidney defects, Down syndrome, and cleft palate. The test is also useful in identifying **neural tube defects** (i.e., abnormalities) of the brain and spinal cord. Two neural tube defects

are spina bifida and anencephaly. In **spina bifida**, the fetal spinal column fails to close completely during the first month of pregnancy. There is usually nerve damage that causes at least some paralysis of the legs. In **anencephaly**, much of the brain does not develop. Babies with anencephaly are either stillborn or die shortly after birth.

For pregnancies where there is a risk of the fetus having a genetic abnormality, tissue for genetic testing can be obtained either by: (1) aminocentesis or (2) chorionic villus sampling. The **amniocentesis** procedure was developed in the early 1960s. The procedure involves withdrawing fluid from the amnion (the fluid-filled sack that contains the fetus). The fluid is taken from the woman's abdomen using a needle cannula (Figure 11.17). The cellular structure of the fluid is then analyzed to determine the karyotype of the fetus. Amniocentesis is performed during the 16th week of pregnancy, carries a low level of risk, and can be accomplished in an obstetrician's office.

FIGURE 11.16. Illustration of ultrasound testing.

FIGURE 11.17. Illustration of amniocentesis in which amniotic fluid is withdrawn and later analyzed.

Chorionic villus sampling was developed in 1975 by Chinese gynecologists as an aid to the early diagnosis of genetic disorders. In this approach, a catheter is inserted through the woman's cervix into the placenta. An abdominal ultrasound is also performed to determine the position of the uterus, the size of the gestational sac, and the position of the placenta within the uterus (Figure 11.18). A small piece of placenta tissue (i.e., chorionic villi) is removed from the uterus and examined microscopically for the existence of chromosomal abnormalities, as well as several hundred genetic disorders, such as cystic fibrosis and sickle cell disease. The main advantage of chorionic villus sampling over amniocentesis is that the test can be performed earlier, generally between 11 and 12 weeks of pregnancy.

TREATMENT OF GENETIC CONDITIONS

Prophylactic Therapy

Prophylactic therapy involves the prevention of symptoms before they occur. One form of prophylactic therapy is the administration of vaccines to immunize against many diseases such as mumps, measles, and chicken pox. An example of prophylactic therapy involves treatment

FIGURE 11.18. Illustration of chorionic villi sampling, involving removal of a small piece of placenta tissue (chorionic villi) from the uterus.

for a genetic condition known as phenyl-ketonuria (PKU). **PKU** is caused by mutations in the gene for phenylalanine hydroxylase, which is responsible for normal brain functioning. An infant's blood can be tested shortly after birth to determine whether PKU is present. If detected early, the baby's diet can be modified to ensure normal development and a normal life span.

Replacement Therapy

Replacement therapy involves replacing the gene product (i.e., protein) that is missing or defective in an affected person with a functioning gene product. For many years, such therapy has been available to individuals with conditions such as diabetes (where insulin is replaced) or growth hormone deficiency (where growth hormone is replaced). These disorders have been relatively easy to treat because the normal gene products are transported around the body in the bloodstream and it is possible to inject the synthetic gene product intravenously. However, even for these disorders, the treatment has the disadvantage of having to be continually repeated.

Treatment of Symptoms

For most genetic disorders, the symptoms of the disorder are treated rather than the actual affected gene/chromosome. Such treatments include surgery, the administration of drugs, and the control of a patient's environment. For example, it is common for people with Down syndrome to be born with heart defects, which can be corrected surgically. For women with Turner syndrome,

hormone-replacement therapy is given to prevent early-onset osteoporosis that occurs because of the absence of estrogen. The excessive eating and weight gain of patients with PWS has to be managed with strict diet control. Treatment of communication disorders among individuals with genetic abnormalities is directed toward underlying causes such as hearing loss or impaired speech motor control. In addition, young children may be placed in early intervention programs to provide optimal input for speech and language acquisition.

CULTURAL CONSIDERATIONS REGARDING GENETICS

It is often assumed that diseases found to occur within a family "tree" must be purely genetic. However, this family trend may reflect a common environment and lifestyle rather than a genetic influence. The term **ethnicity** is a complex construct that includes biology, history, cultural orientation and practice, language, religion, and lifestyle—all of these factors affect an individual's health (Pearce et al., 2004). For example, the Pellagra Commission was established in 1900 to investigate the problem of pellagra (a vitamin deficiency disease) in the southern United States. The Commission concluded that pellagra was purely genetic because it occurred within the same families. Unfortunately, members of the Commission failed to recognize that poverty and malnutrition also were major issues in the same families.

Even for classic genetic diseases, environmental factors usually have an important role. In fact, genetic studies can show the importance of environmental factors. A New Zealand study of alcoholism provides one example of a health-related genetic difference. Marshall et al., (1994) found that the ADH2-2 gene, which is believed to protect against alcoholism, was relatively common in the indigenous Maori people of New Zealand. This same gene is not found in New Zealand Europeans. Yet national statistics have revealed that alcohol-related health problems are more common in Maori, suggesting that the protective genetic factors are being outweighed by social, economic, cultural, and political factors. In summary, although some diseases are found to occur in some groups of people at a higher rate than others, the constant interaction between genes and the environment indicates that few diseases are purely hereditary.

CURRENT RESEARCH IN GENETICS

Human Genome Project

Since completion of the HGP in 2003, a startling finding was that the number of human genes totals approximately 30,000, which is only twice the number of genes found in the fruit fly *Drosophilia*. So what makes humans more complex than a fruit fly? The answer appears to lie in a gene's production of proteins, rather than the total number of genes. Genes exert their effects (traits) by telling the body to make certain proteins. The future of genetics lies in understanding the nature of these proteins and how they work to create an individual person. This new and burgeoning scientific field is known as **proteomics**.

Communication Disorders

In recent years, important advances have been made in genetics that apply to individuals with communication disorders. For example, researchers now understand that many aspects of communication disorders have a genetic component. In addition to the syndromes that have clear genetic etiology (e.g., Down syndrome, Fragile X syndrome), genetics is increasingly being shown to play a role in a variety of disorders previously not thought to be of genetic origin, such as autism, reading difficulties, and specific language impairment (Barkmeier-Kraemer, 2007). Examining the speech and language development in **twins** provides a natural experiment that is ideally suited to examining the relative contributions of nature and nurture to variations in human traits and behaviors (Hayiou-Thomas, 2008). Identical

FYI

Cloning is the creation of an organism that is an exact genetic copy of another. This means that every piece of DNA is the same between the two organisms. Cloning is an asexual process because only one parent is required. Certain plants, such as types of grapes to make fine wines, have undergone cloning for hundreds of years. Only recently has the technology become available to clone animals, and the advent of this technology has sparked ethical debate.

twins (also known as monozygotic, or MZ), share 100% of their DNA, whereas fraternal twins (dizygotic, or DZ) share approximately 50% of the DNA that varies from person to person. The twin method is based on comparing the similarity of the members of a twin pair on a given communication trait, such as vocabulary size, for MZ and DZ twin pairs. If MZ twins have more similar vocabulary scores than DZ twins, we can infer that the extra similarity in MZ vocabulary comes from these twins' extra genetic similarity. On the other hand, if MZ and DZ twins are equally similar, then we can infer that something in the twins' environment is driving that similarity. Results of studies like this seem to suggest that differences in young children's language skills, such as vocabulary and grammar, appear to be due largely to environmental influences. On the other hand, differences in speech skill appear to be mostly due to genetic effects.

GENETICS AND SYNDROMES ON THE WORLD WIDE WEB

Listed below are Web sites that provide further information on the topics of genetics and syndromes. At the time of publication each Web site was freely accessible.

Cracking the Genetic Code of Life Video
http://www.pbs.org/wgbh/nova/genome/program.html

Human Genetics Disorders Videos
http://www.humangenetics disorders.com/

Information on Genetics
http://www.genetics.com

Inheritance of Genetic Disorders Videos
http://www.teachersdomain.org/resource/tdc02.sci.life.gen.lp _disorder/

REFERENCES

Barkmeier-Kraemer, J. (2007). Translating research into treatment efficacy: Genetics and neuroscience applied to communication disorders. *The Asha Leader*, 12(12), 23.

Gerber, A. (1990). *Prevention: The etiology of communicative disorders in children*. Englewood Cliffs, NJ: Prentice-Hall.

Hayiou-Thomas, M. E. (2008). Genetic and environmental influences on early speech, language and literacy development. *Journal of Communication Disorders, 41*, 397–408.

Hook, E. B., Cross, P. K., & Schreinemachers, D. M. (1983). Chromosomal abnormality rates at amniocentesis and in live-born infants. *Journal of the American Medical Association, 249*, 2034–2038.

Marshall, S. J., O'Brien, D., Wheeler, K., Hermans, I. F., Chambers, G. K., Robinson, G. M., & Stace, N. (1994). Genes and alcoholism: A preliminary report. *New Zealand Medical Journal, 107*, 106–107.

Pearce, N., Foliaki, S., Sporle, A., & Cunningham, C. (2004). Genetics, race, ethnicity and health. *British Medical Journal, 328*, 1070–1107.

Shprintzen, R. (1997). *Genetics, syndromes and communication disorders*. San Diego, CA: Singular.

SECTION 4

Audition

HEARING DISORDERS

OBJECTIVES

After reading this chapter, the student should be able to:

- Understand the concepts and terminology of the nature of sound.

- Understand basic audiology terminology.

- Describe various attributes of hearing loss including type, degree, and configuration of loss.

- Identify the primary types, causes, and characteristics of hearing disorders in children and adults.

- Describe common disorders of hearing associated with each part of the auditory system.

- Understand theory and practice of various audiologic diagnostic tests.

- Describe the primary assessment of hearing disorders in children and adults.

INTRODUCTION

As noted in Chapters 1 and 2, communication involves the processes of encoding and decoding. Human communication is the exchange of a message between someone producing speech and someone listening to speech. A major portion of this book thus far has been dedicated to the wide range of communication disorders that result from a breakdown in the process of speech production. We now turn our attention to those communication disorders that result from a disruption in hearing. There is perhaps no other health condition that can have as profound an effect on one's quality of life as a hearing disorder. Loss of hearing makes even routine communication difficult. This may result in frustration, withdrawal from social activities, depression, and marital discord. People lose the ability to appreciate sounds of everyday living such as birds singing, children's voices, and even police sirens.

Hearing loss in adults is usually a condition that develops gradually over the years, and most people are not aware of the extent of their hearing loss until family or friends bring it to their attention. A hearing loss that occurs early in childhood can have devastating consequences to a child's ability to learn. Such impairment also interferes with a child's psychological, emotional, and speech development. Even mild forms of hearing loss can cause great difficulties to people young and old. Loss of the ability to hear can be a serious problem, but in many cases there is help available through medical or surgical treatment or with hearing aids. This chapter provides an introduction to the wide range of hearing disorders found in children and adults. Some disorders are more common than others, and there are unique ways of testing for various hearing disorders. Audiologists are professionals educated in the diagnosis and management of hearing disorders. For those interested in pursuing audiology as a career, this chapter should provide some insight into the complexities of the auditory system and the truly remarkable process of hearing.

TERMINOLOGY AND DEFINITIONS

The ear is one of the most amazing features of the human body, as well as the body of many living creatures. It is one of the smallest and most complex organs in the body and is capable of transforming airborne sound waves into a form the brain can understand. **Sound** results from a disturbance in air particles (i.e., molecules). Such disturbances are typically caused by the vibration of an elastic body such as a stereo speaker, bass drum, guitar string, or the vocal folds. Vibrations cause a disturbance of air particles. These particles bump into the particles close to them, which causes them to vibrate as well. The disturbance of particles move in a back and forth motion creating a **sound wave**. One complete back and forth motion of a particle is called a **cycle** of vibration. The **frequency** of a sound wave refers to how fast the particles vibrate and is measured by the number of complete vibrations that occur per unit of time. If a particle of air undergoes 1000 vibrations in 1 second, then the frequency of the wave would be 1000 cycles per second. The notation used to designate frequency is the **hertz** (Hz) scale (e.g., 1000 Hz). The hertz notation is used in honor of

Heinrich Hertz (see later section). Low frequency sounds are those that have a small number of vibrations per second. These vibrations are perceived as having a low-pitched sound. Alternatively, high-frequency sounds involve a large number of vibrations per second that we perceive as having a high-pitched quality. When a sound consists of only one frequency it is referred to as a **pure tone**. A **complex sound** is one that contains more than one frequency. Sounds that have no consistent vibratory periodicity are referred to as **noise**.

The back and forth motion of a pure tone can be represented graphically as a **waveform** (Figure 12.1). On such a graph, the height of the sound wave is the point at which the particle is at its maximum point of disturbance. The terms used to describe the maximum disturbance of a sound wave are **amplitude** and **intensity**. The scale for measuring intensity is the **decibel** scale (dB). One decibel (1 dB) is considered the smallest difference in sound intensity that the human ear can discern. The decibel was named in honor of Alexander Graham Bell (see also Chapter 2). We perceive the intensity of a sound wave as its **loudness**. All sound waves can be described in regard to their frequency and intensity. For example, a sound wave may be produced with a single frequency of 2500 Hz and an intensity of 40 dB, or frequency components of 50 Hz and 70 Hz with an intensity of 100 dB. The variations in frequency and intensity for types of sound waves are endless. Illustrations of sound waves of varying frequency and intensity are shown in Figure 12.1.

Some facts and figures about hearing loss are provided in Table 12.1. It is estimated that approximately one in

FIGURE 12.1. Examples of sound waves of varying frequency and intensity. (**A**) has the highest amplitude and lowest frequency, followed by (**B**) and (**C**), respectively. (**D**) is a complex sound consisting of these same three sounds combined together.

Table 12.1. Some Facts About Hearing Loss
• 22 million people in the United States have hearing loss.
• 9 million people in the United Kingdom have a hearing loss.
• 3.5 million people in Australia have a hearing loss.
• 4 million people in South Africa with a hearing loss.
• 400,000 New Zealanders have a hearing loss.
• Hearing loss is highly associated with aging.
• Approximately 60% of the hearing-impaired are over the age of 65 years.
• Men are more likely than women to have hearing loss—some 60% of people with hearing loss are men.
• Hearing loss is the third leading chronic disability, following arthritis and high blood pressure.
• The prevalence of hearing loss decreases as family income and education increase.
• People with hearing loss are generally less healthy than those with no hearing loss.
• Four out of five Americans with hearing loss do not use hearing aids.
• About 15% of university graduates have a level of hearing loss equal to or greater than their parents; a significant cause is listening to loud music.
• Minor decreases in hearing, especially of higher frequencies, are normal after the age of 18 years.

seven individuals has impaired hearing. This occurrence is found for countries throughout the world, including Europe, North America, and those in the southern hemisphere. Hearing impairment encompasses individuals who are deaf and hard of hearing. **Deafness** is defined as a partial or complete loss of hearing. Deafness at birth is known as **congenital deafness**, whereas deafness that occurs after birth is called **adventitious deafness**. Some diseases that are known to cause adventitious deafness are meningitis, mumps, and chicken pox. Deafness that occurs prior to an individual learning to speak is called **prelingual deafness** and **postlingual deafness** is hearing loss that happens after a period of language learning. **Hard of hearing** is defined as a hearing loss ranging from mild to profound for which a person usually receives some benefit from a hearing aid. Common causes of hearing loss are excessive noise exposure and aging. Not surprisingly, the frequency of occurrence of hearing loss is highest among the elderly. By the age of 65, one in every 4 individuals has a significant hearing loss. Hearing loss is the third most self-reported health problem of individuals 65 years of age or older, listed after arthritis and hypertension. It is estimated that untreated hearing impairments cost the United States economy $56 billion in lost productivity, special education, and medical care.

HISTORIC ASPECTS OF HEARING DISORDERS

Paleontologists who uncovered ancient skeletal remains have shown that hearing disorders such as otitis media (OM) occurred among early human populations. Skulls dating back to the Bronze Age (2000 BC) have shown evidence of temporal bone decay. Investigations of Egyptian mummies suggest that OM was present in Egyptian populations as far back as the 13th dynasty (1700 BC). Skulls uncovered from prehistoric Iran found evidence of OM among individuals from 1300 to 300 BC. Specific individuals who have either directly or indirectly contributed to our knowledge concerning hearing loss can be traced back approximately 200 years. Some of the more noteworthy contributors are mentioned below.

Prosper Ménière (1799–1862) was a French laryngologist (Figure 12.2), who at the age of 39, was appointed chief physician at the Institute for Deaf-Mutes in Paris, succeeding the renowned Gaspard Itard (noted for his work with the wild boy of Aveyron). Ménière was the first to describe the unusual ear disease that was later named in his honor. In 1861, he published a report entitled *Lesions of the Inner Ear Giving Rise to Symptoms of Cerebral Congestion of Apoplectic Type*. In this report, Ménière identified a condition in the inner ear that affected both hearing and balance. He concluded in this article that the auditory apparatus of the inner ear may be affected suddenly, causing ringing in the ear and loss of hearing. In addition, the balance structures of the inner ear could also be affected suddenly, resulting in attacks of dizziness and unsteady gait, which may be accompanied by nausea and vomit-

FIGURE 12.2. Prosper Ménière. French laryngologist who was the first to describe the unusual ear disease that was later named in his honor.

ing. Ménière died in Paris of influenza pneumonia at the age of 63 years, the year after publication of his most famous work. While Ménière's name is now known around the world, he did not receive the recognition due to him while he was alive.

Hermann von Helmholtz (1821–1894) was a German physicist who made outstanding contributions to the areas of human physiology, particularly in regard to the eye and the ear (Figure 12.3). He invented the ophthalmoscope that was used for inspecting the interior of the eye and the ophthalmometer, a devise used for measuring the eye's curvature. Helmholtz was also an authority on acoustics and hearing. In

FIGURE 12.3. Hermann von Helmholtz. German physicist who made outstanding contributions to the areas of human physiology, particularly in regard to the eye and the ear.

FIGURE 12.4. Heinrich Hertz. German physicist who was the first to send and receive electromagnetic radio waves.

1863, he published *On the Sensations of Tone as a Physiological Basis of the Theory of Music*. In this book he described the placement of the higher frequency fibers at the basal end of the cochlea and the lower frequencies near the apex, which is now referred to as **tonotopic organization**.

Heinrich Hertz (1857–1894) was a German physicist who happened to be one of von Helmholtz's students (Figure 12.4). Hertz was the first to send and receive radio waves. He proved that electricity could be transmitted in electromagnetic waves, which travel at the speed of light. His experiments with electromagnetic waves eventually led to the development of the wireless telegraph and the radio. His name also became the term used for referring to the measure of frequency per unit of time, or the number of cycles per second (Hz). The hertz designation has been an official part of the international metric system since 1933. When we use the Hz notation to refer to a low-frequency or

---

FYI

Gallaudet University, located in Washington DC, was the first university in the world specifically designed to accommodate deaf and hard of hearing students. The university was established in 1864 during the presidency of Abraham Lincoln. The university is named after Thomas Hopkins Gallaudet who was the founder of the first school for deaf students in the United States. Hearing students are admitted to the graduate school and degrees in audiology and speech-language pathology are offered.

high-frequency hearing loss we are acknowledging the pioneering work of Heinrich Hertz.

Hendrik Zwaardemaker (1857–1920) was both an otolaryngologist and a physiologist who was a professor at Utrecht University in the Netherlands (Figure 12.5). He was the first individual to describe the relationship between advanced aging and a high-frequency hearing loss, for which he coined the term **presbycusis**. Zwaardemaker studied various ways of assessing hearing and the use of whispered voice as a hearing test. He also worked on the physiology of speech production and examined acoustic properties of hearing aids. Since Zwaardemaker's initial description of presbycusis, extensive research has attempted to determine the precise physiologic causes of presbycusis, which remain unknown.

Georg von Békésy (1899–1972) was a biophysicist born in Budapest, Hungary (Figure 12.6). His early research interest was focused on telecommunications and finding ways of improving the acoustic quality of long-distance telephone calls. However, he later turned his attention to the physics of sound and the physical processes involved in hearing. Békésy found that sound traveling through the cochlea flows as a series of waves. He demonstrated that these waves provide maximum stimulation of hair cells (i.e., auditory nerve receptors) at different places along the cochlea: low frequencies toward the apical end of the cochlea and high frequencies near its base. He discovered that the location of this maximum nerve receptor stimulation is the most important factor in determining the pitch and loudness of sounds. His work led to advances in ear

FIGURE 12.5. Hendrik Zwaardemaker. Dutch otolaryngologist who coined the term presbycusis.

FIGURE 12.6. Georg von Békésy. Nobel Prize winner for his research on the functioning of the inner ear. From the University of Hawaii. Reprinted with permission.

surgery and the design of better hearing aids. In 1961, Békésy was awarded the Nobel Prize in Physiology and Medicine for his research on the function of the cochlea.

Rita Levi-Montalcini (b. 1909) is a Nobel Prize winning neurologist from Italy who discovered a protein that causes developing cells to grow by stimulating surrounding nerve tissue (Figure 12.7). She named this protein nerve growth factor (NGF). Since her initial discovery, NGF has been shown to play an important role in the growth of nerve fibers throughout the peripheral nervous system. The role of NGF in regenerating nerve fibers damaged in the cochlea of humans has yet to be proven; however, her initial discovery of this protein has opened an area of research that may someday lead to a cure for cochlea-based hearing loss.

FIGURE 12.7. Rita Levi-Montalcini. Nobel Prize winning neurologist from Italy who discovered the protein called nerve growth factor (NGF).

TYPES OF HEARING DISORDERS

Hearing disorders can be described and categorized in a number of ways. For purposes of this introduction, they are presented below according to the categories of: (1) type of hearing loss, (2) degree of hearing loss, (3) location of hearing loss, and (4) configuration of hearing loss.

Type of Hearing Loss

There are three types of hearing loss: (1) conductive, (2) sensorineural, and (3) mixed.

A **conductive** hearing loss is due to problems affecting sound transmission through the outer or middle ear. These problems disrupt the normal flow of sound entering the inner ear. People affected by a conductive hearing loss experience an overall reduction in the loudness of sounds and find it difficult to hear faint sounds. Most conductive losses are not permanent and can be treated medically or surgically. However, if left untreated, conductive hearing losses can result in permanent impairment.

A **sensorineural** loss occurs when there is damage to the inner ear or to the nerve pathways from the inner ear leading towards the brain. In addition to affecting loudness of hearing, a sensorineural loss can also affect the clarity of hearing. For example, normally we can hear sounds between the frequency range of 20 Hz to 20,000 Hz. In the case of a sensorinueral hearing loss, a person may be unable to hear sounds higher than 2000 Hz, which can have a major impact on clearly understanding what is being said. Sensorineural hearing loss results in a permanent hearing disorder that cannot be corrected, although an individual's hearing can be improved by using some sort of hearing aid. A sensorineural hearing loss accounts for 90% of all types of hearing loss.

A **mixed** hearing loss is a combined conductive hearing loss and sensorineural hearing loss. The condition may result from one pathology affecting both the middle ear and inner ear, or two separate independent pathologies. An example of mixed hearing would be a situation where a person may initially have a conductive hearing loss due to an ear infection and later develops a sensorineural hearing loss. Sometimes a mixed hearing loss is a temporary condition because the conductive component of the hearing loss can be successfully treated, leaving only the sensorineural hearing loss.

FYI

There is a bit of debate as to whether chronic snoring actually can cause a noise-induced hearing loss. The noise generated by a person snoring can sometimes exceed 70 dB (comparable to the loudness of a vacuum cleaner), so it is no wonder its relationship to hearing loss is being explored.

Degree of Hearing Loss

Degree of hearing loss refers to the **severity** of the loss. All types of hearing loss are defined by degrees. The severity of hearing loss can range from mild to profound which represents the lowest or softest intensity level at which sound can be heard. A classification system for degree of hearing loss is listed in Table 12.2. Depending on the degree of hearing loss, various treatment options

Table 12.2. Classification of Hearing Loss

Amount of Hearing Loss	Degree of Hearing Loss	Ability to Hear Speech
0–25 dB	None	No significant difficulty in hearing.
26–40 dB	Mild	Difficulty hearing soft speech and conversations, but can manage in quiet environments.
41–55 dB	Moderate	Difficulty understanding conversational speech, especially when there is background noise. Higher volume levels are required for listening to the TV.
56–70 dB	Moderate-to-Severe	Speech clarity is significantly affected. Speech must be loud and the person may have difficulty hearing in group conversations.
71–90 dB	Severe	Normal conversational speech cannot be heard. The person may also have difficulty with loud speech or only be able to understand shouted or amplified speech.
91+ dB	Profound	Unable to clearly understand even amplified speech.

are suggested such as hearing aids, speech therapy, and counseling. The treatment approaches for working with hearing-impaired individuals are addressed in Chapter 13.

Location of Hearing Loss

A portion of Chapter 3 was dedicated to the anatomy of the auditory system. From this chapter we learned that the entire auditory pathway can be neatly divided into two systems, peripheral and central auditory systems. Each of these systems provides an important contribution to the process of audition. Damage to any of the components comprising the auditory system can result in varying degrees of hearing loss. Disorders of hearing that occur at various locations throughout the auditory system are described below.

Disorders of the Outer Ear

When conditions occur that interfere or block the normal transmission of sound through the outer ear, a conductive hearing loss will occur. In most cases, this condition does not result in a severe hearing loss. Examples of outer ear disorders are: (1) atresia, (2) obstruction of the ear canal, and (3) otitis externa. The term **atresia** refers to an absence of a normal opening. Atresia can affect many structures in the body, and one of these structures is the ear canal. The absence of the external auditory canal is a congenital condition and almost always involves abnormalities of the middle ear bones. A moderate conductive hearing loss typically is present in an atretic ear (Figure 12.8).

A common disorder of the outer ear involves an **obstruction** in the ear canal that prevents sound from normally entering the middle ear. The ear canal's natural secretion of ear wax, known as **cerumen** can become impacted to the point where normal hearing is affected, (see Figure 12.8). Impacted cerumen is not unusual, with approximately 2 to 6% of the general population having this condition. A likely cause of impaction is

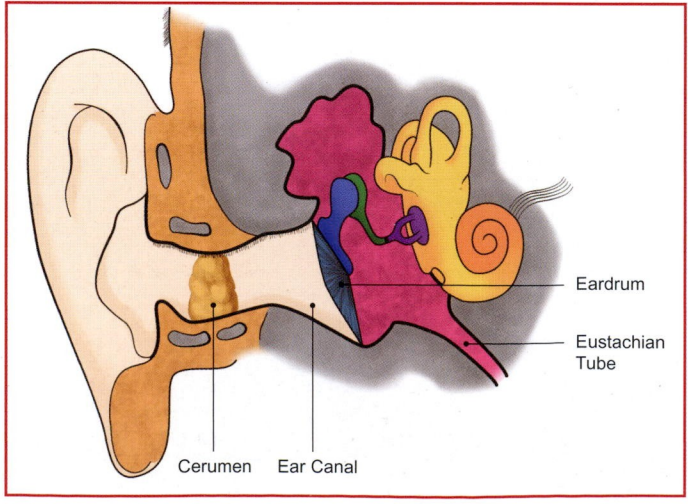

A **B**

FIGURE 12.8. (**A**) is an illustration of atresia, where the ear canal fails to develop. An example of cerumen (earwax) impaction is shown in (**B**).

through the misuse of cotton swabs, where the swab serves to push cerumen towards the tympanic membrane. Cerumen impaction is also prevalent among hearing aid users. Problematic cerumen can be removed with dissolving drops, water jets ("irrigation"), or through the use of special instruments available to a qualified specialist.

Another disorder of the outer ear is **otitis externa**. The term otitis is Latin with *oto* referring to the ear, and *itis* meaning inflammation. So this particular condition is an infection of the outer (external) ear. The common term for otitis externa is **swimmer's ear**. In most cases, bacteria cause this infection in the thin layer of skin lining the canal. Our ear canals work best when they are dry, so if they are exposed to excess moisture, such as from frequent swimming, they are more likely to become infected.

Swimmer's ear can be easily treated with antibiotic ear drops.

Disorders of the Middle Ear

Abnormalities of the middle ear will result in a conductive hearing loss. Examples of middle ear disorders are: (1) a perforated eardrum, (2) otitis media, and (3) otosclerosis. A hole or rupture in the tympanic membrane is called a **perforated eardrum**. This condition is accompanied by decreased hearing because the tympanic membrane ceases to work normally in the transmission of sound waves along the ossicular chain. The causes of a perforated eardrum are usually due to trauma or infection. Instances of trauma include a skull fracture or if a foreign object is pushed too far into the ear canal (Figure 12.9). A perforation can also result from a severe

FIGURE 12.9. Example of a perforated tympanic membrane resulting from damage by a foreign object.

middle ear infection that causes the eardrum to rupture or tear. Most eardrum perforations heal on their own within weeks of the rupture, although some may take several months to heal. During the healing process, the ear must be protected from water to prevent further damage to the middle ear.

Otitis media (OM) refers to an inflammation of the middle ear cavity. OM affects about two-thirds of children at least once before they reach their second birthday. The only childhood illness that occurs more often than OM is the common cold. An earache in children is often an indication of OM. The frequent occurrence of OM in young children is usually attributed to the small size, horizontal position, and immature functioning of their eustachian tube compared to adults, making it easier for infectious organisms in the mouth and nose to gain access to the middle ear (Figure 12.10). OM can be further classified according to longevity and type of condition. **Acute OM** is an infection lasting less than three weeks. **Subacute OM** lasts between three weeks to three months and **chronic OM** lasts longer than three months. **Otitis media with effusion** (OME) is a condition where a watery or mucus-like fluid fills the middle ear cavity. In some countries, the shorthand term used for OME is **glue ear**. Many times, the condition of OM can be diagnosed by examining the coloring of the tympanic membrane through the use of an **otoscope** (Figure 12.11). An otoscope is a standard piece of equipment found in most doctors' offices. Use of an otoscope allows for visualization of the outer ear, as well as a portion of the middle ear. Examination of the ear provides doctors with helpful information regarding a patient's overall health status.

FIGURE 12.10. Depiction of infant and adult eustachian tubes. The horizontal angle of the tubes in infants makes them susceptible to ear infections.

Otosclerosis is the abnormal growth of spongy bone in the middle ear. This bone prevents the ossicular chain of the middle ear from working properly and causes hearing loss. The etiology of otosclerosis is not fully understood, although research has shown that otosclerosis tends to run in families so there may be a genetic component. On average, a person who has one parent with otosclerosis has a 25% chance of developing the disorder. Women are three times more likely to acquire the disease compared to men. There are also differences in regard to ethnicity with Caucasians more susceptible to the disease than Asians or Africans. One way of treating otosclerosis is to surgically repair the ossicular chain.

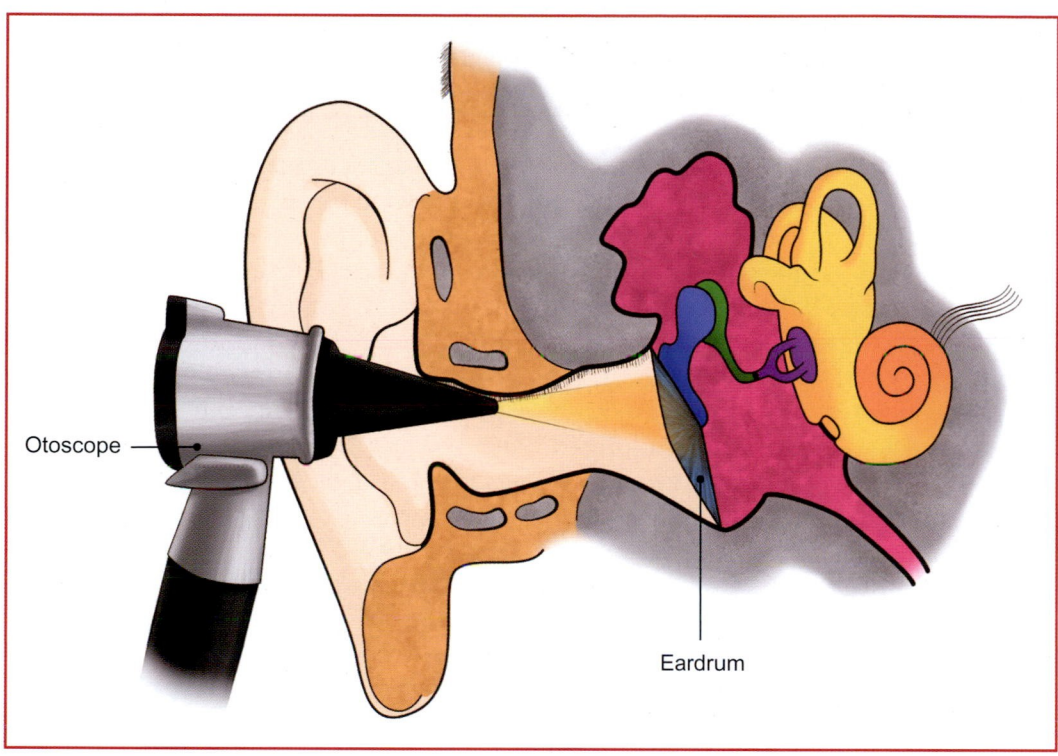

FIGURE 12.11. Example of an otoscope. The device shines a beam of light to help visualize and examine the condition of the ear canal and eardrum.

Many times this involves **stapedectomy**, which is removal of all or a portion of the stapes and substitution of an artificial stapes.

Disorders of the Inner Ear

Damage to the inner ear will result in a sensorineural hearing loss. Problems of the inner ear represent the largest group of hearing disorders. These disorders can affect balance as well as hearing. Examples of inner ear disorders are: (1) prenatal causes, (2) meningitis, (3) ototoxic drugs, (4) Ménière's disease, and (5) presbycusis. Prenatal causes are those that affect the mother and her developing fetus. The mother may acquire a virus during her pregnancy that has an adverse affect on the normal growth

and development of the unborn child's cochlea. **Cytomegalovirus** (CMV) is the most prevalent prenatal disease known to cause hearing loss. CMV is actually a very common viral illness. It belongs to the herpes virus family, which also includes viruses that are responsible for chickenpox, glandular fever, and cold sores. Between 50 and 85% of people in Australia, the United Kingdom, and the United States have had a CMV infection by the time they are 40 years old. CMV infections are rarely serious in otherwise healthy children and adults. When symptoms do appear, they are similar to those seen in mononucleosis ("mono") and last a few weeks. CMV is only a risk when the mother develops a CMV infection during pregnancy and passes this virus to the unborn baby before birth.

The results can be severe with as many as 20% of these children failing to survive. The children who do survive may show intellectual disabilities, visual defects, and hearing loss. The severity of hearing loss can range from to mild to profound.

Meningitis is an inflammation of the thin protective tissue that surrounds the brain and spinal cord, called the meninges. **Viral meningitis** usually does not cause serious illness, although in severe cases, it can cause prolonged fever and seizures. **Bacterial meningitis** is much rarer than viral meningitis but far more serious. Bacterial meningitis usually starts with bacteria that cause a coldlike infection. The infection can block blood vessels in the brain and lead to stroke and brain damage, as well as damage to other organs like the cochlea. Bacterial meningitis may lead to total deafness; however, early treatment with steroids can assist in reducing the severity of hearing loss.

An **ototoxic** hearing loss happens when someone takes or is given a drug that causes hearing loss as one of its side effects. There are roughly 200 prescription and over the counter drugs recognized as ototoxic. Sometimes the drugs are needed to save lives, and hearing loss is the price paid for being able to live. Common medications that are known to be ototoxic include various antibiotics, chemotherapy medications, anesthetics, cardiac medications, steroids, mood altering drugs, and some vapors and solvents. Often an ototoxic hearing loss is reversible simply by discontinuation of the drug. People with an existing hearing loss need to be especially aware of the potential for ototoxic effects, as an ototoxic drug can worsen the hearing loss.

Ménière's disease is an inner ear disorder caused by increased fluid pressure in the chambers of the inner ear. The disease affects both the balance and hearing systems of the inner ear, and usually just one ear is involved. There are various symptoms that are indicative of a person having Ménière's disease. These symptoms include episodes of severe dizziness (i.e., vertigo), nausea, unilateral hearing loss, ringing in the ear (i.e., tinnitus), and a feeling of ear pressure or pain in the affected ear.

FYI

The Dutch artist **Vincent Van Gogh** (1853–1890) created some of the world's most expensive and popular paintings. Was it his madness that prompted him to cut off his ear or was it his reaction to Ménière's disease? Prior to his death, Van Gogh was severely depressed. He suffered from vicious, recurring attacks of dizziness, nausea, and an intense ringing in the ear, all symptoms of Ménière's disease.

The disease may be extremely debilitating. Episodes of dizziness can occur without warning and may last from minutes to several hours or even days. The cause of Ménière's disease is unknown, although some feel it is a result of **endolymphatic hydrops**, which is the oversecretion of endolymph (i.e., the fluid contained within the cochlea). Surgery to drain excessive endolymph is found to help reduce the debilitating aspects of the disease. In extreme cases, the inner ear may be surgically destroyed to help alleviate vertigo and tinnitus, which results in permanent deafness of the affected ear.

Presbycusis is the gradual deterioration in hearing that happens as we grow older. It is likely the hearing mechanism begins to deteriorate shortly after birth, although most experts agree that by the age of 18 years, a natural reduction in the performance of our auditory system begins to occur. As we age, the hair cells within the cochlea become damaged through normal wear and tear of use, particularly those that are found at the entrance (basal end) of the cochlea. This deterioration is synonymous with the entryway into a carpeted room. As years go by, the carpet fibers at the entryway of the room become flattened and damaged, whereas those at the back of the room retain their shape. This form of damage results in a high-frequency hearing loss that can start as early as middle age. The condition is to be expected in men by their early 60s and women by their late 60s. Presbycusis most often occurs in both ears. Because the process of loss is gradual, people who have presbycusis may not realize their hearing is diminishing. Between the ages of 65 to 75 years, about 35% of adults have a hearing loss. After the age of 75 years, hearing loss is found in almost 50% of all individuals.

Whereas presbycusis reflects a natural aging of the auditory system, **noise-induced** hearing loss is a form of impairment that mirrors that of presbycusis somewhat but can be found in people at a much younger age. This hearing loss is not a result of natural aging but rather damage due to exposure to excessive noise, whether at work or play. Among the elderly, it may be difficult to differentiate between presbycusis and noise-induce hearing loss simply because both pathologies affect hearing of high-frequency sounds. Noise-induced hearing loss is a preventable disorder that can be avoided by taking necessary precautions such as noise-reduction headphones or ear plugs.

Disorders of the Central Auditory System

Any damage to the auditory system running from the auditory nerve to the brain is called a **retrocochlear** pathology because the damage occurs beyond (or behind) the cochlea. One type of retrocochlear pathology is a tumor called an **acoustic neuroma** (Figure 12.12). An acoustic neuroma is a noncancerous (i.e., benign) brain tumor. All types of brain tumors are rare and acoustic neuromas account for eight out of 100 primary brain tumors. An acoustic neuroma tends to grow very slowly and normally is not a life-threatening condition. In very rare cases, the tumor can grow large enough to press on the brain. However, most acoustic neuromas can be treated before they get to this stage. Typically, the tumor is only found on one side of the central auditory system. Approximately 50% of acoustic neuromas are treated by surgery where the tumor is removed. About 25% of neuromas are treated with radiation and the remaining 25% are

FIGURE 12.12. Illustration of an acoustic neuroma (tumor), resulting in a retrocochlear hearing loss.

monitored (i.e., left untreated). Regardless of the treatment approach, an acoustic neuroma almost always results in total hearing loss in the affected ear. Every year in the United Kingdom and the United States approximately 13 people out of every million are diagnosed with an acoustic neuroma. Acoustic neuromas occur more often in women compared to men, although the reasons for this are not yet understood. People who are 30 to 60 years of age are usually affected.

Configuration of Hearing Loss

The configuration of a hearing loss refers to the extent of loss at various frequencies of hearing, ranging from low to high. The configuration of hearing loss gives an overall picture of a person's hearing acuity. For example, an individual who is unable to hear frequencies within the range of 2000 to 8000 Hz at a soft loudness level would show a **high-frequency hearing loss**. Some hearing loss configurations are **flat**, indicating the same amount of hearing loss for low, middle, and high frequency sounds. Another aspect of hearing loss configuration is whether or not two ears are affected: a **unilateral** hearing loss means that only one ear is affected by the loss, and a **bilateral** hearing loss means both ears are affected. In addition, a hearing loss can be symmetrical or asymmetrical. A **symmetric** hearing loss means the severity of loss and the frequencies affected are the same for both ears. An **asymmetric** loss means there is loss of hearing in both ears but the severity of loss and frequencies affected are not identical. A final way of describing hearing loss configuration relates to the change in hearing over time. A **progressive** hearing loss is one that becomes increasingly worse. This is found in conditions such as presbycusis. A **fluctuating** hearing loss is one whereby a person's hearing may improve or worsen from one day to next. This is often the case in conditions such as OM and Ménière's disease.

Other Types of Hearing Disorders

There remain other types of hearing disorders that are less easy to classify according to a specific location along the auditory pathway. Two such types of disorder are tinnitus and auditory processing disorder. **Tinnitus** is the medical name used to describe a continuous noise in the ears. The term comes from the Latin word for *ringing*. Some people experience a mild ringing noise, whereas others are troubled by loud, high pitched noises. Tinnitus can occur in one or both ears. Tinnitus is divided into two types: (1) objective and (2) subjective. Objective tinnitus is rare. In this condition, the faint noise generated in the ear can be heard (using special equipment) by somebody examining the patient. In such cases, the talents of an ENT surgeon are required to seek a surgical cure. Subjective tinnitus is by far the more frequently occurring form of the disorder. In this condition, the noise can only be heard by the patient. Subjective tinnitus is not a disease but a problem in the auditory pathway or in the central nervous system of the brain. There are many factors that have been associated with tinnitus including headaches, elevated blood pressure, emotional tension, exposure to loud noises, medications, allergies, and fatigue. Estimates from the United Kingdom, United States, Australia, and New Zealand indicate that tinnitus affects anywhere from 10 to 20% of the general population. Of these, about 1% experience the condition to a disturbing degree.

Auditory processing refers to the way the brain makes sense out of the incoming signals from the auditory pathway. Auditory processing helps us to discriminate between different sounds, pick out sounds or speech from a noisy background, and understand speech when the sound quality is poor. The disorder known as an **auditory processing disorder** (APD) is a condition in which an individual demonstrates normal hearing and normal intelligence but may show a hearing problem in the sense that he or she is unable to process information normally. They can hear perfectly well but have trouble interpreting or understanding what is being said. Examples of the types of processing difficulties demonstrated by individuals with APD

FYI

Prolonged exposure to loud noise has resulted in many well-known musicians acquiring the condition of tinnitus. The list includes Jeff Beck, Bono, Blinda Butcher, Cher, Eric Clapton, Phil Collins, Al Di Meola, Mick Fleetwood, Ted Nugent, Ozzy Ozborne, The Edge, Trent Reznor, Sting, Pete Townsend, and Neil Young.

are shown in Table 12.3. The prevalence of APD in the general population has not been firmly established. Estimates indicate that APD occurs in approximately 3% of people, with a 2-to-1 ratio between males and females. Neurologic disorders account for most instances of APD in adults. Among children, a definitive neurologic cause for APD is found in only 5% of diagnosed cases. The remaining occurrences have an unknown etiology. In these cases, APD has been called an invisible disability as there appears to be nothing physically wrong with the individual. The difficulties these individuals experience are often incorrectly assumed to be the result of an attention deficit or a lack of motivation. There are no established therapies for the treatment of individuals with APD. A general recommendation is to modify the environment by minimizing background noise to facilitate improved auditory processing.

Table 12.3. Types of Difficulties Shown by Individuals With an Auditory Processing Disorder

- Asks for things to be repeated
- Poor listening skills
- Mishears words
- Needs more time to process information
- Difficulty following multistep instructions given orally
- Difficulty hearing in background noise
- Distracted
- Low academic performance
- Language comprehension difficulty

ASSESSMENT OF HEARING DISORDERS

Audiometry is the measurement of hearing. Measurement of auditory function enables the audiologist to determine the type, degree, location, and configuration of hearing loss. Some of the tests performed to evaluate auditory function are: (1) pure-tone audiometry, (2) immittance testing, and (3) electrophysiologic testing.

Pure-Tone Audiometry

In **pure-tone audiometry**, a person's hearing acuity for each ear is measured for tones as low as 250 Hz and as high as 8000 Hz. Although our entire range of hearing extends from 20 Hz to 20,000 Hz, the 250 to 8000 Hz range is tested because this is the frequency range used to hear conversational speech. The device used to generate pure tones is called an **audiometer**. Pure-tone audiometry is usually completed while an individual is seated in a sound isolated booth. During the test, the individual is asked to respond each time they hear the tone. Adult patients usually push a button when the tone is heard and children will raise their hand (Figure 12.13). As part of the test, the audiologist determines the person's threshold for each of the tones. The **threshold** represents the loudness (dB) level at which tones are barely audible. Once determined, the threshold for each frequency is recorded on a graph known as an **audiogram**. The test frequencies (pure tones) are plotted on the horizontal axis of the audiogram, and the loudness threshold for each test frequency is indicated on the vertical axis. The symbols, "o" and "x" are used

FIGURE 12.13. Example of pure-tone audiometry. A hand is raised in response to any sound that is heard.

to indicate the thresholds of the right and left ear, respectively. A score of 0 to 20 dB is considered normal hearing acuity. It is possible to have scores less than 0, which indicate better than average hearing. A wide range of audiograms are presented in Figure 12.14.

Two types of pure-tone testing are: (1) air conduction and (2) bone conduction. During **air conduction** testing, headphones are placed over the outer ear. Small, foam insert-earphones are sometimes used in place of headphones. Insert-earphones are placed directly in the entrance to the ear canals. Air conduction testing is designed to examine a person's hearing of sounds as they travel through the air. The sound (pure tone) leaves the earphone and travels down the ear canal as an airborne acoustic signal. Air conduction testing allows the audiologist to examine a person's hearing as sound travels through the entire peripheral auditory system (Figure 12.15). It is not possible to determine

the precise location of the impairment by air conduction testing alone. If the person's hearing thresholds for air conduction fall outside the normal range of hearing, it is necessary to perform a follow-up test known as **bone conduction** testing. In bone conduction testing, the pure tones are not presented as an airborne (acoustic) signal, but rather via a bone vibrator that is placed on the surface of the skull behind the ear (i.e., mastoid process of temporal bone). These vibrations are transmitted directly to the cochlea, and toward the central auditory system (see Figure 12.15). Bone conduction testing bypasses the outer and middle ear systems. If a person was to show a hearing loss from air conduction testing but normal hearing from bone conduction testing, the hearing loss is likely to be an impairment of the outer or middle ear. This is called a **conductive hearing loss** (see Figure 12.14). A **sensorineural loss** would be indicated if both air conduction and bone

FIGURE 12.14. Audiograms depicting normal hearing and various types of hearing loss. The "x" symbol represents the left ear threshold and the "o" symbol is the right ear. The "<" and ">" symbols represent bone conduction thresholds for the left and right ear, respectively.

conduction hearing thresholds were higher than normal (see Figure 12.14). If both air and bone conduction thresholds were higher than normal but bone conduction was the higher of the two, a **mixed hearing loss** would be indicated.

A

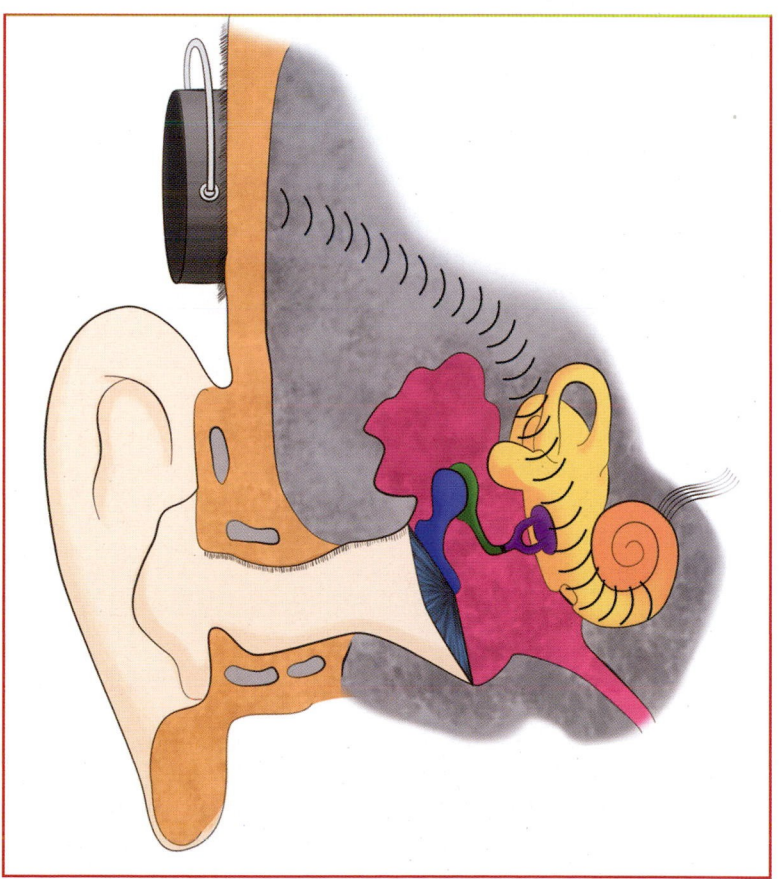

B

FIGURE 12.15. Example of air conduction (**A**) and bone conduction (**B**) pure tone audiometric testing.

FYI

Sound can travel through any medium such as air, water, rock, and steel. Sound cannot travel through a vacuum because it is devoid of matter (i.e., particles). There is no sound in outer space.

Immittance Testing

The term **immittance** refers to ease or compliance of movement. In audiological testing, immittance is the ease with which sound travels from one medium to another, as from air to bone. These tests do not provide a direct measure of hearing loss, but rather provide information about the mobility of the tympanic membrane and functioning of the middle ear. Immittance tests are also considered **nonbehavioral tests** because the individual is not required to push a button or raise their hand for various tones. The response occurs naturally. Two types of immittance tests are: (1) tympanometry and (2) acoustic reflex.

Tympanometry is a testing methodology that provides useful information about the presence of fluid in the middle ear, mobility of the middle ear system, and ear canal volume. It provides a graphic representation of the relationship between air pressure in the external ear canal compared to the movement of the tympanic membrane and middle ear ossicular chain. The test is noninvasive. A **tympanometer** instrument is used to perform the test. The instrument consists of a probe that is fitted snuggly into the ear canal and slowly changes the pressure within the ear canal, at the same time transmitting a tone into the

canal. The tone strikes the tympanic membrane, causing vibration of the middle ear. Some of this sound is reflected back and picked up by the tympanometer (Figure 12.16). The amount of sound that is reflected back from the eardrum as the pressure in the ear canal varies is quantified and plotted on a graph. These **tympanogram** plots are classified as type A (normal middle ear functioning), type B (flat, indicative of middle ear fluid or punctured eardrum), and type C (off-center, indicative of eustachian tube malfunction). Examples of tympanogram plots are shown in Figure 12.16.

The **acoustic reflex** is an involuntary contraction of the stapedius muscle located in the middle ear. The response is obtained by presenting high intensity sounds via a probe at the opening of the ear canal. High-intensity sounds (e.g., 90 dB) are presented and the probe detects the decibel level at which the stapedius muscle contracts. Acoustic reflex testing is completed with the same equipment used for tympanometry. Acoustic reflex testing is done in each ear following tympanometry. We all should show an acoustic reflex to loud sounds. If an acoustic reflex is not present, a middle ear or brainstem disorder would be suspected.

Electrophysiologic Testing

Electrophysiologic tests are nonbehavioral tests that are administered to difficult to assess individuals or to determine the specific site of an auditory lesion. **Otoacoustic emissions** and the **auditory brainstem response** are the most frequently performed electrophysiological tests. They are fast and easy to administer and do not require the individual to give a behavioral response (such as

A

B

FIGURE 12.16. (**A**) is an illustration of tympanometry testing. A probe is inserted into the ear canal and delivers a tone to measure compliance of the tympanic membrane. Part of the probe tone is reflected backwards, and some is admitted into the middle ear. Examples of three types of tympanograms are shown in (**B**).

raising a hand). Otoacoustic emissions (OAEs) are faint acoustic sounds that are generated in the cochlea in response to sounds presented to the inner ear. They are considered to be epiphenomena (i.e., a secondary activity) and a byproduct of a normally functioning cochlea. A healthy cochlea creates internal vibrations whenever it processes sound. Impaired ears usually do not. These sound emissions travel back through the middle ear and into the ear canal where they can be measured with a tiny microphone. Emissions are thought to be generated by the hair cells within the cochlea. Because most forms of hearing involve the loss (i.e., death) of hair cells, the lack of an OAE is a good predictor of hearing loss. OAEs are measured by a probe placed at the opening of the ear canal. An illustration of the OAE setup is shown in Figure 12.17.

In the **auditory brainstem response** (ABR) technique, an **electroencephalograph** (EEG) is used to measure brain wave activity associated with the reception of sound. Prior to the test, three electrodes are attached, one to the forehead and one on each ear. A series of acoustic clicks is then presented to one ear via an earphone. The electrodes pick up the brain's response to those clicks, which appears as a characteristic waveform with five peaks or waves that occur within the first 10 msec of response. The waveform reflects the speed of electrical impulses traveling along the hearing pathway from the inner ear through the brainstem. The person being tested must remain very still during the test and may even be sleeping. An illustration of the ABR setup is shown in Figure 12.18. If the ABR waveform is missing one or more of the five peaks, or there is a time-delay in the appearance of these peaks, the result is indicative of a significant hearing loss or neurologic dysfunction.

Evaluating the hearing abilities of a newborn is a difficult task. Infants cannot respond with words or raise their hand to indicate what they hear and when. However, early detection of hearing problems is important. We have increasing evidence that difficulties in hearing during the infancy period may cause irreparable delays in a child's cognitive and communication development. Currently there is a worldwide emphasis for **universal screening** of newborn hearing. Many countries (e.g., Canada, United Kingdom, United States, and New Zealand) have enacted mandatory screening of newborns shortly after birth. The OAE and ABR tests are the primary instruments for evaluating a newborn's hearing.

CULTURAL CONSIDERATIONS AND HEARING DISORDERS

There are a wide range of cultural and ethnic variables in regard to hearing loss and specific types of hearing disorders. For example, the occurrence of OM among indigenous populations such as New Zealand Maori, Australian aboriginals, and Native Americans is unusually high. The high occurrence is attributed to the general social and physical environment, limited medical attention, allergies and possibly also anatomical predispositions. For many non-indigenous children, especially those with good access to medical treatment, middle ear problems and associated hearing loss have been resolved by the time they arrive at school. For most indigenous children, the ramifications of chronic OM may disadvantage these children throughout the school years and into adulthood.

A

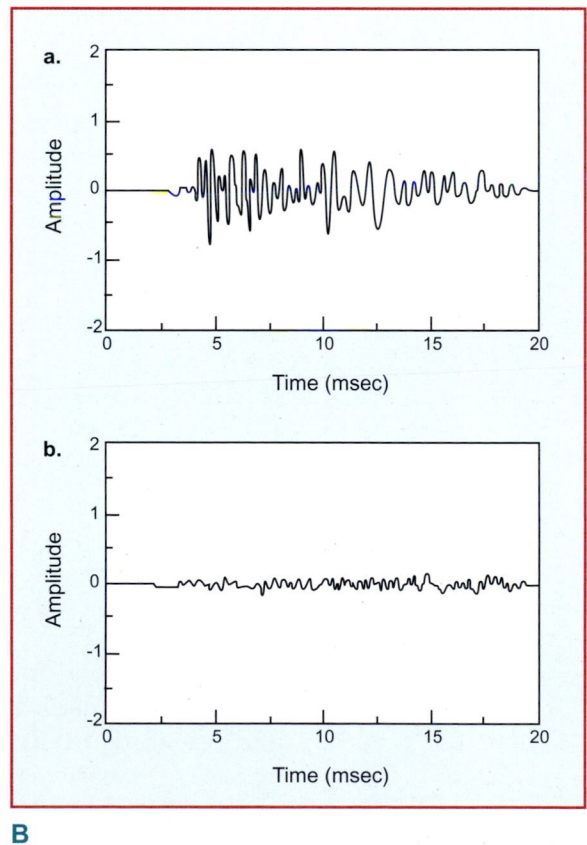

B

FIGURE 12.17. Depiction of the equipment setup for evoking and recording an otoacoustic emission (OAE) (**A**). The figures in (**B**) show (*top panel*) an example of normal OAE and (*bottom panel*) a low emission level, which may indicate cochlear dysfunction.

A

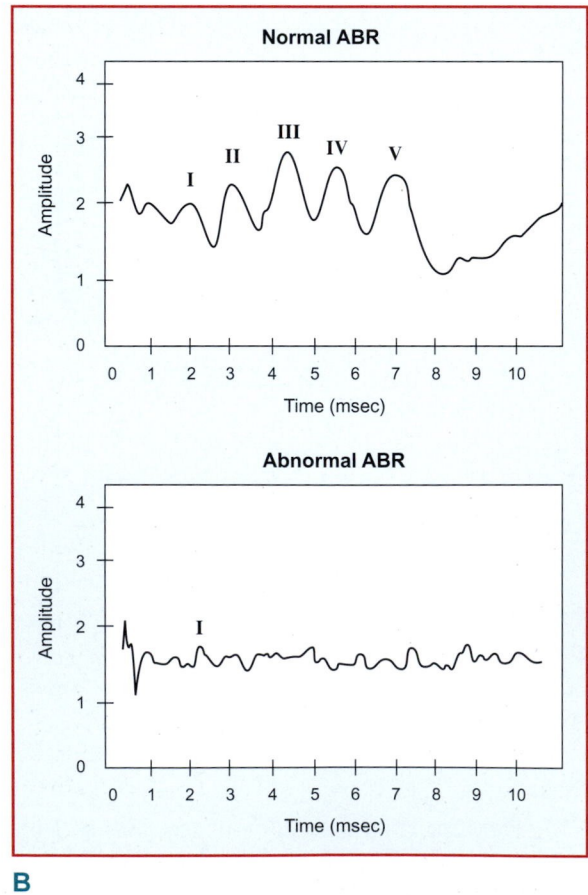

B

FIGURE 12.18. (**A**) Depiction of the equipment setup for evoking and recording an auditory brainstem response (ABR). The figures in (**B**) show an example of normal ABR with five distinct waveform peaks (*top panel*) and an abnormal ABR indicative of a brainstem tumor (*lower panel*).

Epidemiological studies have consistently demonstrated that age related hearing loss is most common in white men, followed by white women, black men, and black women, suggesting that whites are more vulnerable to the harmful effects of noise exposure than non whites (Ishii & Talbott, 1998). Interestingly, tribal people in rural Africa do not seem to experience as much age-related hearing loss compared to adults with European backgrounds. One proposed explanation is that melanin-A pigment is found in higher levels among blacks compared to whites (Helzner et al., 2005). Research has shown that high concentrations of melanin-A within the cochlear hair cells may serve to protect hair cells from damage. In addition to race, gender has also been found to affect one's chances of developing an age-related hearing loss. Men are five times more likely then women to acquire a hearing loss at some point in their lifetime. This gender imbalance is attributed to likely biological differences between men and women, as well as the tendency for men to work in occupations that may increase the chance of acquiring a noise-induced hearing loss.

Finally, hearing loss can affect one's culture in regard to participating in society at large. People with hearing loss are less likely to participate in social activities than people without hearing loss. For example, among people over the age of 65 years, those with a hearing loss are less likely to engage in community volunteer work compared to those without a hearing loss. Hearing loss can also affect an individual's emotional well-being. Among people age 70 and older, those with a hearing loss are more likely to experience bouts of depression compared to those without a hearing loss (Morgan-Jones, 2001).

FYI

A **malingerer** is a person who deliberately lies about a physical or psychological condition for some special gain. The term has found its way into hearing disorders, where an individual may fake a hearing loss as a means of seeking special gain, such as additional financial compensation.

CURRENT RESEARCH IN HEARING DISORDERS

MP3 Players

The baby boomer generation was the first to demonstrate that loud rock music was hazardous to hearing. The development of MP3 players is likely to significantly increase the occurrence of noise-induced hearing loss and tinnitus for Generation X and Y'ers. These devices use earbud earphones, rather than headphones, which are situated directly in the entrance of the ear canal. They efficiently funnel music down the ear canal and enable the user to turn up the volume without disrupting others. As a result, MP3 players easily desensitize the user to dangerously high sound levels. These devices are able to store thousands of songs that can be played continuously for hours without the need for recharging. Most MP3 players produce sound in excess of 100 dB. This situation sets the stage for prolonged exposure to high levels of loudness.

A recent survey at the University of Hong Kong examined the listening habits of 1,000 young adults who were

MP3 users for more than one year (Hong Kong Society for the Deaf, 2007). The results found that that 70% of users would turn up the volume of their music player in noisy surroundings. One-third of the users perceived that their hearing sensitivity had worsened since they started using music players, and 20% experienced ringing in their ears within a short period of time after turning off their music players. Researchers have found that exposure to sounds in excess of 80 dB for only 90 minutes duration is sufficient to cause a hearing loss. Audiologists recommend what is called the **60-60 rule**, which translates to a listening level of 60% (of the maximum volume) for no more than 60 minutes. The full impact of MP3 players on the occurrence of noise-induced hearing loss has yet to be determined. Early indications are that young people are putting themselves at risk for permanent hearing loss by exposing themselves to excessive noise.

Tinnitus

Over the last 10 years, scientists have made tremendous advances in figuring out what causes tinnitus and how to treat it. But the definitive cause of tinnitus has yet to be determined and there is no magic pill for the treatment of tinnitus. We have known for some time that exposure to loud noise appears to be a factor that triggers the onset of tinnitus. Recent research indicates that tinnitus can either originate in the brain or cochlea. Imaging techniques such as functional magnetic resonance imaging (fMRI) and positron emission tomography (PET) have revealed that areas of the brain that process information from the ears are more active in tinnitus sufferers than in people without the condition. As a next stage, researchers are trying to stimulate these overactive areas of the brain to see whether they can reduce people's perceptions of tinnitus. There is also evidence that tinnitus may originate within the cellular structure of the cochlea. Scientists have discovered that a unique set of cells in the cochlea release a chemical called **ATP** (adenosine triphosphate), which causes the hearing system to generate brain activity in the absence of sound. By controlling the release of ATP, it may be possible to reduce or eliminate tinnitus (Tritsch et al., 2007).

Some of the current treatment approaches for tinnitus include devices that look like hearing aids and produce sound that will "mask" or cover up tinnitus. The use of a traditional hearing aid is also found to be useful in some cases. Other, less traditional forms of treatment include use of **medications** such as lidocaine, benzodiazepines, and antidepressant drugs, but so far none has been found to be truly effective. **Cognitive behavioral therapy** (CBT) is a treatment administered by a psychotherapist that seeks to change people's attitudes and behavior. When used to treat tinnitus it seems to improve patients' quality of life, even when the volume of noise from the tinnitus remains the same. Another new therapy is **neuromonics**, which was developed in Australia. This therapy involves the combined use of acoustic stimulation (namely music) with a structured program of counseling and support. The therapy approach is in need of independent assessment to demonstrate its benefits.

Vestibular Prostheses

Neuroprosthetics is an area of considerable scientific and clinical interest. Since the introduction of the cardiac pacemaker in 1932, there have been developments in neuroprosthetic techniques for bladder and bowel control, deep brain stimulation for Parkinson disease (see Chapter 9), restoration of respiration for paralyzed individuals, and the development of cochlear implants to improve hearing (see Chapter 13). Individuals suffering from dizziness and balance disorders may also benefit from the progress made in neuroprosthetics. The inner ear's vestibular system provides information about self-motion and helps stabilize vision during movement. Damage to this system can result in dizziness, vertigo, nausea, blurred vision, and instability in walking. Medical, surgical, and rehabilitative approaches are all used to treat balance problems. Even though all of these approaches have greatly improved over time, they are still not 100% effective in all cases. Vestibular prostheses include a range of approaches to vestibular impairment. All approaches rely on motion detectors that measure head movement and send a signal back to the central nervous system (CNS) to process these motion cues. Both implantable and nonimplantable prostheses are currently being developed. An implantable prosthesis delivers self-motion cues to the CNS via implanted stimulators directly within the vestibular nerve. A nonimplantable prosthesis is a less invasive means of providing some self-motion cues. They are sensory substitution devices that send motion and balance information to the CNS through sound, vision, tactile vibration, or electrostimulation of the tongue. Although not yet available clinically, vestibular prosthetics could provide another option for those with balance problems, as well as for those who are elderly and prone to falling (Wall, 2008).

HEARING DISORDERS ON THE WORLD WIDE WEB

Listed below are Web sites that provide further information on the topic of hearing disorders. At the time of publication each Web site was freely accessible.

Auditory Processing Disorders in Children Video
http://www.webmd.com/video/auditory-processing-disorder-in-kids

The Wonderful Hearing and Sound Activity
http://www.wonderville.ca/v1/activities/hearing_sound/hearing_sound.html

Assorted Hearing Loss and Deafness Videos
http://www.goldbamboo.com/video-t2753.html

Listen to Your Buds
http://www.listentoyourbuds.org/game.php

Pediatric Hearing Loss Videos
http://www.infanthearing.org/videos/index.html

Sound Advice for Farmers Video
http://www.cdc.gov/nasd/videos/v000001-v000100/v000001.html

REFERENCES

Helzner, E. P., Cauley, J. A., Pratt, S. R., Wisniewski, S. R., Zmuda, J. M., Talbott, E. O., . . . Newman, A. B. (2005). Race and sex differences in age-related hearing loss: The health, aging and body composition study. *Journal of the American Geriatric Society, 53,* 2119–2127.

Hong Kong Society for the Deaf. (2007). *A study on the impact of MP3 players on hearing amongst young people*. Retrieved September 22, 2009, from http://www .deaf.org.hk/documents/press_release/ 2005_7/mp3_press_030207_e.pdf

Ishii, E., & Talbott, E. (1998). Race/Ethnicity differences in the prevalence of noise-induced hearing loss in a group of metal fabricating workers. *Journal of Occupational and Environmental Medicine, 40*, 661–666.

Morgan-Jones, R. A. (2001). *Hearing differently: The impact of hearing impairment on family life*. London: Whurr.

Tritsch, N., Yi, E., Gale, J., Glowatzki, E., & Bergles, D. (2007). The origin of spontaneous activity in the developing auditory system. *Nature, 450*, 50–55.

Wall, C. (2008, July 15). Vestibular prostheses: Engineering and biomedical issues. *The ASHA Leader, 13*(9), 14–17.

AUDITORY REHABILITATION

OBJECTIVES

After reading this chapter, the student should be able to:

- Define aural rehabilitation and understand why the service is necessary for those who have hearing loss.

- Describe the components of a hearing aid.

- Understand the different types and styles of amplification or assistive listening devices plus the related advantages and disadvantages of each device.

- Explain the nature and features of various auditory implants.

- Describe the speech and language features that accompany a severe hearing impairment.

- Describe the types of aural rehabilitation programs available to children and adults.

- Discuss, compare, and contrast the different types of communication options, methods, training approaches, and philosophies (e.g. oral/aural, total communication, sign only, ASL/BSL).

- Discuss issues pertaining to Deaf culture.

INTRODUCTION

Hearing loss is referred to as an invisible condition, yet its impact is anything but invisible (Tye-Murray, 2009). Whether the severity of hearing loss is mild or profound, it can have serious consequences on an individual's overall well-being.

A number of devices to improve hearing and various forms of treatment have been developed to assist individuals with a diagnosed hearing loss. Decisions regarding the best approach are guided by factors such as the age of the person and the type of hearing problem they demonstrate, with the ultimate goal of improving an individual's quality of life. The purpose of this chapter is to provide background on the tools and approaches used to help improve hearing and minimize the consequences of a hearing loss.

TERMINOLOGY AND DEFINITIONS

Aural rehabilitation involves techniques used with people who are hearing impaired to improve their ability to speak and communicate. Presumably, these individuals once demonstrated normal hearing earlier in life. Since then, a hearing impairment has occurred, requiring assistance in improving their listening abilities in order to compensate for sounds they no longer hear. People who are hearing impaired at birth also require assistance in compensating for their hearing loss. For these individuals, the more appropriate term is **aural habilitation**. Aural rehabilitation (including habilitation) is all about learning how to take advantage of what a person hears and sees in the environment. The particulars of a rehabilitation program are unique to each individual. A person's age, severity of hearing loss, and daily living environment are taken into consideration. For example, an individual who is **hard of hearing** shows a partial hearing impairment that may range from mild to severe. His needs could be quite different from those of an individual with **deafness**, who has minimal or no hearing. Aural rehabilitation typically is provided by an audiologist, although speech-language pathologists and teachers of the deaf or hard of hearing may also make important contributions. There are various locations where aural rehabilitation occurs, including hospitals, nursing homes, community centers, as well as the classroom.

HISTORIC ASPECTS OF AURAL REHABILITATION

Origins of Aural Rehabilitation

The concept of aural rehabilitation was developed in the 1940s as a response to World War II. Prior to this time, there was no particular program for improving the quality of life for adults with postlingual hearing loss, despite schools for the deaf having been in existence since the late 1800s. Many individuals who served in the war developed severe cases of noise-induced hearing loss. These losses could not be treated using medical or surgical techniques. Military hospitals began to develop aural rehabilitation programs to assist these injured soldiers. Specialists in fields such as speech pathology, psychology, medicine, and deaf education were brought together to design aural rehabilitation programs. Lip reading was stressed as one of the major rehabilitation approaches. During the 1940s, wearable hearing aids were also available and, along with lip reading, became a significant component of rehabilitation.

The need for a specially qualified individual to assist with the needs of people with hearing loss eventually led to creation of the profession of audiology. The establishment of audiology contributed to new techniques for diagnosing and managing hearing impairment for children and adults. However, the major focus of the audiology profession during the period of 1950 to 1980 was on the diagnosis of hearing loss, with far less attention placed on the rehabilitation of hearing loss. The lack of attention to rehabilitation was driven by the view that it was unethical for an audiologist to sell a hearing aid. Such an activity was left to salespeople who had little or no training in audiologic care, which created a situation in which the actual rehabilitation of individuals with hearing loss was performed by individuals far less qualified than audiologists. All of this changed in 1978 when the American Speech and Hearing Association permitted audiologists to dispense hearing aids. Today, audiologists are able to provide comprehensive diagnostic and rehabilitative services to hearing-impaired individuals. This situation has led to enormous improvements in the provision of audiologic care.

History of Hearing Aids

Dating back to the earliest hearing aids, their function has remained essentially unchanged: to increase the loudness of sound. Prior to the 20th century, the only way to provide amplification was to reduce the amount of outside, "distracting" noise. The primary way to accomplish this noise reduction was to filter out other noise by directing the desired sound straight into the ear with some kind of tube or trumpet (Figure 13.1).

FIGURE 13.1. Early hearing aid, known as an ear trumpet. The instrument was designed to reduce the amount of distracting noise.

These trumpets were large and awkward, although some models could be worn on the head attached to a harness. Cupping your hand behind your ear gives a similar (but smaller) amplification effect.

Hearing aid technology has certainly come a long way in past 100 years. Changes in hearing aids were linked to two important milestones in technology: (1) the advent of electricity and (2) Alexander Graham Bell's work on the telephone. Early electric hearing aids used the concept of a **microphone** that picks up sound, an **amplifier** which makes the sound louder, and a **speaker** that delivers the amplified sound to the ear. The first electric hearing aids were created around 1900 and were so large that they sat on a table. The cost of these was far beyond the means of most. In the early 1920s, hearing aid technology incorporated the use of vacuum tubes, which allowed a much more efficient method for amplifying sound. However, the early electric hearing aids were still unwieldy and could not be carried around easily. The miniaturization of batteries in the 1930s led to a significant decrease in the size of hearing aids. Hearing aids were made portable by allowing the user to wear a battery pack. By the early 1950s, vacuum tubes were replaced by transistors and this resulted in a technologic revolution in the design of hearing aids. Early transistor hearing aids were designed to fit within the frames of eyeglasses. Later, they were adapted to fit behind the ear. The 1990s saw a major shift in hearing aid technology from analog to digital circuitry, which led to major improvements in sound quality. In spite of the many changes in hearing aid design and technology over the past 100 years, they still rely on the concept of a microphone, amplifier, and speaker.

Deaf Education

Pedro Ponce de León (1520–1584), a Benedictine monk living in Spain, was the first teacher of the deaf in the modern era (Figure 13.2). His students were mostly children of aristocrats who had the financial means to provide their children with private tutoring. His work with these deaf children focused on helping them to learn how to speak intelligibly. He also instructed the children in sign language. The monks observed daily periods of silence and had developed a series of hand gestures to help communicate during those times. Thus, it was natural for de León to apply this form of communication with his deaf students. The prevailing opinion among most Europeans in the 1500s was that people with deafness were incapable

FIGURE 13.2. Monument of Pedro Ponce de León in Madrid, Spain was the first teacher of the deaf circa 1550.

of being educated. Many even believed that the deaf were too intellectually disabled to be eligible for salvation under Christian doctrine. So de León's work with the deaf was considered quite bold and courageous. He was able to demonstrate that these children could not only learn to speak but could also learn to read and write.

Laurent Clerc (1785–1869) was born in a small village near Lyons, France (Figure 13.3). Although he was French, Clerc is considered by many to be the "Father of Deaf Education" in the United States. He was born hearing, but as an infant fell from his high chair, which resulted in a complete loss of hearing in both ears. He entered the Royal Institution for the Deaf in Paris where he excelled in his studies. His outstanding academic abilities, in spite of a profound hearing loss, caught the attention of a visiting American, **Thomas Hopkins Gallaudet** (1787–1851) (see Figure 13.3).

Gallaudet invited Clerc to visit the United States and the two eventually established the first school for the deaf in Hartford, Connecticut, now known as the American School for the Deaf. Clerc never returned to France and dedicated his life to educating deaf children. The American School for the Deaf remains the oldest existing school in the United States for the education of deaf students. Gallaudet University in Washington, DC is named in honor of Thomas Gallaudet (see also Chapter 12).

Laura Bridgman (1829–1889) was born in Hanover, New Hampshire (United States) (Figure 13.4). At 2 years of age, she developed scarlet fever. The illness killed two of her older sisters and one of her brothers, but she survived, although without vision or hearing. A courageous individual, she was the first deaf-blind individual to be successfully educated in the modern era. She attended the Perkins School for the Blind in Massachusetts,

A

B

FIGURE 13.3. Laurent Clerc (**A**) and Thomas H. Gallaudet (**B**) established the first school for the deaf in the United States.

FIGURE 13.4. Laura Bridgman, the first person with deaf-blindness to be educated in the United States.

where she learned to read, write, and also sew. She eventually became a sewing teacher at the school and remained there until her death. Bridgman was famous for her accomplishments which were described in newspapers and magazines worldwide. Her fame was later eclipsed by that of Helen Keller.

Helen Keller (1880–1968) was born in Tuscumbia, Alabama (United States) (Figure 13.5). Her birth history was quite similar to Laura Bridgman's—Helen had a normal birth but at the age of 19 months developed scarlet fever that left her deaf and blind. Her only companion until the age of 6 years was the family servant, named Martha Washington. As Keller grew older, the family became increasingly frustrated in their attempts to communicate with their daughter. Helen's mother eventually read about the success of Laura Bridgman and later visited

FIGURE 13.5. The student Helen Keller and her teacher Anne Sullivan.

The life of German composer **Ludwig van Beethoven** (1770–1827) was affected by hearing problems. Beethoven did not become suddenly deaf—his loss of hearing was a slow process, spanning approximately 20 years. He was known to use a hearing trumpet. By the age of 50, he was completely deaf and could not hear music. In his years of total deafness, he completed his Ninth Symphony. It is said that after his first public performance of the symphony he cried when he was turned around in order to see the audience's response to the music.

a local expert on the problems of deaf children. This expert was Alexander Graham Bell and he recommended that the family take Helen to the Perkins School for the Blind. It was there that Helen met her teacher **Anne Sullivan** (1866–1936) who would become Helen's companion for the next 50 years. In 1904, Helen graduated from Radcliffe College, becoming the first deaf-blind person to earn a Bachelor of Arts degree. She and Anne went on a series of lecture tours around the world, speaking of her experiences. She became a major advocate for ensuring the rights of the deaf and blind. During her lifetime she was introduced to every U.S. president from Grover Cleveland to Lyndon B. Johnson and met many celebrities as well.

TREATMENT APPROACHES: HEARING REHABILITATION

One feature of aural rehabilitation is to directly treat the hearing loss. Three approaches to treating hearing loss are: (1) surgery, (2) hearing aid fitting, and (3) auditory implants.

Surgical Treatment

Two surgical procedures that address pathology of the tympanic membrane and middle ear are myringotomy and tympanoplasty. **Myringotomy** involves making a small incision in the eardrum to drain fluid which has accumulated in the middle ear space and serves to relieve pressure within the middle ear. The surgery is often performed on children who are prone to otitis media with effusion, although adults occasionally acquire similar problems requiring the myringotomy procedure. The buildup of fluid implies that the eustachian tube is not functioning and is unable to perform its normal role of keeping the middle ear dry and ventilated. The fluid buildup creates a conductive hearing loss and once the fluid is drained, the child's hearing is essentially restored. As part of the surgery, a small **ventilation tube** (also called a **pressure equalization**

tube or **grommet**) is placed in the area of the incision. The tube serves to ventilate the middle ear and to prevent fluid from accumulating (Figure 13.6). Most tubes are made of a synthetic plastic material, such as silicone or Teflon.

A

B

FIGURE 13.6. Myringotomy procedure (**A**) and insertion of a ventilation tube (i.e., grommet) in the tympanic membrane (**B**).

They typically stay in place for around 9 months before they are pushed out by the rapidly healing eardrum. A small scar usually forms in the eardrum, although the scarring does not impair hearing. The surgery is an outpatient procedure, meaning the patient returns home on the same day the surgery took place.

Tympanoplasty is a microsurgical procedure to repair a perforated tympanic membrane or reconstruct the small bones of the middle ear. The procedure can also help treat certain types of hearing loss and prevent infection of the middle ear. Three types of tympanoplasty are: (1) myringoplasty, which is a repair of a tear in the eardrum; (2) tympanoplasty with ossiculoplasty, which is a repair of a tear in the eardrum and correction of a defect in middle ear ossicles; and (3) tympanoplasty with mastoidectomy, which is a repair of an eardrum tear and removal of a bony infection in the area behind the ear. An illustration of tympanoplasty is shown in Figure 13.7.

Hearing Aids

The use of hearing aids to treat hearing loss typically is considered when no medical or surgical option is available to correct the loss. As mentioned earlier, a hearing aid consists of three major components: (1) the microphone, (2) amplifier, and (3) speaker. All components are housed in a plastic case that protects them and allows the hearing aid to be fitted on the ear (Figure 13.8). The microphone serves to transform the incoming acoustic sound into an electrical signal. The amplifier then increases the intensity of the electrical signal. A programmable filter is an additional feature of the amplifier. Filters have the ability to selectively modify sound, so only the sounds needed by the person with a hearing loss are amplified. The speaker converts the electrical signal that has been amplified back into an acoustic sound, which is transmitted down the ear canal. The hearing aid user can regulate loudness with a volume control.

A

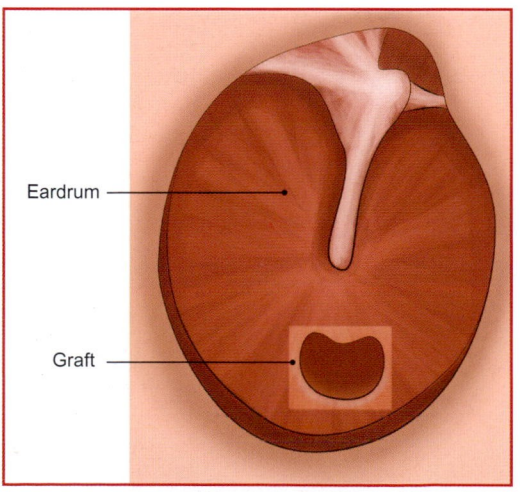

B

FIGURE 13.7. Example of a perforated (punctured) tympanic membrane (**A**) and tympanoplasty involving repair of the puncture (**B**).

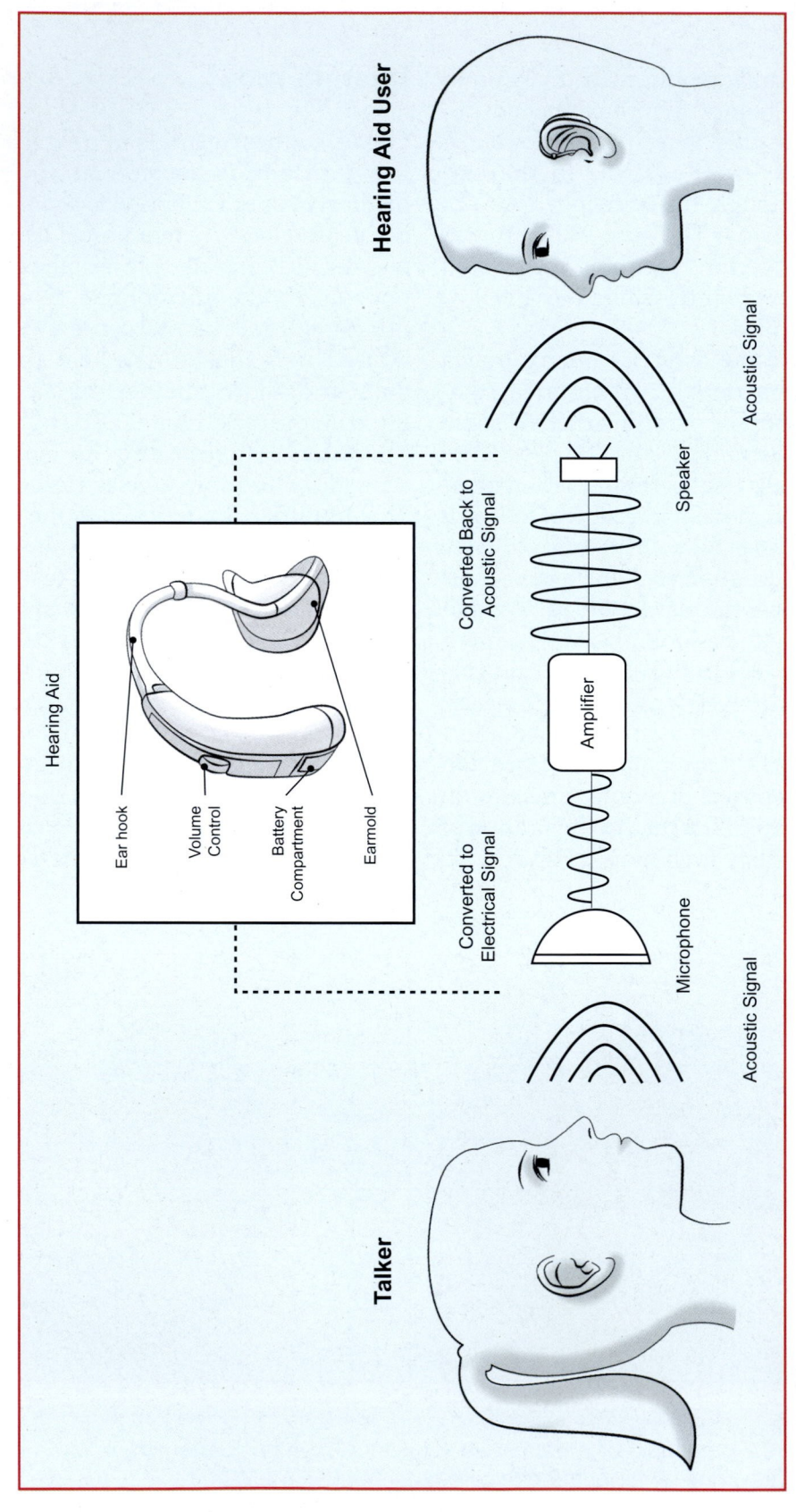

FIGURE 13.8. The transmission of sound between a speaker and a hearing aid user.

Some aids have other controls that can be used to make the signal clearer.

Hearing aids tend to be expensive and the high cost is due to the manufacturing of miniaturized components. They are built to be durable, but like any electronic device, can be broken if dropped on a hard surface. Exposure to water also can lead to damage so they must not be worn in the shower or when swimming. Hearing aids come in various sizes, generally corresponding to the amount of power (or amplification) that can be provided. Large hearing aids usually provide the most amplification and are prescribed for individuals with more severe hearing loss. A listing of the various types of hearing aids follows.

Behind-the-Ear (BTE) Aids

A **BTE** aid consists of two parts (Figure 13.9); one part is the actual hearing aid and this is situated behind the ear, the other part is an acrylic/silicon earmold that fits in the outermost portion of the ear canal. The mold is connected to the hearing aid with a transparent tube which transmits the amplified sound from the hearing aid into the ear canal. People with a wide range of hearing losses, from mild to profound, can be fitted with BTE hearing aids. Because the components are housed outside of the ear, these aids tend to be the most durable. This durability makes them ideal for children and the size of the hearing aid also provides a high level of amplification if needed. Some BTE aids are designed in such a way that it can be fitted in the ear without a mold but with a small plastic tip on the end of the tubing (called an open-ear fitting). The soft silicone tip has holes so that the ear canal is not sealed off. The advantage of an open-fit BTE is the cosmetic appeal, as well as the open feeling in the ear canal.

In-the-Ear (ITE) Aids

All components of an **ITE** aid are built into a custom-made mold (see Figure 13.9)

FYI

Count **Alessandro Volta** (1745–1827) was an Italian physicist born in Como, Italy and is known for his pioneering work in electricity and inventing the voltaic pile, a forerunner of the electric battery, which produced a steady stream of electricity. The electrical unit known as the volt was named in his honor. Volta was the first to note that the auditory system could be stimulated electrically. He inserted an electrical current into his ears via two metal rods. He reported a sensation that was like a "boom within the head" followed by a sound similar to that of "boiling of thick soup."

FIGURE 13.9. The various types of hearing aids currently available to individuals with varying degrees of hearing loss.

that fits snugly in the outer most portion of the ear canal. The mold is normally made to be similar to the color of one's skin. The ITE hearing aid can be used by people who have mild to severe hearing losses. This aid is not recommended for individuals who have a severe to profound hearing loss, or problems with finger or hand dexterity that make manipulating small controls difficult.

In-the-Canal (ITC) Aids

The **ITC** aid is custom designed, smaller in size than the ITE aid, and fits mainly in the ear canal (see Figure 13.9). It has a wide cosmetic appeal because it is less visible than ITE aids. Like the ITE, all components are housed within a single plastic shell. Because they are smaller in size, ITC aids are particularly good for management of mild to moderate hearing losses.

Completely-in-the-Canal (CIC) Aids

A **CIC** aid is small and fits deep into the ear canal (see Figure 13.9). This type of aid has the advantage of sitting very close to the eardrum, which improves sound quality and reduces the "echo" sensation sometimes found in larger aids. The size of the CIC makes it very appealing from a cosmetic standpoint. The small size, however, also has some disadvantages, such as short battery life because the batteries are so small. Some people may not be good candidates for a CIC aid if they have unusually shaped ear canals or if they have a severe hearing loss.

Body-Worn Aids

The earliest forms of modern hearing aids were body worn. This type of aid may seem outdated but they are still in use today. These aids can be clearly distinguished from other hearing aids because they require a battery pack and amplifier that is worn in a harness on the body (or situated in a shirt pocket) (see Figure 13.9). They are much less bulky than the older body aids and are more attractively designed. These days, **body aids** are used by individuals with a profound hearing loss because it is likely to provide the highest level of sound amplification. They also are prescribed for some individuals who do not have the manual dexterity to operate a BTE aid as they are simple to operate with large controls and switches that are easy to handle. Finally, the cost of body aids tends to be substantially less than BTE-style aids.

Assistive Listening Devices

The hearing needs of some individuals cannot be successfully addressed with hearing aids alone. In these cases, devices have been created that are used to facilitate listening in various environments, especially those with excessive noise. Some **assistive listening devices** (ALDs) are designed to be used with hearing aids, whereas others are designed for independent use. ALDs can amplify a sound, but their primary purpose is to separate background (distracting) sounds from speech sounds. They improve what is known as the **signal-to-noise ratio (SNR)**, which is the difference in level between the signal of interest and the background noise. Examples of ALDs include: (1) a telecoil, (2) sound field amplification, and (3) captioning. A helpful feature of most hearing aids is called the **telecoil**, or "t-switch." A telecoil is used when speaking and listening on a telephone. A hearing aid uses a microphone to pick up sound and send it into the ear canal. When the telecoil switch is activated, the hearing aid also can detect a magnetic signal transmitted through the actual telephone device. This magnetic signal serves to further enhance the SNR allowing for better listening over the telephone. **Sound field amplification** systems typically are found in classroom settings and are designed to amplify and broadcast the teacher's voice through loudspeakers. The system consists of a microphone/FM transmitter, amplifier, and one or more loudspeakers. **Captioning** is a form of ALD, in which words that are said on a TV show are embedded in the signal and become visible with a special decoder. The decoder lets a hearing-impaired individual see captions at the bottom of the screen that tell them what is being spoken in the TV program. Most TVs have a built-in option to display closed captioning of broadcasts; however, this feature will only work if the specific TV program has been captioned beforehand.

Auditory Implants

An auditory implant provides a new mechanism for hearing when use of a traditional hearing aid alone is insufficient. An auditory implant is very different from a hearing aid—hearing aids amplify sound, whereas auditory implants compensate for damaged or nonworking parts of the auditory system. There are four principal types of auditory implants: (1) **bone-anchored hearing aid**, (2) **cochlear implant**, (3) **auditory brainstem implant**, and (4) **middle ear implant**.

Bone-Anchored Hearing Aid (BAHA)

We typically think of hearing as a process of air conduction. That is, sound is transmitted through the air, which travels down the ear canal toward the eardrum, middle ear ossicles, and the inner ear. However, sound is also transmitted through bone conduction via the bones in the head that bypass the outer and middle ear going straight to the inner ear (see also Chapter 12). Conventional hearing aids sit in the ear canal and transmit sound via air conduction. Some people cannot use conventional hearing aids due to chronic outer or middle ear infection problems or lack of a functioning ear canal (e.g., atresia). A BAHA is an auditory implant for people with hearing loss who cannot receive benefit from a normal hearing aid. The BAHA works **percutaneously** (i.e., through the skin) by vibrating the skull directly through a small titanium fixture that is implanted in the skull behind the ear (Figure 13.10). The device works by taking the sound from the outside and transmitting it to the inner ear through the temporal bone. This bypasses the ear canal and the middle ear. The BAHA was first used in Europe in 1977 and has been approved for use in the United States since 1996 for conductive and mixed hearing losses.

Cochlear Implant

One of the most groundbreaking biomedical achievements in the last 30 years was the cochlear implant (CI). Prior to 1975, the primary aural rehabilitation device for profoundly deaf or severely hearing-impaired children and adults was a BTE hearing aid. Anyone above 12 months of age, with severe to pro-

A   B

FIGURE 13.10. Illustration of bone-anchored hearing aid (BAHA). The BAHA is attached to a small titanium implant behind the ear (**A**). The sound travels via the bones of the skull to the inner ear (**B**).

found sensorineural hearing loss in both ears (70 dB or greater), who receives limited benefit from a hearing aid is a candidate for a CI. The major components of a CI are located outside, as well as inside the head. The components located outside the head are a microphone that picks up sounds in the environment, and a sound processor that arranges the sounds into an electrical signal that is transmitted through the skull. The transmitted signal sent through the skull is picked up by a receiver located inside the head. This receiver sends the electrical impulses to an array of 22 electrodes that stimulate different regions of the cochlea (Figure 13.11). A CI does not restore normal hearing. Instead, it can give a deaf person a useful representation of sounds in the environment to assist with the understanding of speech. Although sound quality is sometimes described as "mechanical," the cochlear implant provides users with the ability to sense sound that they could not oth-

erwise hear. Nearly 200,000 individuals in more than 120 countries have been fitted with a CI.

Auditory Brainstem Implant

An auditory brainstem implant (ABI) is the first device specifically designed to bypass the cochlea and the auditory nerve to transmit sound directly to the brainstem. Because it bypasses the auditory nerve, the device is most useful for people who have lost or will lose their

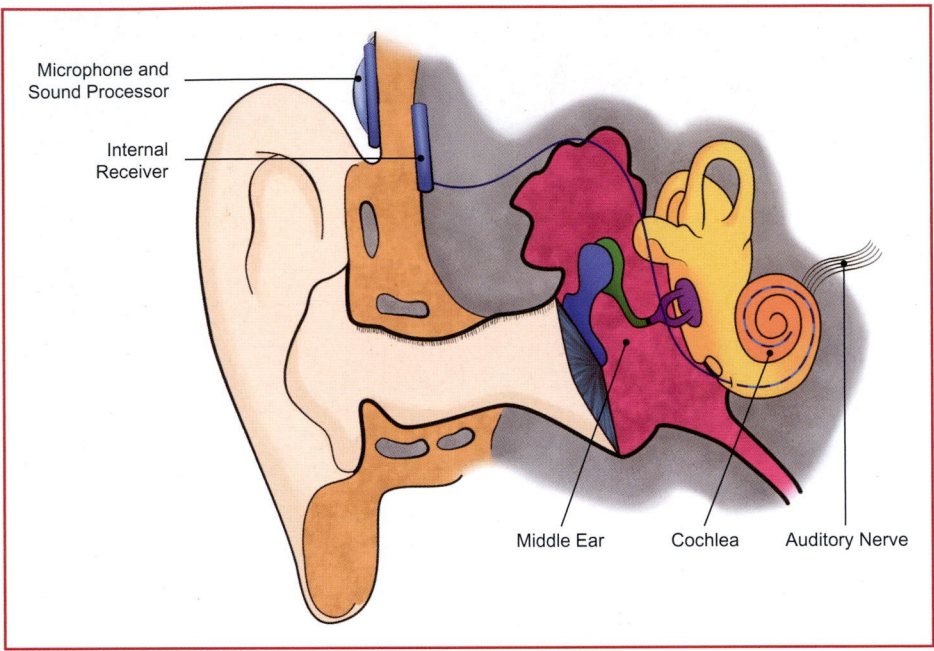

FIGURE 13.11. Illustration of a cochlear implant.

hearing in both ears following the removal of an auditory nerve tumor. Similar to a CI, the device involves components located outside and inside the head. The ABI device consists of a tiny microphone positioned by the ear, a sound processor, and an array of electrodes implanted directly on a nerve center at the base of the brainstem called the cochlear nucleus. The microphone picks up sounds from the environment and transmits them to a receiver inside the skull. This receiver stimulates the brainstem electrodes, allowing for electrical impulses of sound to be transmitted to the brain (Figure 13.12). Most ABI recipients benefit from the device through increased sound awareness. Most patients are able to hear noises like a telephone ringing or horn honking, but the degree of hearing usefulness can vary greatly. At this point in time, few ABI recipients are able to understand

speech without lip reading, but this may improve in the future. However, the environmental and speech sounds that patients receive through the ABI help to significantly improve their communication and quality of life.

Middle Ear Implant

The newest type of implant to be developed is specific to the middle ear. This form of implant is not a hearing aid (i.e., the device does not amplify sounds). Instead, this implant is designed to convert sound into mechanical vibrations that are then delivered to the inner ear. Similar to a CI and ABI, a middle ear implant involves components located outside and inside the head. The external component receives sounds which are then delivered to a transducer implanted in the middle ear that causes

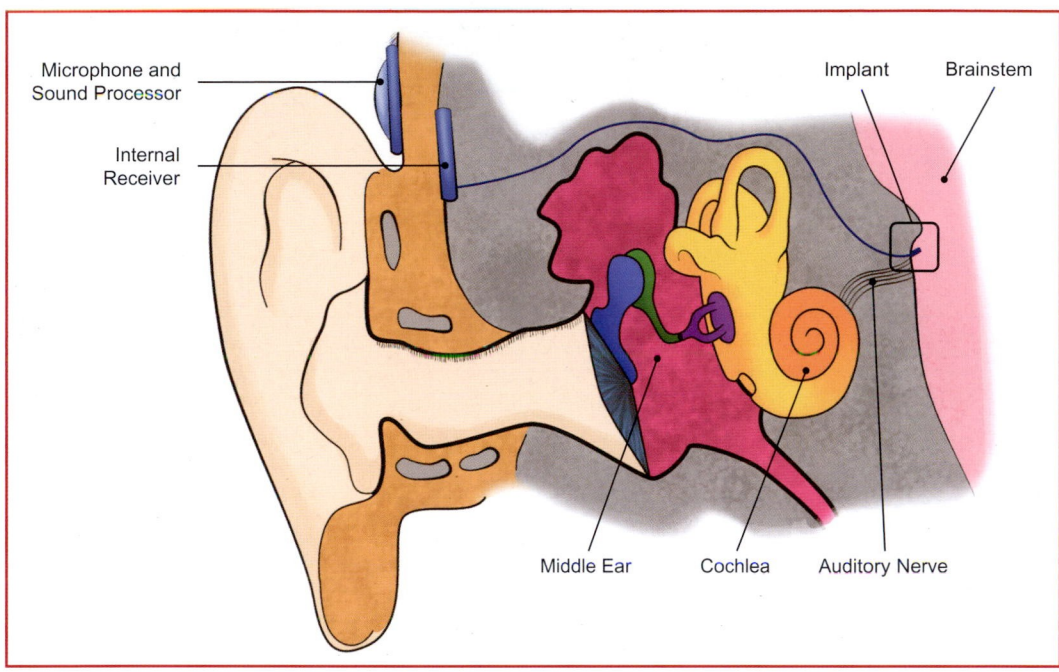

FIGURE 13.12. Illustration of an auditory brainstem implant.

the ossicles to vibrate. A middle ear implant can be used to treat individuals with conductive, mixed, or sensorineural losses. The implant is ideal for individuals who cannot tolerate a traditional type of hearing aid that is inserted to the ear canal.

TREATMENT APPROACHES: SPEECH AND LANGUAGE REHABILITATION

Another aspect of aural rehabilitation concerns treatment of the speech and language abnormalities that may accompany a hearing impairment. Generally, the earlier the hearing loss occurs (e.g., congenital, prelingual) and the more severe the hearing loss (e.g., severe, profound), the greater its impact on speech and language. The presence of a severe hearing loss during the critical periods of speech and language development deprives a child of the opportunities to hear language and can thus affect a child's ability to develop the features of normal communication (i.e., form, content, and use). Some of the primary speech and language disorders which result from a severe hearing loss are provided in Table 13.1. A brief summary of these features is provided below followed by an assortment of treatment approaches.

Speech and Language Characteristics

Phonology

A child with a severe hearing loss is likely to show impaired speech articulation. The child's ability to accurately

Table 13.1. Characteristics of Speech and Language Found in Deaf and Severely Hard of Hearing Individuals

Feature	Characteristics
Phonology	Consonant and vowel omissions, substitutions, and distortions
	Less visible phonemes more likely to be misarticulated
	Acoustic features of phonemes can influence perception and production
Semantics	Vocabulary can range from normal to severely impaired
Syntax	Short and simple sentences
	Incorrect word order and sentence constructions
Pragmatics	Limited understanding of figurative language, idioms, metaphors
	Restricted range of communicative intents such as conversational skills
Voice	Quality is impaired, likely to be hypernasal
	Pitch is likely to be high
	Regulation of loudness may be impaired
Suprasegmental features	Slow speaking rate
	Impaired speech intonation and phrasing

produce consonants and vowels is influenced by two variables: (1) speech **sound visibility** and (2) **acoustic characteristics**. Some speech sounds are more easily perceived on the face of a speaker compared to others. For a severely hearing-impaired child, this visual information can assist in learning to produce speech sounds accurately. For example, the /f/ sound is highly visible compared to the /k/ sound. Not surprisingly, low visibility sounds such as /k/ are likely to be misarticulated more often than highly visible sounds.

All consonants and vowels have unique acoustic characteristics that are differentiated from one another in regard to duration (ms), loudness (dB), and frequency (Hz). Depending on the configuration of a person's hearing loss, some sounds are less likely to be perceived clearly compared to others and this can lead to inaccurate speech sound production. For example, assuming a child has a high-frequency hearing loss, sounds that are naturally produced with a high frequency (e.g., /s/, /sh/) are less likely to be perceived and produced clearly compared to low-frequency sounds (e.g., /m/, /z/). The general acoustic characteristics of speech sounds are shown in Figure 13.13. A hearing loss that falls outside the range of the acoustic characteristics for various speech sounds would presumably be problematic for a hearing-impaired individual to perceive. In turn, the same sounds may be difficult to produce accurately.

FIGURE 13.13. Depiction of the acoustic features of various consonants and vowels overlaid on an audiogram. In the case of an individual with a severe bilateral hearing loss, it is unlikely these sounds would be audible.

Voice

Voice disorders are often found in the severely hard of hearing and deaf populations. Foremost among these voice problems is the production of **hypernasal speech**. This excessive nasality is thought to occur due to a lack of auditory feedback during speaking. Without auditory feedback, a deaf speaker may not learn the motor routines needed to separate the oral and nasal cavities, resulting in inadequate velopharyngeal closure and subsequent speech nasality. A second feature of voice found to be impaired is voice pitch, particularly among individuals with deafness. Attempts to produce voice, without being able to hear one's voice, tend to result in excessive tension in the region of the larynx. This results in abnormally tense vocal fold vibration that leads to the production of a **high pitched voice**.

Language

Deaf children acquire language in the same developmental stages as a child with normal hearing; however, deaf children generally develop language at a slower pace. The primary deficit area is in the area of **language syntax** and includes problems with grammatical markers, articles, and word endings. The deficit likely results from a combination of factors. The syntactic structure of English is both complex and subtle with a number of inconsistencies. For example, consider these three sentences: (1) *"I am going home,"* (2) *"I am going to school,"* and (3) *"I am going to the store."* It is not surprising to find an individual with hearing impairment unable to grasp the subtleties of these differences and say something like, *"I am going to home"* or *"I am going school"* (Schow & Nerbonne, 2007). Another factor influencing an individual's correct use of syntax may stem from the mismatch between the language systems used by deaf and hearing individuals. For example, the language structure of American Sign Language (ASL) is quite different from Standard English. For a deaf child who first learned ASL, the later acquisition of Standard English may prove challenging.

Speaking Rate

There is considerable research confirming that HI individuals speak more slowly than normally hearing speakers. Prelingually deaf children speak at one-fourth the rate of normally hearing children and adults. And even after practice, the deaf child's speaking rate is still half that of normally hearing children and adults (Dwyer et al., 2009).

Rehabilitation Approaches

Speech Reading

For people with deafness, use of their eyes rather than ears provides the critical link with the world. One way of taking advantage of this visual link for communication is the act of speech reading. **Speech reading**, sometimes called lip reading, involves the decoding of language spoken by an individual by paying close attention to the speaker's mouth. The speech reader will also use the speaker's facial expressions, gestures, and hand movements as visual cues. All of this decoding is performed without being able to hear the speaker's voice. Even under optimal conditions, speech reading involves a great deal of guesswork. When we speak English, only 30% of the consonants and vowels are clearly visible on the mouth. For example, compare the highly visible "f" and "th" sounds with the nearly invisible "t" and "k" sounds (Figure 13.14). The speech reader needs to become adept at filling-in the gaps between visible and invisible sounds to read words and

---

FYI

A speech reader's poem by Grace Cleys (1997):

You, who have good hearing
Are mystified, it's true
To watch a group of people
Try to lipread, as we do.

It's exciting, quiet enchanting
And a thrill amid some fears
As we slowly try to listen
With our eyes instead of ears.

At times it can be tricky
And often just plain fun
Success means lots of practice
Perfection's seldom won.

We share each other's troubles
And laugh at our mistakes
It takes a load of practice
And lots of give and takes.

FIGURE 13.14. Various mouth shapes that can be seen during speech reading. Can you identify the sounds being produced by this speaker?

phrases. People with deafness who are experienced speech readers can decode approximately 40% of single words. Speech reading is not normally used as the sole means of aural rehabilitation. Speech reading is a strategy that is used in combination with other assistive listening devices to communicate effectively.

Cued Speech

Cued speech was created as a means of helping to solve the decoding problems related to speech reading. Some speech sounds are not readily visible (e.g., "t," "k") and some speech sounds look almost identical. Consider the differences between the sounds "m," "b," and "p." All of these sounds are produced with the lips closed and could easily be confused by the speech reader when trying to distinguish the words "my," "buy," or "pie." Cued speech is a supplement to spoken language in which the speaker uses a set of sound-related hand shapes while talking to a severely hard of hearing individual. These hand shapes are intended to remove the guesswork from speech reading. It is a phonemically based system that uses eight hand shapes in four locations near the face. A total of 36 different cues are used to clarify 44 different sounds in English (Figure 13.15). Cued speech has not been used widely as a rehabilitation technique. The major limitation is that the system is not applicable to everyday communication situations. Both the speaker and the speech-reader need to be familiar with the cued speech system of communication.

Oral/Aural Approach

The terms **oral** and **aural** refer to the mouth and ear, respectively. Thus, the **oral/aural approach** to speech and language

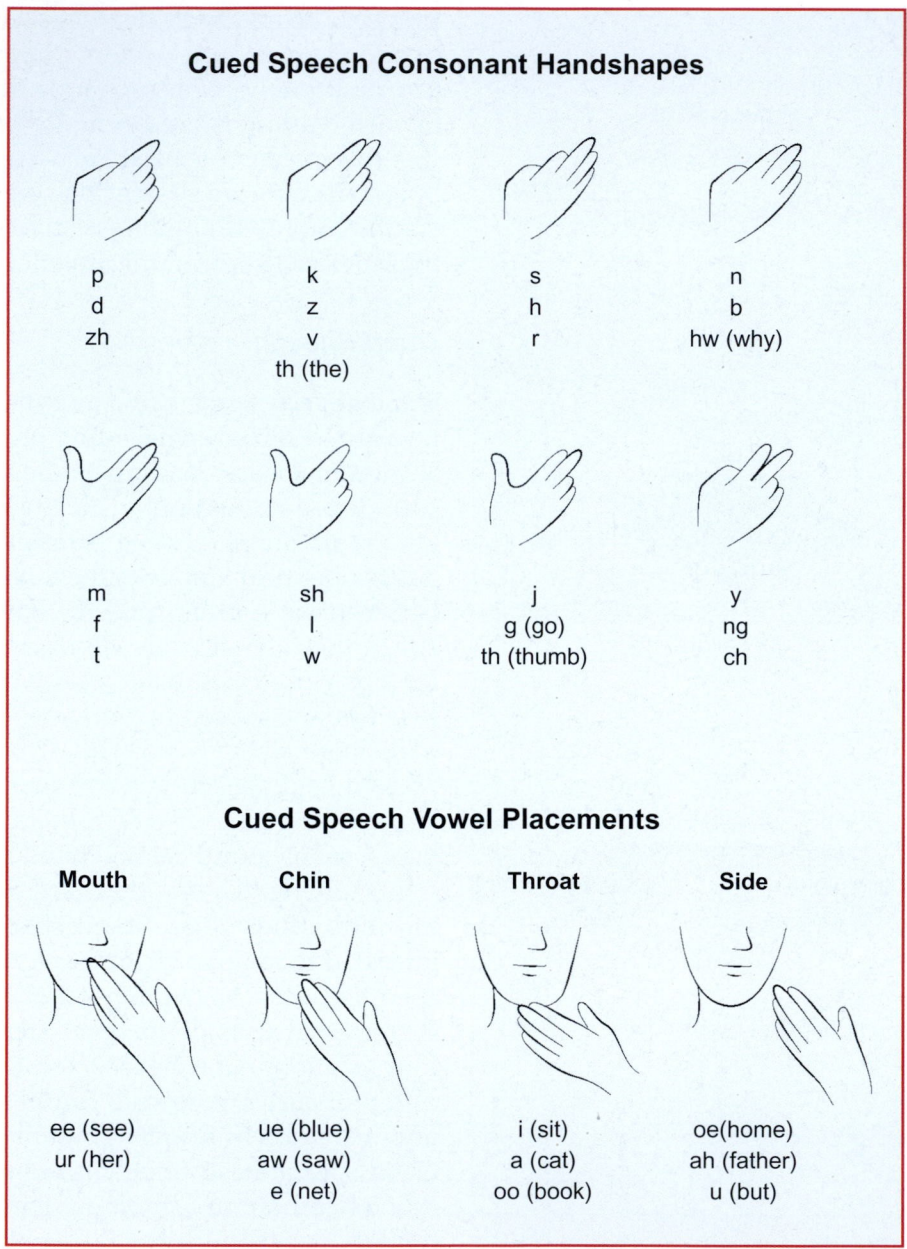

FIGURE 13.15. The hand symbols used for cued speech.

rehabilitation focuses on improving both speech and hearing abilities. This method stresses the use of speech articulation, hearing aids, and speech reading skills. A primary objective is to develop clear spoken language abilities to enable the person to function in a hearing society. People using this method are discouraged from relying exclusively on visual cues (such as sign language).

Manual Approach

Manual communication is often thought of as **sign language**. The language involves movement of the hands, body, face, and head as the primary mode of communication. Advocates of the manual communication approach believe that knowledge and understanding of language is more important than the ability to speak clearly. Because deaf and severely hard of hearing individuals use the visual mode more readily, communicating through the visual mode is a natural form of expression. Two examples of manual communication are **finger spelling** and sign language. Finger spelling is the process of creating words using a finger alphabet and is generally used alongside sign language to spell out names, places, and unusual words which do not have their own, distinct sign. The finger alphabet used in Canada and the United States is based on hand shapes formed using one hand. The finger alphabet used in the United Kingdom, Australia, and New Zealand uses two hands (Figure 13.16). Sign language is the process of forming sentences using various hand shapes that reflect specific words. American Sign Language (ASL) is the visual/gestural language used by many people in the Deaf community in the United States, Canada, and parts of Mexico, although it originated in Europe. It is considered a distinct language and not just a visual representation of English. ASL has its own grammar and syntax and does not follow the word order we would normal use when speaking English. British Sign Language (BSL) is the sign language used in the United Kingdom and is quite distinct from ASL in the hand shapes for various words, as well as grammar and syntax. The Australian sign language (Auslan) and New Zealand sign language (NZSL) systems have evolved from BSL.

Simultaneous Communication Approach (SimCom)

Simultaneous communication (SimCom) is an aural rehabilitation approach that encourages all possible modes of communication to help a hearing-impaired individual communicate effectively. The various modes of communication include using a combination of spoken language, sign language, finger spelling, speech reading, amplification, writing, and gestures. SimCom is a common form of communication used in educational settings for deaf children. Advocates of this approach believe that individuals can learn and use language in a way

---

FYI

In April 2006, the New Zealand government officially declared New Zealand sign language (NZSL) as one of three official languages in the country. The two other official languages of the country are English and Maori. Other countries that have made a similar declaration concerning sign language include Sweden, Denmark, Finland, Norway, Switzerland, Ireland, Portugal, and Greece.

A

FIGURE 13.16. Manual finger spelling alphabet used in America (**A**). *continues*

best suited to their needs, while developing communication skills to function in the hearing world.

The Deaf and Blind Person

A critical feature of most aural rehabilitation programs is to capitalize on an individual's existing communication skills. This includes sound amplification and utilizing visual cues such as speech reading and sign language. Alternatively, an individual with blindness relies primarily on auditory cues to communicate effectively. In the case of an individual who has lost vision and hearing, aural rehabilitation is particularly challenging. **Deaf-blindness** is defined as a combination of both auditory and visual disabilities that can contribute to severe disorders of development, learning, and

B

FIGURE 13.16. *continued* Manual finger spelling alphabet used in Britain (**B**).

communication. The prevalence of deaf-blindness is approximately 1 per 10,000 individuals. For the profoundly deaf and blind individual, the primary means by which he or she experiences the outside world is through touch. One method of communication that has been designed for deaf-blind individuals is the **Tadoma method**, which was developed in Sweden in the 1920s and named after two children (Tad and Oma) who were deaf and blind. The deaf-blind individual places a thumb on a speaker's lips and spreads their remaining fingers along the speaker's face and neck (Figure 13.17). Communication is transmitted through

FIGURE 13.17. Illustration of the Tadoma method used by individuals with deaf-blindness to comprehend spoken language.

vibrations, motions of the jaw, and facial expressions of the speaker. Although the Tadoma method is very difficult and time-consuming to learn, it has proven successful, allowing fluent Tadoma users the ability to comprehend spoken language.

CULTURAL CONSIDERATIONS AND AURAL REHABILITATION

Culture is defined as a system of values, attitudes, beliefs, and learned behaviors shared by a population. Culture is shaped by factors such as geographic location, education, age, and sex. A person's hearing abilities can also be a defining feature of one's culture. This is especially the case among those with a profound hearing loss. Sociologists have identified two opposing perspectives on culture and deafness, which are referred to as the **medical model** and **cultural model**. In the medical model, deafness is viewed as an illness and disability.

The disability can be treated by surgery and/or prosthetic devices like a cochlear implant or hearing aid. The condition can also be treated by allied health professionals including audiologists and speech-language pathologists. The medical model discourages "separatism" from the hearing world; instead, emphasis is placed on encouraging deaf people to acquire oral language skills. The use of sign language is discouraged. In the cultural model, Deaf people are seen as nondefective persons, who are members of a minority culture. Deafness is not an illness or impairment but a difference, so there is no need for surgical intervention. Deaf and hard of hearing people are disabled only by barriers created by other people trying to make them fit into the "hearing" world. The cultural model sees the Deaf community has having its own unique culture. Evidence of Deaf culture is found in a number of ways. Deaf and hard of hearing people produce plays, books, artwork, magazines, and movies targeted at deaf and hard of hearing audiences.

Socialization in the Deaf community takes many forms. A particularly popular means of socialization is meeting at a restaurant, which has come to be known as a *signing supper* or ASL dinner. Another popular social vehicle is the *Deaf coffee*, a meeting at a local café to chat. The Deaf community also has its own online dating sites.

There are also cultural assumptions in regard to the manner in which the word "deaf" is written. The term "deaf," as written with a lower case "d," is used to refer to people who are profoundly hearing impaired and choose to use oral communication as their first language of communication. The term "Deaf," as written with a capital "D," is used to describe people who are profoundly hearing impaired and use sign language as their major mode of communication. Capital "D" deafness denotes the social, political, and cultural strands of members belonging to the Deaf community.

CURRENT RESEARCH IN AURAL REHABILITATION

Telehome Aural Rehabilitation

The use of new technologies to provide remote healthcare is a burgeoning area of rehabilitation. This form of healthcare has been termed **telehome**, and is defined as the use of communication and information technology to deliver health services and exchange health information to and from the home. Telehome care was prompted by the need to access patients in remote geographic areas and the availability of Internet service to these areas. Telehome care does not replace in-person healthcare visits, but is used primarily to augment current services.

Telehome care also is a cost-effective means of providing healthcare in the current environment of sky-rocketing costs. Personal computers and video equipment can transmit data over ordinary telephone lines and allow health providers to monitor patients and provide care at a fraction of the cost. Research is underway that links hearing-impaired individuals with health care professionals to help better manage their hearing loss in the comfort of their own home (Denev, Morris, Velasco, & Mohamad, 2008). The use of an online support system can be tailored to the situational and individual needs of the hearing aid user.

Frequency Transposition

Hearing aids rarely provide sufficient amplification to the high-frequency range of hearing without over-amplifying the low-frequency region. As a result, individuals with a high-frequency hearing loss seem to never be fully satisfied with their hearing aids. They have normal hearing in the low to mid frequencies so amplification of these regions is not necessary. One approach to helping these individuals is to design a hearing aid that delivers high-frequency speech sounds to the lower frequency region. This is referred to as **frequency transposition**. There have been many attempts to do this, going back more than 30 years. However, previous attempts to transpose frequencies ended up obscuring the overall quality of the sound delivered to the ear. Modern day hearing aids use a digital processing technology that allows for improved transposition of frequencies and ultimately may help individuals with a high-frequency hearing loss (Kuk, Keenan, Auriemmo, & Korhonen, 2009).

Neuroimaging and Cochlear Implants

The study of congenitally deaf individuals provides a unique opportunity to understand the organization and potential for reorganization of regions in the brain following cochlear implantation. Cochlear implants provide auditory sensation to parts of the brain that had previously received no sensation. A current line of research is to use neuroimaging techniques such as magnetic resonance imaging (MRI) and positron emission tomography (PET) scans to examine the structural organization of various regions of the brain. In the past, the effectiveness of a cochlear implant typically was evaluated by a subjective appraisal of the individual's speech recognition and speech production abilities. However, these assessments do not provide information regarding sites in the brain that are responsible for good (or poor) results. The use of neuroimaging techniques allows researchers to examine the cortical areas that are used by a cochlear implant user and to evaluate the consequences of electrical stimulation by the cochlear implant (Tobey & Devous, 2007).

Postauricular Muscle Response

The postauricular area is located behind the pinna (i.e., auricle). A number of muscles have their points of attachment in this general area, most notably the auricular muscles. Over 30 years ago, researchers discovered that these muscles could be deliberately activated (and measured) when sound was presented to the ears (Figure 13.18). The phenomenon

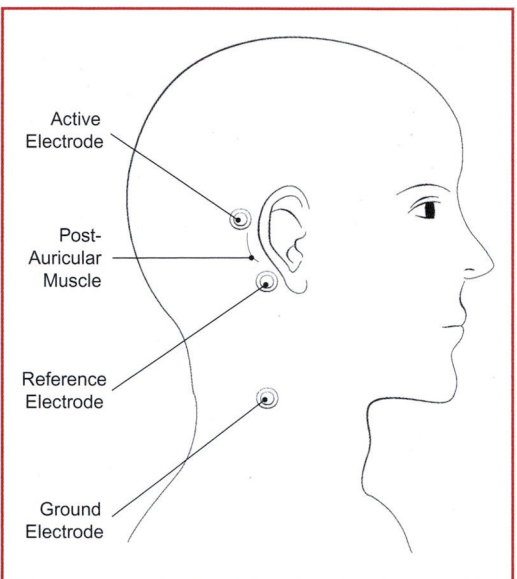

FIGURE 13.18. Electrode placement for measurement of postauricular muscle response (PAMR).

has been referred to as the **postauricular muscle response** (PAMR). This naturally occurring response has prompted a number of researchers to consider using the PAMR as a method of screening for hearing impairment, especially in the infant population (O'Beirne & Patuzzi, 1999). Research currently is underway to refine the method of collecting and measuring the PAMR and it may someday be used as an adjunct to auditory brainstem response (ABR) testing for objective hearing assessment (Purdy, Agung, Hartley, Patuzzi, & O'Beirne, 2005).

AURAL REHABILITATION ON THE WORLD WIDE WEB

Listed below are Web sites that provide further information on the topic of aural rehabilitation. At the time of publication each Web site was freely accessible.

Better Hearing Institute Videos
http://www.betterhearing.org/video/pbs/spotlight.cfm

Cochlear Implant Videos
http://ci4me2007.vodpod.com/

Hearnet.Com Public Service Announcements
http://www.hearnet.com/features/feature_PSA.shtml

Oral Deaf Education Videos
http://www.oraldeafed.org/

Selecting a Hearing Aid Video
http://www.webmd.com/video/choosing-hearing-aid

Sign Language Video Clips
http://www.mydeaflife.com

REFERENCES

Cleys, G. (1997). A lipreaders poem. Retrieved September 23, 2009. from http://www.geocities.com/Heartland/Park/7180/lippoem.html

Denev, D., Morris, S., Velasco, C., & Mohamad, Y. (2008). eRehabilitation: A portal framework for aural rehabilitation. In *Computers helping people with special needs.* Berlin: Heidelberg, Germany: Springer.

Dwyer, C., Robb, M., O'Beirne, G., & Gilbert, H. (2009). The influence of speaking rate on nasality in the speech of hearing impaired individuals. *Journal of Speech, Language, and Hearing Research, 52,* 1321–1333.

Kuk, F., Keenan, D., Auriemmo, J., & Korhonen, P. (2009, Jan 20). Re-evaluating the efficacy of frequency transposition. *The ASHA Leader, 4*(1), 14-17.

O'Beirne, G., & Patuzzi, R. (1999). Basic properties of the sound-evoked post-auricular muscle response (PAMR). *Hearing Research, 138,* 115-132.

Purdy, S. C., Agung, K. B., Hartley, D., Patuzzi, R. B., & O'Beirne, G. A. (2005). The post-auricular muscle response: An objective electrophysiological method for evaluating hearing sensitivity. *International Journal of Audiology, 44,* 625–630.

Schow, R., & Nerbonne, M. (2007). *Introduction to audiologic rehabilitation* (5th ed.). Boston: Pearson Education.

Tabak, J. (2006). *Significant gestures.* Westport, CT: Praeger.

Tobey, E. A., & Devous, M. D. (2007, Sept. 4). Neuroimaging and cochlear implants: A look at how the brain hears. *The ASHA Leader, 12*(12), 6–9.

Tye-Murray, N. (2009). *Foundations of aural rehabilitation: Children, adults, and their family members* (3rd ed.). Clifton Park, NY: Delmar Cengage Learning.

GLOSSARY OF TERMS

AAC: *See* alternative or augmentative communication.

abducted: To move away from the midline position. Vocal fold opening is a form of abduction.

ABR: *See* auditory brainstem response.

accent: A characteristic of speech pronunciation as determined by regional or social background.

acid reflux: Regurgitation of stomach acid into the esophagus.

acoustic neuroma: A benign tumor located on the 8th cranial nerve that may affect hearing and balance.

acoustic reflex: An involuntary muscle contraction that occurs in the middle ear as a result of sudden loudness in sound.

acquired disorder: A communication impairment that results after a period of normal communication. A traumatic brain injury is a form of acquired disorder.

acrocentric chromosome: A chromosome with its centromere located near the end of the chromosome.

acute care hospital: A hospital that provides short-term and highly specialized patient care.

addition: Type of speech sound misarticulation in which one or more consonants or vowels are included in the intended word production.

adducted: To move toward the midline position. Vocal fold closing is a form of adduction.

adenoids: Pairs of lymphoid tissue located in various regions in the back of the pharynx that serve to filter out debris from inhaled air. A related term is tonsils.

adenosine triphosphate (ATP): An adenosine nucleotide that is used during muscle contraction. ATP is thought to provide natural protection from acquiring a noise-induced hearing loss.

adult-centered therapy: Form of speech and language therapy in which the adult plays a dominant and directive role in a child's therapy session.

adventitious deafness: Form of acquired communication disorder where a hearing loss occurred after a period of normal hearing. An acoustic neuroma can result in an adventitious hearing loss.

affricates: A category of consonants classified according to the manner in which they are articulated in the vocal tract. The consonant /ch/ is an example of an affricate.

age of mastery: An approach to determining a child's acquisition of speech sounds. Each sound is expected to be acquired (mastered) by a particular age.

age of suppression: An approach to determining a child's suppression of phonological processes. Each process, for example, final consonant deletion, is expected to disappear by a particular age.

air conduction testing: Form of hearing test where sounds are presented through earphones directly into the ear canal.

alaryngeal speech: A unique form of speaking in the absence of a larynx. Removal of the larynx often is a result of cancer.

ALD: *See* assistive listening device.

alphabet: A standard set of letters used to display spoken language. Each symbol generally assumes a sound (phoneme) of the language.

altered auditory feedback: Collective term for sound masking, delayed auditory feedback, and frequency altered feedback. These forms of feedback are used in the treatment of stuttering.

alternative or augmentative communication (AAC): A unique form of communication to assist people with severe expressive communication difficulties.

alveolar ridge: The gum ridge of the upper jaw (maxilla) located directly behind the teeth.

alveoli: The final (end) branches of the respiratory system in the lungs that function to exchange gas between the lungs and the bloodstream.

ALS: *See* amyotrohpic lateral sclerosis.

Alzheimer, Alois: German psychiatrist who was the first to identify the unique brain disease related to cell death.

Alzheimer's disease: Most common form of dementia characterized by progressive memory loss and intellectual abilities.

amniocentesis: Medical procedure used in the prenatal diagnosis of chromosomal and fetal abnormalities.

amplifier: A key feature of a hearing aid designed to boost the loudness level of incoming sound before entering the ear canal.

amplitude: The height of a sound wave. Related terms are intensity and loudness.

amyotrophic lateral sclerosis (ALS): A progressive and fatal neurodegenerataive disease. Also known as motor neuron disease or Lou Gehrig disease.

anatomy: The science concerning the structure of the body.

anencephaly: Condition present at birth that affects the formation of the brain and the skull bones that surround the head.

ankylogossia: Condition caused by an abnormally short lingual frenulum. The condition is commonly referred to as "tongue tie."

anomic aphasia: An expressive language disorder characterized by a severe problem with recalling words.

anthropometry: The science that relates to the measurement of body dimensions.

aphasia: A disorder which results from damage to the regions of the brain that are responsible for language. A similar term is dysphasia.

aphonia: Medical term used to describe a condition in which a person is unable to speak, or has lost their voice.

approximates: A classification of consonant sounds that have articulatory and acoustic qualities that fall somewhere between true consonants and vowels. Examples include /w/ and /r/.

apraxia: Neurologic disorder which is characterized by an inability to perform purposeful movements on command. Apraxia of speech is a unique form of speech sound disorder.

Aristotle: Greek philosopher who contributed important writings in the areas of logic, art, psychology, and nature.

articulation: The location at which two structures make contact. Speech articulation refers to the manner in which various anatomic structures work together to create speech sounds.

articulation disorder: Mispronunciation of speech sounds.

arytenoid cartilages: A pair of triangular-shaped cartilages within the framework of the larynx that serve as points of attachment for the vocal folds.

Asperger, Hans: Austrian pediatrician and child psychiatrist who was the first to describe "autistic psychopathology," which was later named Asperger syndrome.

aspiration: Inhalation of foreign material such as food or fluids in the lungs.

assistive listening device (ALD): Any type of device that helps an individual to function better in their daily communication. Closed captioning on a TV is a form of assistive listening device.

asymmetric hearing loss: A hearing loss in both ears, however the degree and configuration of hearing loss is not identical.

ATP: *See* adenosine triphosphate.

atresia: Absence or incomplete development of the ear canal.

audiogram: A graph used to depict an individual's hearing according to frequency (Hz) and loudness (dB).

audiologist: Professional who specializes in the diagnosis and management of disorders of the auditory and vestibular portions of the ear.

audiology: Branch of science that is concerned with balance, hearing, and related disorders.

audiometer: Machine (typically a computer) which is used for measuring hearing sensitivity.

audition: The act of hearing.

auditory brainstem response (ABR): An electrical signal evoked from the brainstem in response to an auditory signal. This response is often used as a test of hearing in difficult-to-test populations such as infants and the intellectually disabled..

auditory cortex: Region of the brain responsible for the processing of auditory (sound) information. Also called Heschl's gyrus, which is located in the temporal lobes of the cerebrum.

auditory nerve: The nerve that caries auditory and balance information from the inner ear to the brainstem. Also known as the cochlear nerve or the eighth cranial nerve.

auditory processing disorder: Broad term used to describe a variety of problems with the brain that can interfere with the understanding of auditory information in the absence of a hearing loss.

aural: Relating to the ear or to the sense of hearing.

aural rehabilitation: The management of hearing loss.

auricle: The outer ear, also known as the pinna.

autism spectrum disorders: Group of autistic conditions with similar features that may vary in symptoms and severity.

badge: A visual display to communicate status or accomplishment.

barium: Soft metallic element that is silvery white in its purest form. If swallowed, the substance is clearly visible during x-ray examination.

basilar membrane: Anatomical structure located in the cochlea that separates the cochlear duct from the scala tympani.

behaviorist theory: Theory based on the assumption that a child's speech and language development is shaped

by individuals and events in the child's environment.

behind-the-ear aid (BTE): A type of hearing aid where the primary components of the aid are situated and fit behind the ear.

Bell, Alexander Graham: Inventor of the telephone.

Bell, Alexander Melville: Scientist with interests in speech and deafness. Father of Alexander Graham Bell.

beneficence: The act of doing good or being charitable.

Berners-Lee, Timothy: British computer scientist known as the inventor of the World Wide Web.

between-word disfluencies: Speech disfluencies that occur across words, such as a phrase repetition or an interjection.

bilabial: A class of consonants categorized according to the place of articulation in the vocal tract. Examples of bilabial consonants are /b/ and /m/.

bilateral cleft lip: A cleft that involves separation of the lip on both sides of the mouth, often shown as a large open gap.

bilateral hearing loss: An impairment of hearing that occurs in both ears.

bilingualism: The ability to communicate in two languages, which may include speaking, listening, reading, and writing.

biofeedback: An approach to teaching an individual to control various functions of the body through relaxation, visualization, and cognitive control processes.

birth defect: An abnormality of structure, function, or body chemistry usually present at birth that can result in physical or intellectual disability.

Blackwell, Elizabeth: First woman in the United States to graduate from medical school and practice medicine.

blogging: Contraction of the terms web and log. A Web site, usually maintained by an individual, which contains regular entries and personal commentaries.

Bloom, Lois: American professor of speech-language pathology who developed the framework of form-content-use to define communicative competency.

body aid: Type of hearing aid which involves a battery pack and amplifier worn in a harness that delivers sound to the ears. A very powerful hearing aid.

body language: A form of nonverbal communication that involves use of various parts of the body. Arm crossing is a simple example of body language.

bolus: Food that has been chewed and mixed in the mouth with saliva.

bone conduction testing: Test of hearing that bypasses the outer and middle ear by sending sound vibrations through the skull bones toward the cochlea.

bone-anchored hearing aid (BAHA): A surgical implant for the treatment of hearing loss that works through bone conduction.

bound morphemes: A morpheme that cannot stand alone as an independent word while carrying lexical meaning when attached to another morpheme.

brachycephaly: Condition in which the head is disproportionately wide (or flattened).

bradykinesia: An abnormal slowness in the execution of movement.

brainstem nuclei: A cluster of sensory or motor nuclei located in the brainstem.

breathy voice: Quality of voice production where excessive air accompanies the voice.

Bridgman, Laura: First deaf-blind child in the United States to gain a formal education.

Broca, Paul: French neurosurgeon responsible for naming the region in the left frontal lobe responsible for speech production (Broca's area).

Broca's aphasia: Expressive language disorder in which a person is able to comprehend language but has difficulty executing the motor movements to produce words. A form of nonfluent aphasia.

Brodmann, Korbinian: German neurologist who mapped the cerebral cortex into 52 distinct functional areas.

Brodnitz, Friedrich: Well-known medical specialist in the treatment of vocal disorders, particularly those associated with singing.

bronchial tubes: Series of subdivided tubes that carry air to and from the mouth and the lungs. The smallest of these tubes are called bronchioles.

Brown, Hallie Quinn: The American daughter of former slaves who was a black civil rights leader, teacher, and elocutionist.

Bryngelson, Bryng: Pioneer in the speech-language pathology profession in the United States. He had a particular interest in the area of stuttering.

BTE: *See* behind-the-ear aid.

Butler, Margaret F. An American pioneer in the area of otolaryngology.

Campbell-Swinton, Alan Archibald (A. A.): Engineer from the United States who was the first to envision the development of a television signal.

captioning (closed): An assistive listening device that provides a visual display of text on a television screen.

Carhart, Raymond: The "Father of Modern-Day Audiology" in the United States.

Carter, Henry Vandyke: English anatomist who was responsible for drawing all of the anatomic illustrations in the famous textbook, *Gray's Anatomy*.

CAS: *See* childhood apraxia of speech; central auditory system.

case history: A detailed account of facts gathered about an individual or family that have analytic value for assessing medical, educational, or psychological conditions.

Casserius, Julio: Italian anatomist who made an important contribution to the study of voice.

castrato: An adult male with a singing voice equivalent to a soprano that occurs as a result of castration (removal of testicles) or an endocrine disorder.

CBT: *See* cognitive behavioral therapy.

cell: The basic unit of life.

cellular anatomy and physiology: The microscopic study of cells and tissues. Also called histology.

central auditory system (CAS): Portion of the auditory system consisting of the auditory nerve, brainstem, and brain.

central nervous system (CNS): Portion of the nervous system consisting of the brain, brainstem, and spinal cord.

centromere: Region of a chromosome where the arms of a chromosome intersect.

cerebral palsy: A nonprogressive disorder that effects muscle tone, movement, and motor skills.

cerebrovascular accident: A condition where the blood supply to the brain is disturbed in some way resulting in brain cell death. Also called stroke.

cerebrum: The largest portion of the brain divided into two hemispheres.

Certificate of Clinical Competency: A qualification granted by the American Speech-Language-Hearing Association to audiologists and speech-language pathologists who meet the educational and clinical criteria for independent practice.

cerumen: A normally extruded product of the ear canal. Also known as earwax.

cervical (neck) auscultation: Use of a stethoscope placed on the neck to listen to sounds produced during swallowing.

chemical communication: Form of communication where an animal species produces a chemical that is interpreted by other members of the same species.

child-centered therapy: Approach to working with a communicatively impaired child in which the therapist provides treatment to the child that is geared around the child's naturally occurring play activity.

childhood apraxia of speech (CAS): A type of speech sound production disorder characterized by inconsistent misarticulations patterns. Considered to be a rare and poorly understood disorder.

Chomsky, Noam: American linguist who proposed the nativist theory of early language acquisition.

chorionic villus sampling: A medical procedure used in the prenatal diagnosis of chromosomal and fetal abnormalities.

chromosomes: A threadlike strand of DNA and proteins that are found in every cell nucleus of a living organism.

CIC: *See* completely-in-the-canal aid.

circumlocution: A roundabout manner of talking rather than using specific, direct language.

Class I malocclusion: Normal alignment of the upper and lower jaw, with the exception of some minor dental abnormalities.

Class II malocclusion: Abnormal alignment of the upper and lower jaw, indicative of a severe overbite.

Class III malocclusion: Abnormal alignment of the upper and lower jaw, indicative of a severe underbite.

cleft lip or palate: The lack of fusion of the lip and/or palate during embryonic development.

cleft palate team: A collective group of specialists in various aspects of medical, health, and educational care who work together to assist individuals with a cleft lip/palate.

Clerc, Laurent: The "Father of Deaf Education" in the United States.

cliché level: A form of communication between individuals that involves low level of intimacy.

cloning: The process of producing a genetically identical organism.

cluttering: A fluency disorder characterized by excessively fast speaking rate and word formulation difficulties.

CNS: *See* central nervous system.

cochlea: Snail-shell shaped structure that serves as the hearing organ of the inner ear.

cochlear implant: Surgically implanted device in the cochlea that provides individuals with a sense of sound. The implant does not restore normal hearing.

cochlear nucleus: The location in the central auditory system where the auditory nerve inserts to the base of the brainstem.

code of ethics: A series of broad statements created by a professional body to guide members of the association in their ethical decision making.

cognitive behavioral therapy (CBT): A psychotherapy approach that focuses on correcting patterns of thinking that are maladaptive.

cognitive-communication disorder: Broad term used to describe a wide range of communication problems that result from damage to regions of the brain that control the ability to think.

columella: Fleshy portion of skin under the nose that separates the left and right nostrils.

concussion: Direct blow to the head which may result from violent shaking of the head, or a whiplash type of injury.

contrecoup: Head injury that involves a secondary injury that is opposite to the primary injury whereby the brain essentially rocks back and forth.

coma: A state of extreme unresponsiveness in which the individual exhibits no voluntary movement.

communication: The process of transferring information from one source to another.

communication disorder: An inability to understand or use speech and language to relate to others in society.

complete cleft lip: The complete separation of the lip extending to the nostril.

complete cleft palate: The complete separation from the palate extending from the alveolar ridge to the uvula.

completely-in-the-canal aid (CIC): A miniaturized hearing aid that fits entirely into the ear canal. Typically used by individuals with mild to moderate hearing losses.

complex sound: A sound that contains more than one frequency component.

conductive hearing loss: A hearing loss associated with a problem in the transmission of sound through either the outer or middle ear.

congenital deafness: A profound hearing loss that is found at birth.

congenital disorder: An abnormal physical, cognitive, or medical condition that is found at birth.

connectionism: A theory regarding locations in the cerebrum that are responsible for specific body functions.

connotative: Denotes or implies an attribute.

consecutive bilingualism: Form of bilingualism in which the primary language was learned first followed by learning of another language.

consonant voicing: A classification of consonants based on the presence of vocal fold vibration during articulation of the sound. The sounds /b/ and /z/ are examples of voiced consonants. The sounds /p/ and /s/ are examples of voiceless consonants.

continuous phonation: A stuttering therapy technique that involves constant use of vocal fold vibration across word and phrase boundaries as a means of maintaining speech fluency.

cooing: An early vocal behavior produced by infants that involves use of k-like and g-like sounds during comfort vocalizations. Also known as gooing.

Cooper, Herbert K: Physician from Pennsylvania who was a pioneer in the development of cleft palate teams to assist those with a cleft lip/palate.

cortex: The surface area of the cerebrum.

Corti, Alfonso: Italian anatomist who provided a detailed description of the inner ear, with particular reference to the cochlea. The organ of Corti is named in his honor.

covert repair theory: A theory of stuttering that attributes the disorder to a temporal impairment in the phonological encoding of words prior to actual speech production.

cranial nerves: A series of 12 sensory and motor nerves that emerge directly from the brainstem.

craniectomy: Surgical removal of a portion of the skull.

craniofacial abnormality: A congenital disorder that primarily affects the skull and facial bones.

craniosynostosis: Premature fusing of the cranial sutures that results in restricted growth of the skull.

Cri du Chat syndrome: A syndrome resulting from genetic material missing from chromosome 5. Also known as chromosome 5p-deletion syndrome or Cry of the Cat syndrome because of the distinctive vocal features.

Crick, Francis: British physicist and Nobel Prize winner for discovering the double-helix structure of DNA. His colleague who assisted in the discovery was James Watson.

cricoid cartilage: A part of the laryngeal framework, consisting of a ring-shaped cartilage that sits on top of the trachea.

Crouzon, Louis Octave: French neurosurgeon who was the first to describe the craniosynostosis syndrome, later named Crouzon syndrome.

Crouzon syndrome: Genetic disorder caused by mutations on the long arm of chromosome 10. A distinctive feature of the syndrome is the premature fusion of the cranium sutures. Also called craniofacial dystosis.

crying: The earliest vocal behavior demonstrated by infants.

cued speech: A means of communication in which a speaker uses hand signals to clarify ambiguous mouth movements for lip readers.

culture: A set of attitudes, values, beliefs, and goals shared by a group.

Cupid's bow: The curve of the upper lip indicated by a slight dip, said to resemble the bow of Cupid, the Roman god of love.

cycle: One complete back and forth movement of vibration.

cycles approach: Treatment approach for working with severely phonologically disordered children. The approach emphasizes a wide range of sound productions by the child that are addressed in a series of repetitive cycles.

cytomegalovirus: A form of the herpes virus that rarely causes serious illness in healthy adults. However, the disease can have devastating effects on a newborn.

Darwin, Charles: English naturalist who laid the foundations of the theory of evolution.

de León, Pedro Ponce: Spanish monk who is often credited as being the first teacher of the deaf.

dB: *See* decibel scale.

deaf-blind: A condition in which both sound and sight are profoundly impaired.

deafness: Complete or partial loss of hearing.

debate: Form of communication that involves engagement in argument by discussing opposing points of view.

decibel scale (dB): The unit of measure for loudness.

decode: To extract the underlying meaning of a signal.

deep brain stimulation: Surgical treatment involving the implantation of a brain pacemaker that sends electrical signals to specific parts of the brain. Used as an approach to the treatment of Parkinson disease.

deglutition: The medical term for swallowing.

Déjerine-Klumpke, Augusta: Pioneering French neurologist known for her contributions to neurology and neuroanatomy.

Demands and Capacities theory: A theory of stuttering that views moments of disfluency as resulting when a child's capacities for fluency are not equal to speech performance demands.

dementia: A progressive decline in cognitive function due to damage or disease in the body.

denotative: A word that has distinct meaning.

dentition: The type, number, and alignment of a set of teeth.

deoxyribonucleic acid (DNA): The genetic material found in the cells of all living organisms.

developmental disorder: A condition that is assumed to have been present at birth; however, in some cases the manifestation of the disorder is not visible until the child matures.

dialect: A variety of language this is spoken among a particular group. A dialect is rule-governed and has distinct linguistic features.

dialogue: A form of communication that involves a conversation between two or more people.

diaphragm: A dome-shaped muscle that sits below the lungs. The muscle is most active during the process of inspiration.

Dieffenbach, Johann Friedrich: German physician who performed pioneering surgery for maxillofacial disorders.

direct laryngoscopy: Procedure in which an otolaryngologist uses an instrument such as a flexible scope to examine the vocal folds.

discourse: A type of communication that involves a verbal exchange.

discussion: A formal discourse on a topic.

disfluency: A disruption in the forward flow of speech.

disfluency cluster: The occurrence of two or more disfluencies on the same word and/or adjacent words.

displays: Form of visual communication used by animals to attract or warn off a predator.

dissection: The process of disassembling and observing an anatomic structure to determine its internal structure.

distortion: Type of speech sound misarticulations in which a consonant or vowel is misarticulated to such and extent that the sound produced is unrecognizable.

DNA: *See* deoxyribonucleic acid.

Down, John Langdon: English physician who is best known for his description of what is now called Down syndrome.

Down syndrome: Chromosomal disorder caused by the presence of an extra 21st chromosome. Also known as trisomy 21.

drug therapy: An approach to the treatment of disease by the administration of drugs, chemicals, and antibiotics.

DuMont, Allen B: American inventor of the picture tube that allowed for mass production of television sets.

Dutrochet, Henri: French physiologist who is credited with identifying the cell.

dysarthria: A motor speech disorder characterized by poor speech sound articulation.

dysphagia: Medical term for the symptom of difficulty in swallowing.

dysphonation: An unusual form of voice production, often characterized by moments of chaotic vocal fold vibration.

echolalia: The repetition of words or phrases made by an individual. A feature of speaking often associated with autism. The manner of echolalia can be either immediate or delayed.

echolocation: A sensory system used by animals such as dolphins and bats using high-pitched sounds to determine the direction and distance of objects. Also called biosonar.

edema: Medical condition in which abnormally large volumes of fluid enter muscle tissue.

elective therapy: Form of speech-language therapy that is based on helping an individual improve their communication abilities, although there is no diagnosed communication disorder. A person who speaks English as a second language may seek elective therapy to help reduce their accent.

electroencephalograph (EEG): The recording of electrical activity along the scalp produced by the firing of neurons within the brain.

electrolarynx: Device that is intended to reproduce the role of the vocal folds in patients who have had their larynx removed. A hand-held device that produces audible vibrations is placed against the neck and the person "mouths" speech sounds.

electromyography (EMG): A technique for testing and recording the electrical activity of muscles.

electropalatograph (EPG): Device that records the timing and location of tongue contact with the hard palate during speaking activities. Also called a palatometer.

Elocutionary Movement: Approach to speaking in the 18th century concerned with the skill of communication in public settings, such as poetry readings, speeches, or plays.

embolism: An obstruction in a blood vessel due to a blot clot.

embryo: An organism in its early stages of development, especially before it reaches a recognizable form.

embryology: Branch of biology that deals with the formation and early development of living organisms.

Empedocles: Greek philosopher who speculated on the origins of life and human development.

encode: The process of creating a message into code.

endolymph: Thick fluid that fills the cochlear duct of the inner ear.

endolymphatic hydrops: An over-accumulation of endolymph in the inner ear. Often found to be a cause of Ménière's disease.

English as a second language (ESL): A person who first acquired a language other than English.

ENT: *See* otolaryngologist.

enteral tubes: A tube used for the delivery of nutrition that bypasses normal ingestion of food through the mouth.

epidemiology: Branch of medicine that deals with the causes, distribution, and control of disease within a population.

epiglottis: A leaf-shaped flap of cartilage that covers the trachea during moments of swallowing.

ESL: *See* English as a second language.

esophageal dysphagia: A disorder of swallowing that is due to abnormal function in the esophagus.

esophageal speech: An alternative approach to producing speech without using the vocal folds. A form of speaking used by people having undergone a laryngectomy.

esophageal stage: The third and final stage in the process of swallowing.

esophagitis: Inflammation of the lining of the esophagus.

esophagus: The muscular tube that connects the throat to the stomach.

ethical behavior: Behavior that conforms to accepted professional standards of conduct.

ethnicity: Term that represents social groups with a shared sense of identity, geography, culture, and history.

ethology: The study of animal behavior with special interest in genetically programmed behaviors known as instincts.

etiology: The study of causation.

Eustachi, Bartolomeo: Italian anatomist who described structures of the human body including the eustachian tube of the ear.

eustachian tube: Hollow structure of bone and cartilage extending from the middle ear to the back of the upper throat (nasopharynx).

evidence-based practice: A decision-making process based on considering the best available research. In medicine, it is used to help make informed, clinical decisions for patient care.

exhalation phase: The outward flow of air comprising one phase of the breathing cycle.

external auditory meatus: A cartilaginous and bony tube that runs from the outer ear to the tympanic membrane. Also called the ear canal.

fact level: Form of communication between individuals that involves a low level of intimacy, such as the simple exchange of factual information.

Fairbanks, Grant: American Professor in the field of communication disorders who developed techniques for treating speech sound disorders.

falsetto: Voice register of males that is above (higher than) the normal speaking range.

fast mapping: A mental process whereby a new concept can be learned based on a single exposure to the concept.

feedback loops: Information about the result of an event or action is sent back to the original input of the system. In the case of communication, the speaker obtains feedback from the listener regarding the original message uttered.

feeding tube: Medical device used to provide nutrition to a person who is unable to obtain nutrition through normal swallowing.

feelings level: Form of communication between individuals that involves a high level of intimacy between speakers.

FEES: *See* fiberoptic endoscopic evaluation of swallowing.

Ferrein, Antoine: French anatomist known for his work concerning the physiology of the voice. He is credited with coining the term vocal cords.

fetal alcohol syndrome: Birth defect that affects physical and cognitive development resulting from mothers who consumed alcohol during pregnancy.

fetus: Unborn child, spanning the period from 8 weeks following conception to the moment of birth.

fiberoptic endoscopic evaluation of swallow (FEES): Procedure for evaluating the oral stage of swallowing based on examination of the oral/pharyngeal cavity with the use of a fiberoptic endoscope.

finger spelling: The representation of letters and numbers of a writing system with the use of one or two hands. A system of communication commonly used by individuals with severe and profound hearing loss.

fissure: A long narrow opening. Fissures along the cerebral cortex provide points of demarcation for the various lobes of the brain.

fixed articulators: Speech articulators that have no movable action. Examples of fixed articulators include the teeth and hard palate.

fluctuating hearing loss: Condition in which a person's hearing may improve or worsen from one day to the next.

fluency: The effortless flow of speech that includes proper use of rhythm, rate, pausing, and language formulation.

fluency shaping: A comprehensive therapy for the treatment of stuttering that focuses on changing all speaking behavior, not just moments of stuttering.

fluent aphasia: Language disorder in which a person has difficulty comprehending spoken and written language, although their ability to speak seems to remain relatively intact.

FOXP2: Gene located on chromosome 7 which has been implicated in the development of normal speech and language skills.

Fragile X syndrome: Most common form of inherited intellectual disability that results in a mutation of a gene located on the X chromosome. Also called Martin-Bell syndrome.

Franco, Pierre: 16th century Swiss surgeon known as the "Father of Cleft Palate Surgery."

free morpheme: The smallest unit of language that can occur by itself.

frequency: The number of vibrations that occur per second.

frequency transposition: Technique used in the programming of hearing aids that extends the audibility of higher frequency sounds for people who cannot receive this information from a conventional hearing aid.

fricatives: A category of consonant sounds classified according to the manner in which they are articulated in the vocal tract. The /s/ and /f/ consonants are examples of fricatives.

frontal lobes: The front of the cerebral cortex. Primarily involved in the execution of motor movement, as well as mental reasoning.

front-back confusion: Impairment in the ability to perceive the origin (direction) of a sound source.

functional disorder: Any disorder that results in the absence of a known anatomic, physiologic, or neurologic cause.

functional dysphagia: Form of dysphagia that has no identifiable, organic cause.

fundamental frequency: The lowest frequency component of a complex sound.

Gage, Phineas: One of the earliest documented cases of a severe brain injury and its impact on mental function following recovery. Gage resided in Vermont (United States).

Galen, Claudius: Second century physiologist who is often considered the founder of laryngology and voice science.

Gall, Franz Joseph: German anatomist and pioneer in the study of brain functions. Developed a system for studying the brain by noting the shape of the skull called phrenology.

Gallaudet, Thomas: American educator and founder of the first American school for the deaf in Hartford, Connecticut (United States).

García, Manuel: Spaniard who developed the laryngeal mirror.

gastroesophageal reflux disease (GERD): A chronic condition in which stomach acid is regurgitated resulting in heartburn and indigestion.

gastronomy tube: Feeding tube used in situations when a person is unable to swallow normally. The tube is placed directly into the stomach and is used to deliver nutrition to the body. Also called a percutaneous endoscopic gastrostomy (PEG) tube.

gaze-coupling: An early form of communicative exchange between a young infant and parent where the infant turns toward the speaker and gains eye contact.

gene mutation: A permanent change in the DNA that makes up a gene.

gene splicing: Form of genetic engineering where specific genes are inserted into the genome of a different organism.

genes: Hereditary unit that occupies a specific location on a chromosome and determines a particular characteristic in an organism.

genetic counseling: A service that is designed to help families who may be at risk for an inherited disease or abnormal pregnancy outcome, and discussing the chances of having children who are affected.

genetic syndromes: A disorder caused by abnormalities in one or more genes.

genetics: Branch of biology that deals with hereditary and the transmission of characteristics among organisms.

genome: The total DNA sequence that characterizes a species, including humans.

genotype: The genetic makeup of an organism.

geographic dialects: Variations in the style of speaking according to geographic region. A New England dialect is an example of a geographic dialect.

GERD: *See* gastroesophageal reflux disease.

glides: A category of consonants sounds classified according to the manner in which they are articulated in the vocal tract. The /w/ is an example of a glide.

globus: The sensation of a lump in the throat.

glossectomy: Surgical removal of all or a portion of the tongue.

glottal stop (?): A speech sound produced by a momentary complete closure of the glottis followed by an explosive release.

glottis: The space between the open vocal folds.

Goodall, Jane: Renowned English primatologist and ethologist. One of the world's foremost authorities on the behavior of chimpanzees.

Gray, Henry: 19th century English anatomist whose classic publication regarding human anatomy, *Gray's Anatomy*, is still used today.

grommet: See pressure equalization tube.

gross anatomy: Study of organs, parts, and structures of a body that are visible to the naked eye.

group communication: The interactive exchange of information that occurs among more then 3 people, and usually no more then 20 people.

Gutenberg, Johann: German inventor of the printing press in the 15th century.

Gutzmann, Hermann: German physician who studied speech disorders from a medical point of view.

gyri: A bump or ridge like those found along the surface of the cerebral cortex.

habitual pitch: The speaking voice that is most commonly used.

hair cells: Sensory receptors that are found in the inner ear (cochlea and vestibular apparatus).

hard of hearing: A person who has any level of hearing impairment other than deafness.

hard palate: Bony roof of the mouth that separates the nasal cavity from the oral cavity.

Hawk, Sara Stinchfield: First individual in the United States to obtain a PhD in speech-language pathology.

hearing aid: Device that can amplify sound waves in order to help a hard-of-hearing person perceive sounds more clearly.

helix: The cartilaginous rim of the outer ear.

hemispheres: The two halves of a circle. The cerebrum (brain) is divided into a left and right hemisphere.

hemorrhage: Excessive loss of blood from blood vessels.

Henry, Joseph: American scientist of the 18th century whose early work in electromagnetism eventually led to the development of the telegraph.

heredity: The genetic transmission of characteristics from parent to offspring.

Hertz, Heinrich: German physicist who was the first to send and receive radio waves.

hertz (Hz) scale: Notation used to refer to frequency, or the number of vibrations per second. Developed in honor of Heinrich Hertz.

hieratic: A cursive form of Egyptian hieroglyphics.

hieroglyphics: System of writing using pictorial symbols to represent sounds or meanings.

high-frequency hearing loss: A configuration of hearing loss where a person is unable to clearly perceive sounds that are in excess of 1000 to 2000 Hz.

Hippocrates: Greek physician who described the importance of the lungs, trachea, lips, and tongue in phonation in the early 5th century BC.

hoarse voice: A description of voice quality, involving an unusually low-pitched voice.

Hooke, Robert: English philosopher who coined the term "cell" to refer to the basic unit of life.

Human Genome Project: An international scientific undertaking to determine the complete structure of the human genetic material known as DNA.

Husson, Raoul: French physiologist who proposed one of the earliest modern theories of normal voice production known as the Neurochronaxic theory.

hyoid bone: A horseshoe-shaped bone located high in the neck. The most superior portion of the laryngeal framework.

hyperfunctional voice: Speaking with excessive muscular effort and force resulting in a tense, high-pitched voice. A form of spasmodic dysphonia.

hypernasal speech: Abnormal speech characterized by the excess flow of sound through the nasal cavity.

hypnotherapy: Approach to the treatment of a variety of health conditions by hypnotism or by inducing prolonged sleep.

hypofunctional voice: Refers to inadequate muscle tone of the laryngeal mechanism during the production of voice often resulting in weak, low-pitched voice that may also sound breathy. Found in some conditions associated with muscle weakness such as amyotrophic lateral sclerosis (ALS).

hypotonia: Decrease of normal muscle tone or tension.

idioglossia: Term used to describe a unique, specialized language thought to be indicative of the early speech spoken by twins.

idioms: Words or phrase that cannot be taken literally. *A drop in the bucket* is one such example.

idiopathic: A condition that is of unknown origin.

immittance testing: Form of audiologic testing that provides information regarding eardrum mobility and ear drum function. Often called tympanometry.

in-the-canal aid (ITC): Type of hearing aid where all components of the aid are situated directly within the ear canal.

in-the-ear aid (ITE): Type of hearing aid where all components of the aid are situated within the entrance of the ear canal.

incidence: The number of new cases that occur during a particular period of time.

incomplete cleft palate: A cleft that does not encompass the entire hard and soft palate structure, only a portion is affected.

incomplete cleft lip: A cleft that does not penetrate the nostrils.

incus: The middle bone of the three small bones (ossicles) of the middle ear. Also known as the anvil, reflecting its unique shape.

indirect laryngoscopy: Procedure in which an otolaryngologist uses an instrument, such as a mirror, to examine the vocal folds.

infant: A child under the age of 12 months. Derived from the Latin word meaning "without speech."

inhalation phase: The inward flow of air comprising one phase of a breathing cycle.

instant messaging: Form of real-time communication between two or more people based on typed text over the internet.

intelligence quotient (IQ): A measure used to estimate intellect, usually calculated by examining the ratio of a person's mental age compared to their chronological age.

intelligibility: Term used to describe the clarity of a person's speech sound productions.

interactionist theory: The theory that language learning is influenced by the desire of children to communicate with others. Interactionists believe language development involves a combination of behavioral and nativist processes.

International Classification of Functioning (ICF): Framework developed by the World Health Organization that classifies health according to a number of domains.

International Phonetic Alphabet (IPA): System of phonetic notation developed by the International Phonetic Association that can be used to represent the sounds of any language.

Internet: An interconnected system of networks that allows for communication between computers around the world.

interpersonal communication: Form of communication that occurs between two or more people.

Iowa Scale for Rating the Severity of Stuttering: Scale used for determining the severity of speech disfluency based on noting the number and type of speech disfluencies occurring within a conversational speech sample.

Itard, Jean-Marc Gaspard: French physician known for his work with deaf and intellectually impaired individuals, particularly Victor, the wild boy of Aveyron.

ITC: *See* in-the-canal aid.

ITE: *See* in-the-ear aid.

itinerant SLP: A speech-language pathologist who works in a number of settings. SLPs who are employed by an educational system tend to work in more than one school setting.

Janssen, Zaccharias: Dutch spectacle-maker who is believed to be the inventor of the microscope.

Jefferson, Thomas: Third President of the United States and a follower of the Elocutionary Movement.

Johnson, Wendell: American speech-language pathologist known for his work in stuttering.

Kanner, Leo: Austrian psychiatrist known for his work in autism. First individual to define autism based on examination of 11 self-absorbed children who had "autistic disturbances of affect contact."

karyotype: The arrangement of chromosomes within a cell.

Keller, Helen: American who was the first deaf-blind person to achieve a university education, and later became an advocate for individuals with disabilities.

King Louis II: King of France during the period of 843 to 879 who was known to stutter.

L1: Abbreviation used to designate the first or dominant language.

L2: Abbreviation used to designate the second or less dominant language.

labiodental: A class of consonants that are categorized according to their place of articulation within the vocal tract. The /f/ and /v/ are examples of labiodental consonants.

laceration: A wound or cut which involves direct tearing of tissue.

Lahey, Margaret: American professor who developed a framework for describing the various strands of language according to form, content, and use.

Lahsley, Karl: American psychologist who was interested in the brain mechanisms contributing to learning and memory.

language: The expression of human communication through which information can be experienced, explained, and shared.

language acquisition device: Proposed by Noam Chomsky as a special biological brain mechanism that humans are born with that enables them to learn language.

language content: Aspect of language that concerns meanings of individual words and words in combination. Another name for language content is semantics.

language delay: A language disorder indicating that the child's language system is similar to younger, nondisordered children.

language deviance: A language disorder in which the child exhibits a linguistic system that is unlike that of younger nondisordered children.

language difference: Situation in which the language features of a community differ from the majority. The grammatical rules are normal for the smaller community.

language expansions: Language therapy approach in which the therapist restates the child's utterance using a fuller and grammatically correct language model.

language form: Aspect of language that concerns the features of phonology, morphology, and syntax.

language sampling: Feature of a language assessment in which a representative sample of the child's typical expressive language behavior is collected and later analyzed.

language use: Aspect of language in a social context. Another name for language use is pragmatics.

Larsen, George L.: American speech-language pathologist who was one of the first individuals to develop specific treatment techniques for individuals with dysphagia.

laryngectomy: Partial or complete removal of the larynx, including the vocal folds. The most common form of surgery to treat laryngeal cancer.

laryngitis: Inflammation of the vocal folds, associated with symptoms of sore throat and swallowing difficulty.

larynx: Structural framework that consists of a number of muscles and cartilages that work cooperatively to produce voice.

late talker: a group of children who have an impoverished expressive vocabulary, usually within the age range of 16 to 30 months of life.

Lee Silverman Voice Treatment (LSVT): A structured programmatic approach to voice therapy. The premise of the approach is to encourage a full, loud speaking voice to improve overall voice quality as well as speech clarity.

Lejeune, Jerome: French geneticist who discovered the chromosome abnormalities in humans that causes Down syndrome, as well as Cri du Chat syndrome.

Lidcombe Program: Stuttering treatment program developed in Australia and designed for children younger than 6 years of age.

limbic system: A region deep within the cerebrum that includes part or most of the other lobes (i.e., frontal, parietal, and temporal). The limbic system is involved in affective behaviors such as emotion and motivation.

lingua-alveolar: A class of consonants categorized according to their place of articulation within the vocal tract. Examples of lingua-alveolar consonants are /t/ and /s/.

linguadental: A class of consonants categorized according to their place of articulation within the vocal tract. An example of a linguadental consonant is /th/.

lingual frenulum: Tendon that extends from the floor of the mouth to the underside of the tongue.

linguapalatal: A class of consonants categorized according to their place of articulation within the vocal tract. An example of a linguapalatal consonant is /sh/.

linguavelar: A class of consonants categorized according to their place of articulation within the vocal tract. Examples of linguavelar consonants are /k/ and /g/.

lips: Two bands of muscular tissue encircling the mouth.

liquids: A class of consonant sounds organized according to the manner in which they are articulated in the vocal tract. The consonants /r/ and /l/ are examples of liquids.

lobule: An anatomic extension such as that found at the base of the outer ear.

Logemann, Jeri A.: American professor and speech-language pathologist who is a pioneer in the assessment and treatment of dysphagia.

loudness: The psychological perception of the intensity of an acoustic signal.

lower respiratory tract: The cavities of the body which include the trachea, bronchial tubes, and lungs.

LSVT: *See* Lee Silverman Voice Treatment.

lungs: Two spongy organs encased within the ribcage that function to remove carbon dioxide from the body and provide it with oxygen.

magnetic resonance imaging (MRI): Test that uses a magnetic field and pulses of radio wave energy to make a high resolution picture of organs and structures inside the body.

malingerer: Someone who intentionally fakes or exaggerates a psychological or physical condition for personal gain.

malleus: Outermost of the three small bones (ossicles) of the middle ear. Also known as the hammer, reflecting its unique shape.

malocclusion: An uneven alignment between the upper and lower teeth.

mandible: Anatomical name for the lower jaw.

manner of articulation: Classification of consonant sounds in regard to how they are articulated in the vocal tract.

manual communication: Use of hand gestures to transfer information between individuals. Hand waving and hand shaking are simple forms of manual communication.

Marconi, Gugliemo: Italian inventor who is generally credited with creating the radio.

mastication: The act of chewing.

maximal contrast approach: Treatment approach for phonological disorders that is designed to enact widespread change. Rather than targeting early developing sounds, later developing sounds are the focus of therapy.

mean length of utterance (MLU): A measure that examines a child's increasing ability to combine words and produced complex utterances by noting the average length of utterances according to grammatical morphemes.

medical model: Approach to the identification of disorders on the basis of an identifiable physical cause.

Mendel, Gregor: Austrian botanist who is known as the "Father of Modern Genetics" based on his work with pea plants.

Ménière, Prosper: French otolaryngologist who was the first to describe a form of vertigo (dizziness) that is now known as Ménière's disease.

Ménière's disease: Disorder of the inner ear that can affect balance and hearing.

meningitis: Infection of the fluid that surrounds the brain and spinal cord. The condition is cause by either viral or bacterial infection.

metacentric chromosome: A chromosome with a centrally placed centromere that divides the chromosome into two arms having approximately equal length.

metalinguistic awareness: The ability to reflect consciously on the nature and properties of language.

microcephaly: Abnormal smallness of the head.

microform cleft: Rare anomaly that can appear as a small scar on the lip.

micrognathia: A condition of abnormal smallness of the upper and lower jaws, usually the mandible.

microphone: A transducer designed to transform acoustic energy into an equivalent electrical representation.

middle ear implant: A surgical procedure designed to stimulate movement of the ossicles of the middle ear to incoming sound, as a means of improving hearing.

minimal pair: Refers to a situation where two words differ in pronunciation by only one sound, and the change in sound results in a change in word meaning. The words "dear" and "gear" are examples of minimal pairs.

misarticulation: Any deviation, great or small, in the pronunciation of a consonant or vowel.

mixed (or global) aphasia: Communication disorder that involves impairment in both comprehension and production of language. Generally considered the most severe form of aphasia.

mixed hearing loss: Simultaneous occurrence of both a conductive hearing loss and sensorineural hearing loss.

MLU: *See* mean length of utterance.

modal register: The middle range of one's speaking voice.

monotonic voice: Lack of natural melodic voice inflection. A condition associated with the speaking voice of individual's with Parkinson disease.

Morgan, Thomas Hunt: American pioneer in the area of genetics. Received the Nobel Prize for his work on hereditary traits of fruit flies.

morphology: The smallest meaningful units of language.

Morse code: Alphabetic system for the telegraph that uses a combination of short and long acoustic clicks to create words.

Morse, Samuel: American creator of the telegraph in the 19th century.

mosaicism: Condition in which the cells comprising an organism are not identical, having differing genotypes.

motor speech disorders: Impaired speech sound production ability resulting from nervous system pathway damage affecting the muscles responsible for producing speech.

mouth breathing: Process of inhalation and exhalation through the oral cavity rather than the nasal cavity.

movable articulators: Anatomical structures involved in speech production that are capable of moving. Examples of movable articulators include the lips, tongue, and soft palate.

MRI: *See* magnetic resonance imaging.

multilingualism: Individual who has knowledge of two or more languages. This knowledge may include the ability to speak, understand, read, or write more than one language.

multiple sclerosis (MS): Disease in which the nerves of the central nervous system degenerate causing an impairment of movement, sensation, and body functions.

Mutual Recognition of Credentials Agreement: Pact signed by various speech-language pathology professional organizations worldwide that provides a framework for professionals from one country to practice as therapists in another country.

myelin sheath: The insulating envelope that surrounds the core of a nerve fiber (axon) to facilitate the transmission of nerve impulses.

Myoelastic aerodynamic theory: Well accepted theory of voice production that involves coordination of muscle tension and breath pressure.

myringotomy: Surgical incision into the tympanic membrane (eardrum) that is usually performed to relieve pressure or fluid buildup in the middle ear.

nares: The external openings of the nose. Also called nostrils.

nasal cavity: The cavity lying between the base of the skull and the roof of the mouth and extending from the nostrils to the pharynx.

nasals: A class of consonant sounds categorized according to the manner in which they are articulated in the vocal tract. The consonants /m/ and /n/ are examples of nasal consonants.

nasogastric tube (or NG tube): Type of feeding tube used on a short-term basis and involves passing a tube through the nose, pharynx, and esophagus directly into the stomach.

nativist theory: A theory of normal language acquisition proposed by Noam Chomsky, which suggests that humans are born with the biological makeup to learn language.

natural theory: A theory of phonological development proposed by David Stampe based on the natural occurrence and suppression of phonological patterns (or processes).

needs level: The level of communication that occurs between two people who know one another intimately. They seem to know intuitively what the other person thinks.

Negus, Sir Victor: British laryngologist who was a pioneer in detailing the anatomy of the human and animal larynx.

neural plasticity: Refers to the ability of the brain and/or certain parts of the nervous system to change in order to adapt to new conditions, such as an injury.

neural tube defects: Congenital abnormality of the brain and spinal cord resulting from incomplete closing of the neural tube during embryonic development. Spina bifida is an example of a neural tube defect.

Neurochronaxic theory: A theory proposed in 1950 that viewed the frequency of vocal fold vibration as being dependent upon excitation of nerve cells from the laryngeal nerve.

neurogenic: Refers to having its origin or starting with the nervous system.

neurogenic stuttering: Form of stuttering characterized by a high number of involuntary repetitions or prolongations of speech that do not seem to be a result of poor (hesitant) language formulation difficulties or as a result of psychiatric problems. A condition sometimes found in Parkinson disease.

neuromuscular electrical stimulation (E-Stim): An electrical current is used to simulate the same electrical impulses that are activated during normal exercise. By passively activating the muscle, the body responds in much the same way as during normal exercise.

neuroprosthetics: The design and manufacture of neural prosthetics which can serve as a substitute for a motor or sensory modality that may have been damaged. A cochlear implant is a form of neuroprosthetic device.

Neuropsycholinguistic theory: A theory of stuttering based on the assumption that producing fluent speech involves sophisticated timing between the formulation of language and the actual motor execution of speech movement. Stuttering results in a situation where there is a disruption in the timing (integration) of linguistic formulation and speech movement.

noise: Acoustic sound wave that has random variations in amplitude and frequency. A lack of periodicity (back and forth vibration).

noise-induced hearing loss: Hearing impairment that results from exposure to excessively loud sounds.

nonbehavioral tests: Form of audiology testing that does not require the person to push a button or raise their hand in response to sounds. Rather, the tests are designed to measure natural physiological responses to sounds. The auditory brainstem response is a nonbehavioral test.

nonfluent aphasia: Language disorder in which an individual has difficulty expressing himself when speaking or writing, although their ability to understand language seems to remain relatively intact.

nonmaleficence: Ethical principle in health sciences and public health practice in which the professional strives to do no harm to the patient.

nonstandardized testing: Form of assessment in which there is no consistent or standardized manner to perform the assessment. This generally provides the examiner with more flexibility. The collection and analysis of a conversational language sample is a common form of nonstandardized testing.

nonverbal communication: Form of communication in which the exchange of information occurs without the use of spoken words. The use of eye contact is a form of nonverbal communication.

norms: A standard, model, or pattern regarded as typical. Norms are often used to assess individuals who are suspected of having a communication disorder by comparing their performance to that which is expected of normal communicators of the same age.

nucleus: The central part of a cell that contains hereditary material.

obturator: A prosthetic device serving to close an opening in the body, such as a cleft palate.

occipital lobes: The posterior lobe of each cerebral hemisphere that contains the visual centers of the brain.

OD: *See* other disfluencies.

odynophagia: Pain associated with the act of swallowing.

omission: Pattern of speech misarticulations whereby the intended speech sound is deleted.

onomatopoeia: Use of sounds to signify a word based on the sound associated with the particular word. For example, "beep-beep" would be a form of onomatopoeia to signify the word, car.

Operation Smile: International charity program for the surgical treatment of facial deformities such as cleft lip and palate.

opinion level: The level of communication that occurs between two people on a somewhat personal level and includes comments, concerns, expectations, and personal goals.

Optimality Theory: A theoretical approach to describing the structure of grammar in a given language.

optimum pitch: The level at which we can produce our strongest voice.

oral cavity: The space inside the mouth that runs from the inside of the lips to the back of throat.

oral stage: The first stage in the three-stage process of swallowing.

oral-facial examination: A routine assessment of the structure and function of the mouth and face in regard to their influence on speech sound production.

organ of Corti: Specialized structure located within the scala media of the cochlea. The organ contains hair cells that assist in the transfer of sound through the auditory system.

organic disorder: Medical or health condition with a known physical cause.

organizational communication: Type of communication that occurs in environments such as workplace offices and corporations.

oropharyngeal dysphagia: Most common form of dysphagia that reflects an impairment in the transfer of liquid or food from the mouth and pharynx to the opening of the esophagus.

orthognathic surgery: Procedure that is designed to correct conditions of the jaws and face related to structure and growth.

Orton, Samuel: American physician who was interested in the area of learning disabilities, particularly those associated with reading. The Orton Dyslexia Association was originally named in his honor.

ossicular chain: The three tiny bones the comprise the middle ear, consisting of the malleus, incus, and stapes.

other disfluencies (OD): Class of speech disfluencies that are found to occur in the general population of people who do not stutter, as well as those who do stutter. An example of an OD is a phrase repetition.

otitis externa: Infection of the ear canal, often associated with persistent exposure to water. Also called swimmer's ear.

otitis media: Infection of the middle ear space behind the eardrum. The duration of a bout of otitis media can range from acute, to subacute, or chronic.

otitis media with effusion: Form of otitis media characterized by buildup of fluid in the middle ear space. Also called glue ear.

otoacoustic emissions: Tiny sounds that emerge from the inner ear either spontaneously or shortly after the ear is exposed to an external sound. A screening test for newborn hearing.

otolaryngologist: Surgeon who specializes in the diagnosis and treatment of disorders of the ear, nose, or throat. Also called an ENT.

otosclerosis: Hereditary disorder that results in abnormal growth in the middle ear that causes hearing loss.

otoscope: Instrument consisting of a light and magnifying lens that is used for examining the external auditory meatus (ear canal) and tympanic membrane (eardrum).

ototoxic hearing loss: A hearing impairment (both temporary and permanent) that can result from high doses of certain drugs.

pagoclone: Antianxiety drug that is currently being evaluated as a treatment for stuttering.

papilloma: Benign wartlike tumors that form over muscle tissue. Papillomas have been found to form on the vocal folds.

papyrus: Thick paperlike material produced from the papyrus plant. Used by ancient Egyptians as an early form of paper.

paralanguage: The nonverbal features that accompany speech and help convey meaning.

parallel talk: Language therapy approach in which the therapist describes out loud what the child is seeing, hearing, or thinking during a play activity.

Pare, Ambroise: French surgeon in the 16th century renown for his skill.

parent-directed therapy: Feature of speech and language therapy where parents play an active and integral part of the child's therapy program.

parenteral tube: Feeding tube in which nutrition is delivered to the body intravenously. Also called an IV tube.

parietal lobes: The lobes located at the top of the cerebral cortex that are largely responsible for sensation.

Parkinson disease: Degenerative neurologic syndrome of the central nervous system that is characterized by rhythmic muscular tremors.

particulate theories: Early theories of genetics which posited that information from each part of the parent had to be transferred to create the corresponding body part in the offspring.

Passavant, Philip Gustav: German surgeon who was one of the first to propose a series of surgical solutions to help reduce hypernasal speech in cleft lip and palate.

pediatric dysphagia: A swallowing disorder in children.

Penfield, Wilder: American brain surgeon who made contributions to mapping brain function.

percentage of consonants correct: Measure used to determine the severity of an individual's speech sound disorder. The percentage is calculated by examining the total number of consonants comprising a speech sample in comparison to the number of consonants produced accurately by the speaker.

perforated eardrum: Puncture in the tympanic membrane.

perilymph: Fluid that is located in the scala vestibuli and scala media ducts of the cochlea.

peripheral auditory system: Portion of the hearing anatomy which consists of the outer, middle, and inner ear structures.

peripheral nervous system (PNS): Portion of the nervous system that lies outside the brain and spinal cord.

peristalsis: Rippling, wavelike muscle contractions, which occur when food is digested.

Personality and Emotional Adjustment Theory: A theory that considers an individual's personality and subsequent behavioral patterns in the causation of a voice disorder.

pervasive developmental disorder: Group of disorders characterized by delays in development of social, language, motor, and/or cognitive skills.

PET: *See* positron emission tomography.

pharyngeal cavity: See definition for pharynx.

pharyngeal flap: Surgical procedure designed to reduce hypernasality. A flap of skin creates a bridge between the back of the throat and the soft palate to help close off the nasal cavity during speaking.

pharyngeal fricative (ʕ): A unique consonant that is articulated with the root of the tongue against the pharynx.

pharyngeal stage: The second stage in the three-stage process of normal swallowing, where the tongue transports material toward the back of the throat.

pharyngoplasty: Form of surgery to reduce nasality in speech by narrowing the pharynx.

pharynx: Hollow muscular tube that runs from the back of the nose to the top of the trachea (windpipe) and esophagus (food tube). Also called the throat.

phenotype: The observable physical characteristics of an organism.

phenylketonuria (PKU): Genetic disorder characterized by an inability of the body to utilize the amino acid, phenylalanine, which is essential for delivering protein to the body.

pheromones: Chemical secreted by the body that triggers a natural behavioral response in another member of the same species.

philtrum: Shallow groove or depression running down the center of the outer surface of the upper lip.

phonation: Sound made by the vibration of the vocal folds and modified by the resonance of the vocal tract.

phonatory disorder: An abnormality in the ability to produce one's voice.

phonemes: The consonant and vowel sounds spoken in a language.

phonetic inventory: A list of consonant and vowel sounds that a person is able to accurately articulate.

phoniatrics: The medical research and treatment of organs involved in the production of voice.

phonological approach: Form of treating phonological disorders based on a linguistic (as opposed to motoric) approach.

phonological awareness: An understanding of the sounds of words and word parts, including the ability to identify and manipulate larger parts of the spoken language such as words, syllables, and rhyme.

phonological difference: Pattern of speaking found in bilingual speakers where the individual's dominant language affects the pronunciation of the less dominant language. The patterns are predictable based on the phonological features of the dominant language, and therefore not considered to reflect a phonological disorder.

phonological disorder: Impairment in the accurate production of speech sounds.

phonological interference: Pattern of speech sound production found in bilingual speakers, where the phonological patterns of one language affect (interfere with) the pronunciation patterns in another language.

phonological processes: Systematic pattern of speech sound production that affects an entire class of speech sounds. Stopping of fricatives is an example of a phonological process.

phonology: The study of the speech sounds of a language.

phonosurgery: Medical operation designed to repair damage to the vocal folds.

phonotrauma: Any form of abuse to the vocal folds.

phrenology: The study of the shape of the skull that was once thought to reveal a person's personality and mental capacity.

physiology: The biological study of the function of living organisms and their parts.

Piaget, Jean: Swiss psychologist known for his study of the intellectual growth of children.

picture-naming task: Common method of sampling a person's speech sound production skills in which a person is asked to name a picture containing specific consonant and vowels sounds.

pinna: Most visible portion of the outer ear. Also known as the auricle.

pipe speech: Manner of speaking where the upper and lower jaws are immobilized. This effect can be achieved by biting the end of a pipe and speaking at the same time.

pitch: Perceptual impression of the vocal fundamental frequency of an individual's speaking voice.

place of articulation: Description of consonant sounds in regard to the location in the vocal tract where the sound was articulated.

Plato: Ancient Greek philosopher.

PNS: *See* peripheral nervous system.

positron emission tomography (PET) scan: Method of body scanning in which a small amount of radioactive-labeled compound is injected or inhaled in the tissue to be studied.

postauricular muscle response: Electrophysiologic method of testing hearing sensitivity based on detecting muscular activity located behind the outer ear in response to sound.

postlingual deafness: Profound hearing loss that occurred after a person learned to talk.

Prader-Willi syndrome: Genetic disorder caused by deletion of portions of chromosome 15.

pragmatics: The study of language as it is used in a social context.

prelingual deafness: Profound hearing loss that was present before a child learned to talk.

prelinguistic: Refers to the vocal behaviors a child demonstrates prior to producing first words (language). The production of babbling is a prelinguistic vocal behavior.

premorbid state: An individual's health status before the occurrence of a physical disease or emotional illness.

presbycusis: Type of hearing loss which gradually occurs as people grow older.

pressure equalization tube: Small tube that is inserted through the tympanic membrane (eardrum) to provide ventilation to the middle ear. Also known as a grommet.

prevalence: Total number of cases of a disease in a given population at a specific time.

primary auditory center: Region in the temporal lobe of the brain that is responsible for the sensation of sound. Also called Heschl's gyrus.

progressive hearing loss: A hearing loss that gets worse over time. Persistent exposure to loud noise can result in a progressive hearing loss.

proteomics: Branch of genetics that studies the proteins expressed by the genome of an organism.

proxemics: The study of cultural, behavioral, and sociologic aspects of spatial distance between individuals.

psychogenic disorder: A disorder that stems from mental or emotional problems as opposed to having a known physiological cause.

psychogenic stuttering: Type of stuttering thought to be caused by emotional trauma or problems with thought or reasoning. A rare disorder.

puberphonia: Unusually high-pitched speaking voice that persists beyond puberty.

public communication: Form of communication that is used to promote ideas and social causes.

pulse register: Lowest range of speaking voice. Also known as vocal fry register.

pure tone: A sound composed of a single frequency.

pure-tone audiometry: Use of single-frequency sounds (tones) in the evaluation of a person's hearing sensitivity.

race: Group of people classified on the basis of common history, nationality, geographic distribution, or genetically transmitted physical characteristics.

radio: The wireless transmission of electromagnetic waves that are decoded into audible sounds.

reflux: A flowing back of fluid, often associated with the human digestive system and the reflux of gastric juices.

register of voice: The range of voice produced by humans including low, medium, and high-pitched sounds.

rehabilitation hospital: A hospital that is devoted to providing rehabilitation care to patients with various neurologic or orthopedic conditions on an inpatient basis.

residual errors: Pattern of speech sound misarticulations that are related to the production of either a fricative (such as /s/) or liquid (such as /r/) consonant.

respiratory cycle: One complete breath, including an inspiratory phase and expiratory phase.

retrocochlear pathology: Abnormality of the auditory system that occurs beyond the cochlea, most often seen as tumor of the auditory nerve or brainstem.

reverse swallow: See definition for tongue thrust.

rhetoric: The art or study of using language persuasively and effectively.

rib cage: A set of 12 bones that encloses the lungs and heart.

Rustin, Lena: British professor and speech-language pathologist who was an expert clinician in the area of stuttering management.

S * T = P: Abbreviation for the source-filter theory of phonation.

SALT: (systematic analysis of language transcripts) Computer software program designed to provide a detailed grammatical analysis of a sample of spoken (and transcribed) English.

savant: A scholar or learned person.

scala media: The middle chamber of the cochlea located between the scala tympani and scala media. The chamber is filled with endolymph. Also called the cochlear duct.

scala tympani: The lower chamber of the cochlea that is filled with perilymph.

scala vestibuli: The upper chamber of the cochlea that is filled with perilymph.

Schulthess, Rudolf: Swiss scientist who theorized that stuttering was due to spasms of the larynx.

Scripture, Edward Wheeler (EW): American psychologist who was one of the first trained in the field of psychology. He was interested in various aspects of disordered speech production and developed skills in hearing measurement such as threshold testing and magnitude estimation.

Seashore, Carl: American psychologist interested in music, voice, and hearing. He built the first audiometer.

self-talk: The internal dialogue we use to view the world, explain situations, and communicate to ourselves.

semantics: The study or science of meaning in language.

semicircular canals: Three tiny circular tubes of the inner ear that are positioned at right angles to each other. They serve as the body's balance organ.

semiotics: The theory and study of signs and symbols, especially as they relate to communication.

sensorineural hearing loss: Most common type of hearing loss resulting from damage to the inner ear, or regions of the central auditory system.

SES: *See* socioeconomic status.

sign language: A rule governed language that uses a system of manual, facial, and other body movements as a means of communication.

signal-to-noise ratio: A measure of signal strength relative to background noise. The ratio is usually measured in decibels (dB).

simultaneous bilingualism: An individual who has acquired two or more languages with equal skill in both.

simultaneous communication: Combined use of sign language and speech to communicate.

single words: Earliest identifiable language form produced by children, which usually begin to emerge by the age of 12 months.

Skinner, B. F. American psychologist who published significant scientific works in the analysis of behavior.

SLD: *See* stutteringlike deficiencies.

SLI: *See* specific language impairment.

Smile Train: International charity that provides cleft lip and palate surgery to children in need, as well as medical training to doctors in their native countries.

socioeconomic dialect: A manner of speaking that is associated with an individual's financial and/or social status.

socioeconomic status (SES): A measure based on financial and social indicators.

soft palate: The soft tissue that comprises the back of the roof of the mouth. Also known as the velum.

sound: Vibrations that are transmitted through a medium. Sound can be described according to its duration, amplitude, and frequency of vibration.

sound field amplification: System often used in classrooms for hearing-impaired children, whereby the teacher's voice is transmitted through a microphone and loudspeaker.

sound-to-symbol relationship: The relationship between a specific speech sound and the corresponding letter in the alphabet for that sound. In general, the English language has a poor sound-symbol relationship. The phonetic alphabet provides an exact sound-symbol relationship.

sound visibility: Notion that some consonant and vowel sounds are more readily visible on a talker's face compared to others. For example, the /f/ sound has high visibility, whereas the /h/ sound has low visibility.

sound wave: A pressure wave that is propagated through air (or other media) that is generally audible to the human ear.

spasmodic dysphonia: Voice disorder that is caused by involuntary muscle movements in the vocal folds.

speaker: One of two individuals required for successful communication. Another name for a speaker is encoder. The term is also a component of a hearing aid that delivers an acoustic signal to the ear.

speaking rate: Speed at which a person speaks. Speaking rate is typically reported according the number of words (or syllables) spoken per minute.

specific language impairment (SLI): Preschool child who shows difficulty with language that is not caused by a known neurologic, sensory, intellectual, or emotional deficit.

speech delay: Communication disorder in which the speaking behavior demonstrated by the individual is quantitatively (as opposed to qualitatively) different from normal.

speech reading: Deciphering of spoken language on the basis of visual cues provided by the speaker. Also known as lip reading.

speech-language pathologist: Professional educated in the field of speech-language pathology.

speech-language pathology: The study of disorders which affect a person's speech, language, and swallowing behavior, including methods of assessment, treatment, and prevention.

speech recognition: Process whereby a computer learns to identify and understand discrete words and phrases. Also known as automatic speech recognition or computer speech recognition.

spina bifida: Serious birth abnormality in which the spinal cord is malformed during fetal development. The spinal cord lacks its usual protective skeletal and soft tissue covering.

spinal nerves: Collection of 31 pairs of nerves that enter and exit the spinal cord. The nerves provide motor, sensory, or combined input to various parts of the body.

spontaneous recovery: Natural reappearance of function following a period of lessened response. A concept associated with the recovery of

communication skills shortly after a stroke.

spoonerism: The unintentional transposition of sounds within or across words that occurs when speaking. The phrase *Beeping Sleuty* (Sleeping Beauty) is one such example.

stammering: See definition for stuttering.

standardized testing: Form of assessment in which a test is administered and scored in a consistent manner.

stapedectomy: Surgical removal of the stapes bone within the middle ear as a means of improving hearing.

stapedius: Smallest skeletal muscle of the human body whose purpose is to stabilize the stapes bone that is inserted into the oval window of the cochlea.

stapes: Innermost of the three small bones (ossicles) of the middle ear. Also known as the stirrup, reflecting its unique shape.

statistical learning theory: A theory that focuses on the statistical aspects of learning such as that related to the acquisition of language.

stem cell: An unspecialized cell that gives rise to a specialized cell, such as a blood cell.

Stevens, Nettie Maria: American biologist and geneticist who discovered that chromosomes determine the sex of a species.

stoma: Surgically created opening in the surface of the body, usually in the region of the trachea.

stops: A group of consonants that are organized according to their manner of articulation, namely the complete obstruction of forward airflow followed by a sudden release of air. The consonants /p/, /t/, and /k/ are examples of stops.

stuttering: Disorder in which the flow of speech is disrupted by involuntary repetitions and prolongations of sounds, syllables, words, or phrases, and involuntary silent pauses or blocks. Also known as stammering.

stuttering modification: Treatment technique in which the main goal is to stutter more easily as opposed to speaking more fluently.

stutteringlike disfluencies (SLD): Speech disfluencies that are most indicative of a stuttering disorder. Examples of an SLD include a syllable repetition and a sound prolongation.

submetacentric chromosome: A chromosome whose centromere lies between its middle and its end but slightly closer to the middle.

submucous cleft: Condition in which a cleft of the palate is not visible as a result of the cleft being covered by a mucous membrane lining.

substitutions: Pattern of speech misarticulation whereby the intended speech sound is replaced (substituted) by another speech sound.

sulcus: A deep, narrow groove in tissue. Various landmarks of the cerebral cortex are demarcated on the basis of sulci.

Sullivan, Anne: American teacher and friend of Helen Keller.

swallowing center: Region in the brainstem that is involved in the coordination and regulation of essential swallowing activity.

Sweet, Henry: English linguist who made a significant contribution to the field of phonetics.

symmetric hearing loss: A hearing loss of both ears in which the configuration and severity of the loss are identical.

syndrome: Group of symptoms that collectively characterize an abnormal condition or disease.

syntax: The study of the form of language such as grammatical rules.

syrinx: The vocal organ of a bird.

tactile communication: Form of nonverbal communication in which touching (e.g., handshaking, kissing) conveys a message from sender to receiver.

Tadoma method: Form of communication used by deaf-blind individuals to assist with comprehension of speech. The method involves placement of the hands on the speaker's face to decipher facial movements.

telecoil: Hearing aid device that can amplify sound waves transmitted through a telephone.

telecommunications: The science and technology of communication at a distance by electronic transmission of impulses, as by telegraph, cable, telephone, radio, or television.

telegraph: Basic communication system that is able to transmit and receive simple electric impulses.

telehome care: Emerging field of health care that utilizes web-based Internet communication for the delivery of health care information to a patient.

telephone: Instrument which converts voice and other acoustic signals into a form that can be transmitted to a location where it is reconverted into an acoustic signal.

television: Electronic (and digital) apparatus that is able to receive the simultaneous transmission of images and sounds.

temperament: The manner in which a person thinks, behaves, and reacts.

Templin, Mildred: American professor and pioneer in speech-language pathology known for her research in the area of phonological development.

temporal bone: A bone that forms the sides and base of the skull.

temporal lobes: Side regions of the cerebral cortex. Primarily involved in the processing of sensory input.

temporomandibular joint (TMJ): A joint that connects the mandible (lower jaw) to the temporal bone of the skull.

tensor tympani: Small muscle located in the middle ear that influences the mobility of the tympanic membrane (eardrum).

teratogenic: Relating to, or causing a malformation of an embryo or fetus.

text-messaging: Means of communicating using a mobile phone where short text messages can be sent and received. Also called short message service (SMS).

Thelwall, John: Best known as the radical orator during the movement for parliamentary reform in Britain in the late 18th century.

threshold: Point that must be exceeded in order to elicit a response. A person's hearing threshold represents the lowest level of loudness necessary to perceive a sound.

thrombosis: Formation of a blood clot inside a blood vessel that obstructs blood flow.

thyroarytenoid muscle: Anatomic name for the vocal folds.

thyroid cartilage: Largest of the cartilages comprising the framework of the larynx. A landmark of the thyroid cartilage is a notch, also known as the Adam's apple.

tinnitus: The perception of ringing in the ears without an external cause.

Titze, Ingo: American voice scientist who has made significant contributions to vocal fold physiology and voice rehabilitation.

TMJ: *See* temporomandibular joint.

tongue: The fleshy, movable, muscular organ attached to the floor of the mouth. The primary organ for taste, swallowing, and speech production.

tongue advancement (or carriage): Cat-egorization of vowels according to the horizontal location of the tongue within the oral cavity.

tongue elevation (or height): Categorization of vowels according to the vertical location of the tongue within the oral cavity.

tongue thrust: Forward movement of the tongue, especially in the initial stage of the swallowing process. An infantile swallowing pattern that should diminish with age.

tonotopic organization: Cellular structure of the inner ear whereby the frequencies represented along the basilar membrane of the cochlea are organized from high to low.

trachea: Tubelike cartilaginous structure that is a portion of the respiratory tract. Also called the windpipe.

tracheoesophageal speech: Technique for speaking following laryngectomy. Air is diverted to the esophagus causing it to vibrate and create sound.

traditional approach: Term used to describe a method of treating speech sound disorders. The approach begins with teaching the sound at an isolated level and gradually progressing to the production of the same sound in conversational speech.

tragus: Projection of skin-covered cartilage in front of the ear canal.

transfer function: Transformation that is used to describe the output of a device as a function of the input of the device. Speech production involves the transformation of the original source (vocal folds) into a specific sound resulting from changes in vocal tract configuration. Also noted in the formulat $S * T = P$.

transmission model: Conceptualization of communication that involves encoding (a speaker) and decoding (a listener).

traumatic brain injury (TBI): An injury that occurs when a sudden outside force causes damage to the brain.

Travis, Lee Edward: The father of speech-language pathology in the United States. He was particularly interested in the area of stuttering.

Turner, Henry: American physician who was the first to describe a genetic condition in women caused by the absence of one of the X sex chromosomes.

Turner syndrome: Medical disorder in females as a result of an absent X (sex) chromosome.

Twain, Mark: American humorist and author whose actual name was Samuel Clemens.

Twitter: Internet-based form of social messaging involving short text messages of up to 140 characters in length.

two-word combinations: Early language utterances produce by children at approximately 2 years of age.

tympanic membrane: Thin concave-shaped membrane that separates the outer ear canal from the middle ear. Also called the eardrum.

tympanometer: Instrument used to measure the compliance (sometimes called admittance) of the tympanic membrane. The results of the test are displayed on a graph called a tympanogram.

tympanometry: Test performed to evaluate eardrum (tympanic membrane) mobility and middle ear functioning.

ultrasound: Use of high-frequency sound waves to create an image of internal body structures.

unilateral cleft lip: Failure of the lip to form during fetal development on one side of the nose.

unilateral hearing loss: Type of hearing loss where one ear has normal hearing and the other ear is impaired.

universal newborn screening: Approach to the screening of hearing in newborn infants whereby all children receive a hearing test shortly after birth, preferably before being discharged from the hospital.

upper respiratory tract: The cavities of the body that include the nose, mouth, and throat.

uvula: Small fleshy mass of tissue that suspends from the back of the soft palate.

van den Berg, Janwillem: Dutch scientist who proposed the myoelastic-aerodynamic theory of phonation.

Van Gogh, Vincent: Dutch painter during the 19th century.

Van Riper, Charles: American pioneer in the field of speech-language pathology. He made significant contributions to the areas of stuttering and speech sound disorders.

velopharyngeal closure: Contact between the soft palate (velum) and the back of the throat (pharynx) that normally occurs during swallowing and the production of speech.

velopharyngeal inadequacy (VPI): Malfunctioning of the physiological relationship between the soft palate (velum) and the back of the throat (pharynx), in which a lack of contact between the two structures occurs.

ventriloquism: Art of projecting voice to give the illusion of it coming from another source, such as a dummy or doll figure.

verbal communication: Basis of expressive (vocal) communication that is one way for people to communicate face-to-face.

verbalizations: Production of vocal sounds that express meaning.

vermilion border: Region of redness that surrounds the lips.

vestibular apparatus: Region of the inner ear that is important for maintaining balance and spatial orientation. Consists of the utricle, saccule, and semicircular canals.

videofluoroscopic swallowing study: Radiologic imaging procedure used for the evaluation and treatment of swallowing disorders. Also known as modified barium swallowing.

videofluoroscopy: Motion x-ray of the body that combines traditional fluoroscopy (x-ray) with video technology.

viral meningitis: Infection of the protective membranes surrounding the brain or spinal cord that results from a virus. This form of meningitis is quite common and a relatively mild illness compared to bacterial meningitis.

virgules: A diagonal (/) mark that serves as a form of written punctuation. The individual phonemes of a language are usually depicted using virgules (e.g., /t/, /m/, /f/, etc.).

visual communication: The transfer of information between individuals on the basis of vision.

vocal abuse: Any behavior that strains or injures the vocal folds, thus affecting their normal functioning.

vocal folds: Two muscular bands located within the framework of the larynx that protect the trachea from the entrance of foreign matter. These muscular bands also vibrate for the generation of voice. Also known as the thyroarytenoid muscle.

vocal hygiene: The science of vocal health and steps taken to ensure proper care of the vocal mechanism.

vocal nodules: Small inflammatory or fibrous growth that develops on the vocal folds.

vocal polyp: Small swelling in the mucous membranes covering the vocal folds. Also known as Reinke's edema or polypoid degeneration.

vocal tract: Anatomical cavity in animals, including humans, where sound is produced.

vocalizations: Any sound produced through the action of a vocal apparatus.

vocology: The science and practice of voice rehabilitation.

voice disorder: Condition in which the natural generation of voice and voice resonance is impaired.

voice feminization: Voice therapy procedure that involves the change of voice from masculine to feminine, usually as a result of gender transformation.

voice masculinization: Voice therapy procedure that involves the change of voice from feminine to masculine, usually as a result of gender transformation.

voice rest: Therapy procedure that involves complete cessation of speaking (including whispering) as a means of healing the vocal folds.

von Békésy, Georg: Hungarian physiologist who received the Nobel Prize for his research on the functioning of the inner ear.

von Graefe, Karl Ferdinand: German pioneer of plastic and reconstructive surgery.

von Helmholtz, Hermann: German physicist who made important contributions in acoustics and optics.

von Leden, Hans: American otolaryngologist who coined the term phonosurgery to refer to the restoration of voice using surgical techniques.

von Langenbeck, Bernard: Skilled German surgeon who developed a procedure for the closure of the hard palate.

von Siebold, Carl Casper: One of the first surgeons to recognize the importance of speech therapy for individuals with cleft lip and palate.

VPI: *See* velopharyngeal insufficiency.

Waldyer, Wilhelm: German anatomist who identified the material residing within a cell nucleus that he termed chromosome.

Wallace, Alfred: 19th century British anthropologist who, together with Charles Darwin, supported the concept of natural selection.

Watson, James: American geneticist and Nobel Prize winner for discovering the double-helix structure of DNA. His colleague who assisted in the discovery was Francis Crick.

waveform: Graph obtained by plotting the amplitude of a sound wave as a function of time.

Wernicke, Karl: German neurologist who deduced that the left temporal lobe region of the brain was localized for understanding language. This region became known as Wernicke's area.

Wernicke's aphasia: Language disorder that impacts the comprehension of spoken and written language, resulting from damage to the left temporal lobe (Wernicke's area) region of the brain. Also known as a form of fluent aphasia.

whistle register: Highest range of the human voice. Also known as flageolet register.

wild boy of Aveyron: Feral child, known as Victor, who was found wandering in the woods in France. His lack of speech provided early insight to the role of the environment in learning language.

Wilson, Matthew: American Revolutionary War minister and physician who wrote a compendium of medicine called the Therapeutic Alphabet.

within-word disfluencies: Disruptions in the forward flow of speech that occur within the boundary of a single word. Examples include the repetition or prolongation of a consonant at the beginning of a word.

World Health Organization (WHO): Branch of the United Nations that is concerned with public health.

World Wide Web: The complete set of documents residing on all Internet servers at a given time that is accessible to users via a simple point-and-click system of retrieval.

written language: Form of communication based on the representation of language by means of a writing system.

Wundt, Wilhelm: German physiologist and psychologist who has been referred to as the father of experimental psychology.

Yearsley, James: British surgeon who advocated removal of the tonsils as a form of treatment for stuttering.

Yperman, Jehan: Medieval surgeon who developed a variety of procedures for repair of facial defects.

Zemlin, Willard R.: American professor and speech-language pathologist who was interested in the basic anatomy and physiology of speech and hearing mechanisms.

Zwaardemaker, Hendrik: Dutch otolaryngologist who coined the term presbycusis.

zygote: The cell (organism) that results from fertilization.

INDEX

G